Comprehensive Systematic Review
for
Advanced Nursing Practice

Cheryl Holly, EdD, RN, is associate professor and chair of the Department of Capacity Building Systems, and codirector of the New Jersey Center for Evidence-Based Practice at the University of Medicine and Dentistry of New Jersey (UMDNJ) School of Nursing. At UMDNJ, she teaches doctor of nursing practice (DNP) program courses including information technology for evidence-based practice; quantitative methods of inquiry and program evaluation, which includes meta-analysis; and clinical inquiry seminars and works with DNP students in their capstone residency course. Dr. Holly holds a BS in Nursing degree from the Pace University, Lienhard School of Nursing, Pleasantville, NY; an MEd in Adult Health and Physical Illness; and EdD in Research and Evaluation in Curriculum/Teaching, both from Columbia University. Dr. Holly has completed postgraduate work in financial administration at the New York Medical College School of Public Health, and in economics, accounting, and comprehensive meta-analysis at the Pace University School of Business. She is certified as Train-the-Trainer in Comprehensive Systematic Review by the Joanna Briggs Institute and has offered workshops on Comprehensive Systematic Review across the country. Dr. Holly is the coordinator of the Eastern Nursing Research Society's Research Interest Group on Comprehensive Systematic Review and Knowledge Translation, and a member of the Committee on Directors of the Joanna Briggs Institute of Nursing and Midwifery, and the Evidence Translation Group, Cochrane Nursing Care Field, and a member of the Cochrane Injuries Group. She has published extensively and presented internationally and nationally in the areas of EBP, systematic review, knowledge translation, and critical care nursing.

Susan W. Salmond, EdD, RN, CTN, CNE, is a dean and professor, and codirector of the New Jersey Center for Evidence-Based Practice at the UMDNJ School of Nursing in Newark, where she also has served in various other positions since 2005, including vice dean, associate for administration and planning, and associate dean for graduate studies. Dr. Salmond received a BSN from Villanova University, an MEd in Adult Health and Physical Illness, and EdD in Nursing Administration both from Columbia University. She is certified in nursing education and transcultural nursing. In addition to teaching and administrative responsibilities at UMDNJ, Dr. Salmond has taught at Seton Hall University and at Columbia University. At UMDNJ, Dr. Salmond teaches Qualitative Methods of Inquiry and Program Evaluation, which includes metasynthesis in the DNP program and works with DNP students on their capstone residency projects. She is the North American co-convenor of the Nursing Care Field of the Cochrane Collaboration and certified as a Train-the-Trainer in Comprehensive Systematic Review by the Joanna Briggs Institute of Nursing and Midwifery. Dr. Salmond has coauthored three editions of *Orthopaedic Nursing* and has authored two other books, and numerous book chapters and peer-reviewed journal articles. She is a highly sought after conference presenter and workshop leader, both nationally and internationally, in the areas of cultural competence, qualitative research, EBP, and systematic review.

Marie K. Saimbert, BPharm, MLIS, MSN, RN, is a reference librarian at the George F. Smith Library of the Health Sciences at the UMDNJ, a pharmacology instructor at the UMDNJ School of Nursing, and nurse/pharmacist informatics consultant at the Valley Health System in Ridgewood, NJ. She holds a MSN in Nursing Informatics (2008), MS in Library and Information Science (2003), BS in Pharmacy (1997), BS in Nursing (1994), and BS in English Literature (1994). She serves as an active member of the NY/NJ chapter of the Medical Library Association, the Nursing and Allied Health and Pharmacy and Drug Information Sections, the Health Science Library Association of NJ, the EBSCO Biomedical Advisory Board, and a liaison to the UMDNJ School of Nursing. Ms. Saimbert informs development, use, and maintenance of clinical information systems used by health professionals, and has spent more than 4 years facilitating systematic reviews and searching skills with nurses and nursing students. She has published nine articles and had nine recurring columns in the Health Sciences Library Association of New Jersey (HSLANJ) *ePULSE*. Research interests include library resource integration in health science courses; evidence-based nursing research and infusion of research into practice; nurses' use of electronic technologies; integration of library tools; and decision trees into electronic systems to support EBP and life-long learning. She has practiced in both nursing (pediatrics) and pharmacy (community practice) disciplines.

Comprehensive Systematic Review for Advanced Nursing Practice

Cheryl Holly, EdD, RN

Susan W. Salmond, EdD, RN, CTN, CNE

Marie K. Saimbert, BPharm, MLIS, MSN, RN

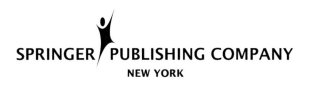

SPRINGER PUBLISHING COMPANY

NEW YORK

Springer Publishing Company, LLC
11 West 42nd Street
New York, NY 10036
www.springerpub.com

Acquisitions Editor: Margaret Zuccarini
Cover Design: DePinho
Composition: Absolute Service, Inc.

ISBN: 978-0-8261-1778-6
E-book ISBN: 978-0-8261-1779-3

11 12 13 14 / 5 4 3 2 1

The author and the publisher of this Work have made every effort to use sources believed to be reliable to provide information that is accurate and compatible with the standards generally accepted at the time of publication. Because medical science is continually advancing, our knowledge base continues to expand. Therefore, as new information becomes available, changes in procedures become necessary. We recommend that the reader always consult current research and specific institutional policies before performing any clinical procedure. The author and publisher shall not be liable for any special, consequential, or exemplary damages resulting, in whole or in part, from the readers' use of, or reliance on, the information contained in this book. The publisher has no responsibility for the persistence or accuracy of URLs for external or third-party Internet websites referred to in this publication and does not guarantee that any content on such websites is, or will remain, accurate or appropriate.

Library of Congress Cataloging-in-Publication Data

Holly, Cheryl.
  Comprehensive systematic review for advanced nursing practice / Cheryl Holly, Susan W. Salmond, Marie K. Saimbert.
    p. ; cm.
  Includes bibliographical references and index.
  ISBN 978-0-8261-1778-6 — ISBN 978-0-8261-1779-3 (e-book)
  1. Nurse practitioners. I. Salmond, Susan Warner. II. Saimbert, Marie K. III. Title.
  [DNLM: 1. Advanced Practice Nursing. 2. Review Literature as Topic. 3. Evidence-Based Nursing—methods. 4. Meta-Analysis as Topic. WY 128]
  RT82.8.H65 2011
  610.73--dc23
                          2011029339

Printed in the United States of America by Gasch Printing

*For Bebe, Grace, and the guys for allowing me the time to
complete this project.   CH*

*For my former, current, and future DNP students to help them through the
process of systematic review, and to my family, who have always been
supportive of my professional endeavors.   SS*

*For Mom, Dad, John, and those believing in the power of discoveries
to shape and positively impact the way we care for ourselves
and others.   MKS*

Contents

Contributors

David Anthony Forrester, PhD, RN, ANEF, Professor, University of Medicine and Dentistry of New Jersey (UMDNJ) School of Nursing (SN), Professor in Residence: Interdisciplinary Health Research Consultant, Morristown Memorial Hospital (MMH-AH), Staff, New Jersey Center for Evidence-Based Practice, University of Medicine and Dentistry of New Jersey (UMDNJ) School of Nursing (SN), Newark, NJ

Pam Hargwood, MLIS, Information and Education Librarian, University of Medicine and Dentistry of New Jersey (UMDNJ) Robert Wood Johnson (RWJ) Medical School Library of the Health Sciences, New Brunswick, NJ

Cheryl Holly, EdD, RN, is an associate professor and chair of the Department of Capacity Building Systems, and codirector of the New Jersey Center for Evidence-Based Practice at the University of Medicine and Dentistry of New Jersey (UMDNJ) School of Nursing

Ronell Kirkley, DNP, CRNA, APN-Acute Care, Chief Nurse Anesthetist, The Department of Anesthesiology, The New York Methodist Hospital, Brooklyn, NY

Jos Kleijnen, MD, PhD, Director, Kleijnen Systematic Reviews, Ltd., London, England

Rita M. Musanti, PhD, APN-C, AOCNP, Clinical Nurse Researcher, MMH-AH, Clinical Assistant Professor, University of Medicine and Dentistry of New Jersey (UMDNJ) School of Nursing (SN), Staff, New Jersey Center for Evidence-Based Practice, University of Medicine and Dentistry of New Jersey (UMDNJ) School of Nursing (SN), Newark, NJ

John T. Oliver, MLIS, Reference and Instruction Librarian, Augustus C. Long Health Sciences Library, Columbia University, New York, NY

Lisa M. Paplanus, DNP, RN-C, CCRN, ACNP-BC, ANP-BC, Vascular Nurse Practitioner, Langone Medical Center, New York University Medical Center, New York, NY

Jenny Pierce, MS, Public Services Librarian, University of Medicine and Dentistry of New Jersey (UMDNJ) Robert Wood Johnson (RWJ) Medical School Library of the Health Sciences, Stratford, NJ

Patricia Polansky, MS, RN, Assistant Commissioner, Department of Health and Senior Services, State of New Jersey, and Clinical Assistant Professor, University of Medicine and Dentistry of New Jersey (UMDNJ) School of Nursing (SN), Newark, NJ

Marie K. Saimbert, BPharm, MLIS, MSN, RN, Reference librarian at the George F. Smith Library of the Health Sciences at the UMDNJ, Pharmacology Instructor at the UMDNJ School of Nursing, and Nurse/Pharmacist Informatics Consultant at the Valley Health System, Ridgewood, NJ

Susan W. Salmond, EdD, RN, CTN, CNE, Dean, Professor, and Codirector of the New Jersey Center for Evidence-Based Practice at the UMDNJ School of Nursing in Newark

Foreword

I am delighted to have been invited to introduce this very comprehensive text on systematic review and evidence-based health care. Medical practitioners, nurses, and allied health professionals are afforded much status in most societies because they are seen to possess a specialized knowledge base. This knowledge base—which is the foundation for the increasingly complex decision making that characterizes health care delivery—is best described as a set of beliefs, ideas, and hypotheses that are sometimes (but not always) drawn from adequate, and preferably strong, evidence. The more convincing the evidence to support it is, the more trustworthy is the knowledge.

Basing practice on evidence has been claimed to be a feature of modern health care—but this claim is by no means the norm in everyday practice. Many health care practitioners continue to base their practice on what they learned in medical, nursing, or allied health schools; on trial and error in practice; or on reading single study reports in a small number of journals. None of these approaches to practice are appropriate in an age of rapidly changing knowledge. The material learned as undergraduate students becomes outdated very quickly, and the results of a single study, or of trial and error, do not stand up to the rigorous standards that are expected by society. Hence, the emergence of the evidence-based practice movement—a movement designed to capture, summarize, and provide useable information to busy practitioners to inform them when they make clinical decisions.

So, what counts as evidence? Whenever health professionals engage in practice, they make numerous clinical decisions. In making such decisions, practitioners draw on a wide range of knowledge—from knowledge of the basic biological and behavioral sciences; their assessment of the current context and of the individual patient; their own experience; and their own current understandings of research reports they may have recently read. All of this knowledge used to make a clinical decision can be referred to as evidence, and the validity of this evidence may be variable.

When making decisions, clinicians (often quite subconsciously) are often trying to select an appropriate activity or intervention, and assess the degree to which the decision will meet the need at hand. Health professionals seek evidence to substantiate the worth of a very wide range of activities and interventions, and, thus, the type of evidence needed depends on the nature of the activity and its purpose (Pearson, Wiechula, Court, & Lockwood, 2005).

This "ranking" of evidence based on study design is often referred to as an "evidence pyramid." Starting at the base of the pyramid is "bench" research conducted in laboratories, and more often than not, performed on animals. This is where most research into ideas, techniques, and therapies starts. Case series and case reports represent collections of reports on the treatment of individual patients or a report on a single patient, respectively. Case control studies represent studies in which patients who have an existing specific condition are compared with people who do not. Further up the pyramid are cohort studies. Cohort studies commonly investigate a large population of patients over time who have a specific condition/treatment and compare them with another group that has not been affected by, or exposed to, the condition or treatment of interest. Randomized controlled clinical trials (RCCTs) represent the studies that carry the most weight when translating evidence into practice. All aspects of RCCTs are carefully planned to study the effect of a therapy (and "only" the therapy or intervention of interest) on patients—this is done by comparing intervention and control groups. This study design necessarily includes methodologies that reduce the potential for bias (e.g., blinding and randomization). Systematic reviews are at the peak of the evidence pyramid. They take the form of an exhaustive search of the scientific literature, usually focusing on a specific aspect of a clinical topic, to identify all relevant and methodologically sound studies. The studies are appraised and reviewed, and the results are summarized. A systematic review may also contain a meta-analysis. If several valid studies on a topic are sufficiently similar in one or more of the aspects of interest to the review question, the results of these studies can be combined and analyzed statistically as if they were from one large study.

On the other hand, one cannot forget the growing importance of qualitative study to the emerging paradigm of evidence-based health care. A naturalistic approach is used to examine context. Subjects are observed in their natural environment in hopes of expanding and illuminating phenomenon to discover associations for generating and/or refining theory (Bradley, Curry, & Devers, 2007).

Evidence-based health care practice focuses on the need for all health professionals to use those interventions that are supported by the most up-to-date evidence or knowledge available. The evidence-based approach acknowledges the difficulties faced by busy practitioners in keeping up-to-date with an ever-growing literature in health care, and emphasizes the importance of providing them with condensed information on a given topic, gathered through the systematic review of the international literature and accessible at the point of care.

Online information systems that provide appropriate, up-to-date evidence at the point of care are potentially among the most effective interventions to support evidence-based practice (Westbrook, Coiera, & Gosling, 2005). Online information systems have been shown to significantly improve the quality of clinicians' answers to clinical problems and, if used effectively, the speed at which they can attain the information necessary to deal with a clinical problem correctly (Coiera, Westbrook, & Rogers, 2008; Magrabi, Coiera, Westbrook, Gosling, & Vickand, 2005; Westbrook et al., 2005). Summarized evidence sources represent an efficient way of disseminating evidence to doctors and nurses, and are becoming an increasingly popular tool used by health care workers consistently inundated with research, opinion, and information in general.

This book comprehensively and concisely examines the complexities related to asking clinical questions, searching for the evidence, appraising and summarizing the evidence, and getting the evidence into practice. *Best practice* in health care is practice that is based on the best available evidence, and it is surely the goal of all health professionals to deliver the very best they can to patients, families, and communities. I commend this book to health professionals who are seeking to do the best they can in health care.

> *Alan Pearson*, AM
> Professor of Evidence-Based Health Care
>   and Executive Director
> The Joanna Briggs Institute
> Faculty of Health Sciences
> The University of Adelaide
> Adelaide, South Australia

REFERENCES

Bradley, E. H., Curry, L. A., & Devers, K. J. (2007). Qualitative data analysis for health services research: Developing taxonomy, themes, and theory. *Health Services Research*, *42*(4), 1758–1772.

Coiera, E. W., Westbrook, J. I., & Rogers, K. (2008). Clinical decision velocity is increased when meta-search filters enhance evidence retrieval. *Journal of the American Medical Informatics Association*, *15*(5), 638–646.

Magrabi, F., Coiera, E. W., Westbrook, J. I., Gosling, A. S., & Vickand, V. (2005). General practitioners' use of online evidence during consultations. *International Journal of Medical Informatics*, *74*(1), 1–12.

Pearson, A., Wiechula, R., Court, A., & Lockwood, C. (2005). The JBI model of evidence-based health care. *International Journal of Evidence Based Healthcare*, *3*, 207–215.

Westbrook, J. I., Coiera, E. W., & Gosling, A. S. (2005). Do online retrieval systems help experienced clinicians answer clinical questions? *Journal of the American Medical Informatics Association*, *12*(3), 315–321.

Preface

How do we understand the millions of research studies published each year? How do we deal with the conflicting and contradictory results we find? How do we know that the content is of high quality? And, finally, how do we know what to do with the findings? The answer, of course, is related to systematic review, a secondary research method that uses primary research studies to identify, appraise, and interpret available research for a focused clinical question. Evidence-based health care is grounded on the premise that although practitioners may become experts in their discipline, the explosion of scientific information has created a situation where knowledge is often not current. Systematic reviews are an efficient answer to the dilemma of too many papers to read in too little time, because they provide reliable evidential summaries of past research. By pooling results from multiple studies, findings are based on multiple populations, conditions, and circumstances. The pooled results of many small studies can have more precise, powerful, and convincing conclusions.

Increasingly, health care practitioners seek systematic reviews for point-of-care guidance. When done following the rigorous procedures presented in this book, systematic reviews are exemplars that bring research closer to practice—narrowing the gap for clinicians. Systematic reviews are not the end. Well-thought out care for patients, families, and communities is the goal. Toward those ends, results from systematic reviews require translation into interventions, policies, guidelines, and programs to serve populations.

Systematic reviews are often compared to traditional narrative review articles. However, narrative articles typically do not use explicit, systematic approaches in the review process and are more subjective. In narrative reviews, search strategies are not described, reasons for inclusion and exclusion of studies are not specified, critical appraisal is not done, and methods for synthesizing evidence are not clearly defined. Transparency is missing. Consequently, narrative reviews are more biased with a higher likelihood for inaccurate or unsubstantiated conclusions. Systematic reviews, on the other hand, are a form of research that aims to identify, evaluate, and summarize the findings of all quality, relevant individual studies on a topic systematically (Centre for Reviews and Dissemination, 2009), thereby relieving the end user of this time-consuming task. It requires the reviewers to have expertise in both the subject matter and the review method. Rigorous systematic reviews are completed by at least two reviewers and key steps, such as screening for inclusion criteria, critical appraisal, and data extraction, are done independently and compared to minimize potential for bias. With methods training, expert practitioners are assuming the critical task of performing systematic reviews.

The importance of systematic review is underscored by the recent publication of an Institute of Medicine report, "Finding What Works in Health Care: Standards for Systematic Reviews" (Eden, Levit, Berg, & Morton, 2011), written as a result of a congressional mandate (Public Law 110-275, Section 304). The report focuses on the development and reporting of systematic reviews of publicly funded comparative effectiveness research acknowledging that these 21 standards are aspirational. It is essential to recognize that the tacit knowledge of clinical expertise and qualitative research is a valuable component of evidence-based practice that cannot be overlooked. We have attempted in this text to do justice to all aspects of systematic review: qualitative evidence, experimental evidence, observational evidence, and economic evidence, in keeping with the way in which advanced nursing practice will use evidence.

Our intent in writing this book is to provide a guide for understanding and conducting systematic reviews. In this book, we discuss the basic components of systematic reviews—planning, conducting, and reporting—and importantly, the relationship of systematic review to clinical practice and policy making. Chapters 1–3 address the steps in the systematic review process and development of a proposal and a clinical question. Chapter 1 relates the emerging paradigm of evidence-based practice to its research antecedent, the systematic review. Chapter 2 presents the steps to follow in conducting a systematic review, although these steps are discussed in depth in later chapters of the book. Chapter 3 outlines the process for developing a systematic review proposal and presents an example of a proposal for a comprehensive systematic review. Chapters 5–7 inform on finding and selecting the best available evidence. Chapter 5 presents the key principles for conducting an exhaustive search. Chapter 6 presents resources and useful tips to actually conduct a search and a description of the most commonly used databases. Chapter 7 describes how to appraise the quality of studies that have been selected to be in the review. Chapters 8–11 provide information on specific types of systematic review, such as those using experimental evidence, observational evidence, economic evidence, and qualitative evidence. Each chapter presents the common research designs within the context of a systematic review. The final section, Chapters 12–14, discusses the current and future use of systematic review. Chapter 12 discusses the use of systematic review in health policy formulation. Chapter 13 presents the systematic review process as the foundation for development of clinical guidelines. Chapter 14 provides a reflection on the future of systematic reviews. A toolkit for conducting a systematic review can be found in the Appendices. At the end of each chapter, we provide suggested readings and exercises for those who wish to learn more about the process of systematic review.

Upon completion of this book, nurses and other clinicians should see systematic reviews as approachable research with great potential to advance clinical practice toward evidence-based care. It all starts with questioning practice, and then methodically reviewing research to discover evidence for translation.

Cheryl Holly
Susan W. Salmond
Marie K. Saimbert
Newark, NJ

REFERENCES

Centre for Reviews and Dissemination. (2009). *Systematic reviews: CRD's guidance for undertaking reviews in health care.* Retrieved from http://www.york.ac.uk/inst/crd/pdf/Systematic_ Reviews.pdf

Eden, J., Levit, L., Berg, A., & Morton, S. (2011). *Finding what works in health care: Standards for systematic reviews.* Washington, DC: National Academy of Sciences, Institute of Medicine.

Acknowledgments

A book is never just the work of one person. For this book, I had the unique opportunity of working with two others who challenged and inspired me throughout the process.

I was also fortunate to work with two former students on this project: Dr. Ronell Kirkly and Dr. Lisa Paplanus, both contributors to this book whose continued and future work in systematic review I look forward to reading. —*Cheryl Holly*

A heartfelt thank you for all of those who see the value of systematic review in advancing nursing practice. —*Susan W. Salmond*

Thank you Dean Salmond and Dr. Holly for always seeing librarians as cocollaborators in nursing research, and allowing me to take on this challenging project. A heartfelt thank you goes to librarians and staff at UMDNJ libraries who supported my efforts on this publication, especially Judy Cohn, Roberta Bronson Fitzpatrick, Pam Hargwood, Anna Huang, Kerry O'Rourke, Jenny Pierce, and Jan Skica. Much thanks is extended to John T. Oliver, a great cocollaborator with an inspiring skill set; Michelle Brewer; Barbara Gladson; Susan Gould-Fogerite; Julie Quain; Patricia May; Leslie-Faith Morritt Taub; Robin Siegel; Maura Sostack; Rick Wright from SCILS; Debby Magnan for the unwavering support; my writing mentors: Robert Deischer (Bloomfield College, NJ), Kathleen Cirillo (St. Mary's High School, Elizabeth, NJ), Lorraine Steefel, DNP, RN, CTN (UMDNJ-School of Nursing, Newark, NJ), and Christine Karch, RN, for your generous heart—always leading by example—and for the professional and personal guidance since nursing school; all your support is definitely appreciated. Thank you for the faith, Mom, Dad, and John; I would not persevere through life as well without your cradle of love and understanding. —*Marie K. Saimbert*

Reviewers

Sarah Cantrell, MLIS, Education Services Librarian, Dahlgren Memorial Library, Georgetown University Medical Center, Washington, DC

Mercedes Echevarria, DNP, ANP-BC, PNP-BC, Assistant Professor and Director of the Doctor of Nursing Practice Program, University of Medicine and Dentistry of NJ, Newark, NJ

Mary C. Kamienski, PhD, FNP-BC, FAEN, Associate Professor and Chair, Department of Primary Care, University of Medicine and Dentistry of NJ, Newark NJ

Ross Ljungquist, MSLS, CSS, AHIP, Expert Searcher, Medical Research Library of Brooklyn, SUNY Downstate Medical Center, Brooklyn, NY

Marybeth Lyons, RN, MS, Clinical Nurse Specialist, Pediatrics and PICU, Westchester Medical Center, Valhalla, NY

Mike McGraw, MLIS, Reference and User Services Librarian, Cleveland Health Sciences Library, Case Western Reserve University, Cleveland, OH

Becky McKay, MA, MLIS, AHIP, Associate Professor, TAMHSC Bryan Campus Librarian Medical Sciences Library, University Libraries, Texas A&M University, Bryan, TX

Lisa M. Paplanus, DNP, RN-C, CCRN, ACNP-BC, ANP-BC, Vascular Nurse Practitioner, Langone Medical Center, New York University Medical Center, New York, NY

Cynthia J. Vaughn, MLIS, AHIP, Clinical Information Librarian, Assistant Professor, Preston Medical Library, University of Tennessee Graduate School of Medicine, Knoxville, TN

PART I

Introduction

CHAPTER ONE

Systematic Review as the Basis for Evidence-Based Practice

Susan W. Salmond and Cheryl Holly

OBJECTIVES

Upon completion of Chapter 1, you will be able to:

- Differentiate between expert-driven health care and evidence-based health care
- Define the components of evidence-based practice (EBP)
- Understand the process of evidence-based health care and the value of systematic reviews as a quality source of evidence
- Define filtered and unfiltered evidence

IMPORTANT POINTS

- The evidence-based care paradigm calls for the integration of best research evidence, along with clinical expertise and the opinions and values of patients and their families, as a component in clinical decision making.
- The EBP process includes *asking* a question, *acquiring* evidence to support the question, *appraising* the evidence, *applying* the evidence to a patient or group, *acting* to put the evidence to use for patients/groups, and *assessing* if the evidence leads to desired patient outcomes.
- Systematic reviews are at the top of the evidence hierarchy because they provide a summary of research findings available on a particular topic or clinical question. Using an explicit, rigorous process to comprehensively identify, critically appraise, and synthesize relevant studies, findings from a systematic review have greater validity than a single research study.

INTRODUCTION

A paradigm is a traditional way of thinking, a traditional theory or model that guides behavior or practice. Paradigms are not static, and over time do undergo minor changes and adaptations. On occasion, significant agents of change drive new ways of thinking, which are not minor changes, but represent significant shifts in perception, knowledge, and ways of behaving. The coexistence of the old and the new paradigm creates tension because the paradigms are incommensurable.

Health care today is in the midst of a paradigm shift from expert-driven health care to evidence-based health care. Expert-driven care is generally seen as a hierarchical system grounded in expert opinion and clinical skills. The rituals and traditions of this paradigm view the experienced practitioner as the source of knowledge and, as such, expert opinion and intuition, tradition, unsystematic clinical experience, and pathophysiologic rationale are primary influencers of practice and clinical decision making (Swanson, Schmitz, & Chung, 2010). Evidence-based health care is grounded on the premise that although practitioners may become expert in the art of their discipline, the explosion of scientific information has created a situation where one's knowledge of the science of the discipline is often not current.

Acknowledging the lag between discovery and actual practice and the significant variation in care and care outcomes, Iain Chalmers, editor of the James Lind Library, wrote "Although science is cumulative, scientists rarely cumulate scientifically" (as cited in Swanson et al., 2010, p. 287). The evidence-based care paradigm calls for the integration of best research evidence, along with clinical expertise and the opinions and values of patients and their families, as a component in clinical decision making. The aim of EBP is improving patient outcomes by a systematic approach to identifying and promoting practices that work, and eliminating those that are ineffective or harmful (Akobeng, 2005).

This chapter will present an overview of the emergence of evidence-based health care as the driving paradigm of health care today, highlighting the new knowledge and skill required to be successful. Through this overview of EBP, the central role of systematic reviews will be seen as a valuable source of evidence that contributes to clinical decision making.

EVIDENCE-BASED PRACTICE DEFINED

In this text, the term *evidence-based practice* is used to reflect a problem-solving approach to the delivery of health care that crosses all disciplines (Melnyk, Fineout-Overholt, Stilwell, & Williamson, 2009). An early definition of evidence-based medicine provided by Sackett and colleagues from the McMaster Medical School involved the conscientious, explicit, and judicious use of current best evidence in making decisions about the care of an individual or groups of patients (Sackett, Rosenberg, Gray, Haynes, & Richardson, 1996). This was subsequently expanded with clarifications that best evidence must be integrated with individual clinical expertise, patient/family preferences and values, and the clinical context. Figure 1.1 illustrates that EBP is a dynamic process that combines the four components of clinical decision making with the aim of improving patient outcomes. Understanding the components of the process and the constant interaction of the components is important. There is no rule for what is most important; rather, the weight given to each component varies according to the clinical situation (Melnyk et al., 2009). When EBP is put in action,

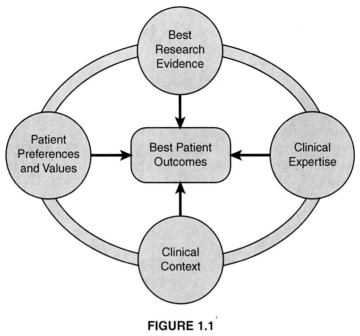

FIGURE 1.1

Components of evidence-based practice.

evidence, expertise, context and preferences, and values inform each other in a positive way (Kitson, 2002).

COMPONENTS OF EVIDENCE-BASED PRACTICE

Best Research Evidence

Use of the evidence-based paradigm emphasizes the need for practitioners to make clinical decisions guided by quality information. Quality or best evidence refers to timely, useful clinical evidence from research-based literature (Cook, Mulrow, & Haynes, 1997). New skills are needed for this to happen. Practitioners need skills to search for the best evidence because research evidence is constantly evolving. What is "best evidence" differs by the clinical question. Clinicians practicing from an evidence-based paradigm need to know what is the best research design to answer a specific clinical question as well as the skills to critically appraise published research for its rigor and trustworthiness. Awareness of the strength and the rigor of the actual study guides the decision making about whether the evidence should be incorporated into the clinical plan.

Clinical Expertise

Best evidence by itself is not sufficient to direct practice; rather, best evidence should inform clinical judgment. Knowledge gained through clinical practice is sometimes referred to as practical knowledge, professional-craft knowledge, or practical "know-how" (Rycroft-Malone, Seers, Titchen, Harvey, Kitson, & McCormack, 2004), and includes the proficiency and judgment acquired through clinical experience and clinical practice (Sackett, 1998). Practitioners use their professional-craft knowledge, which is the proficiency and judgment acquired through clinical experience, to determine whether best evidence applies to the patient or group, and whether the evidence should be integrated into the clinical decision. This tacit knowledge is used to assess the course and effects of implemented interventions.

Once new practices based on best evidence are implemented, the clinician assesses the course and effects of the intervention and uses his or her clinical acumen to make necessary adjustments (Shah & Chung, 2009). This dynamic balance between evidence and expertise is captured by Sackett and colleagues as they describe the dangers in practice that is guided only by clinical expertise or only by best evidence. Without clinical expertise, practice risks becoming tyrannized by evidence, for even excellent external evidence may be inapplicable to or inappropriate for an individual patient. Without current best evidence, practice risks becoming rapidly out of date, to the detriment of patients (Sackett, Rosenberg, Gray, Haynes, & Richardson, 1996). As this text focuses on the systematic review process, it will consequently emphasize best practice using empirical research; however, it is essential to recognize that the tacit knowledge of clinical expertise is a valuable component of EBP.

Patient/Family Preference and Values

It is insufficient to simply blend expertise and evidence, for at the heart of EBP is the patient. Practicing from an evidence-based perspective requires the clinician to recognize the uniqueness of the patient and family, and value the client as a codecision maker in selection of interventions or approaches toward his or her improved health. Best evidence on treatments should be adapted to be congruent with the distinct needs of the patient and family. Needs are influenced by many factors including patient values and beliefs, and the social, emotional, and physical environment. Making the patient central to the decision-making process involves the following:

1. Developing a relationship with the client
2. Listening to the client's expectations, concerns, and beliefs
3. Learning about the patient's experiences in managing his or her illness or treatment regimen
4. Informing the client of the evidence and one's clinical assessment/judgment
5. Explicitly incorporating preferences into clinical decision making (Rycroft-Malone et al., 2004)

Clinical Context

Clinical care takes place within contexts and systems that may dictate their nature, because they affect both patients and professionals (Dieppe, Rafferty, & Kitson, 2002). Sources of evidence in the clinical context may include audit and performance data, patient stories and narratives, knowledge about the culture of the organization and the individuals within it, social and professional networks, and information from stakeholder evaluation and local and national policy (Rycroft-Malone et al., 2004). These sources of data can be used to inform practice decisions, practice changes, as well as inform about the need for research-based evidence.

EVIDENCE-BASED PRACTICE PROCESS

Figure 1.2 depicts the EBP process and links it to Sackett, Straus, Richardson, Rosenberg, and Haynes's (2000) "A" Steps Model. The process will be defined here and its components (ask, acquire, appraise, apply, act, and assess) explained in depth.

Practicing from an evidence-based paradigm calls for clinicians to adopt a mind-set of informed skepticism. Instead of simply accepting tradition, hierarchy, and expert opinion, the EBP clinician questions "why" things are being done as they are, "whether" there is a better way to do it, and "what" the evidence suggests may

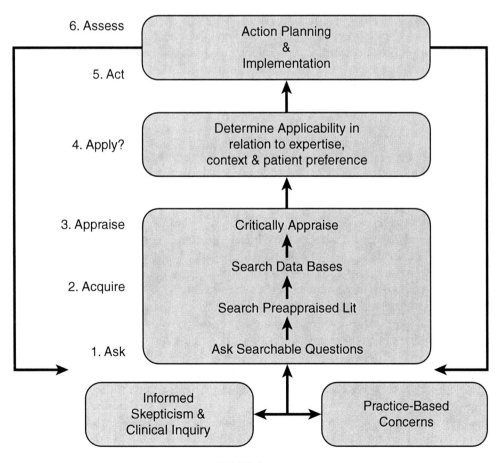

FIGURE 1.2

Evidence-based practice process.

be best in the specific clinical situation (Salmond, 2007). This clinical inquiry stance, along with concerns generated from evidence at the practice level (clinical expertise, patient values, and contextual issues), leads the clinician to recognize the need to ask for further information. A lifelong, self-directed learning process of clinical questioning, searching for and appraising information, and incorporating relevant information into daily practice is central to evidence-based health care (Akobeng, 2005).

Ask

There is both an art and science to *asking* clinical questions to efficiently obtain needed information for informed clinical decisions regarding patients. Information needs from practice are converted into focused, structured, searchable questions that are relevant to the clinical issue by using the population, intervention, comparison, outcome (PICO) approach or similar approaches described in further detail in Chapters 3 and 4. The PICO approach provides a systematic way to identify the components of the clinical issue and structure the question in a way that will guide the search for evidence (Stillwell, Fineout-Overholt, Melnyk, & Williamson, 2010). These four components of a good clinical question can be thought of as data fields that will aid in the search for evidence and answers. How the question is framed or whether the question will include all the components of PICO, such as a "C" or comparison, will depend on the type of question. For example, a PICO for a prognosis question usually has no "C" or comparison.

Acquire

After the question is framed, the next step in the process is to *acquire* the evidence. Practitioners should first search sites where research has already been critically reviewed and summarized and deemed of sufficient quality to guide clinical practice. These resources are sometimes referred to as filtered resources. Filtered resources feature the latest evidence-based literature on a clinical question. Filtered resources containing EBP information can be part of the clinical information systems (CISs) at a health care facility for use by health professionals. They collect and synthesize evidence from various sources, and they typically offer some interpretation and appraisal. Other sources with filtered information include websites such as Best Evidence (http://www.bestevidence.org/) and Bandolier (http://www.medicine.ox.ac.uk/bandolier/), journals such as *Evidence-Based Nursing*, and repositories in institutions and organizations where one can find critically appraised topics (CATs) or summaries of the best available evidence that provide readily accessible evidence. One good site for CATs is the Centre for Evidence-Based Medicine in Toronto, available through the Knowledge Translation (KT) Clearinghouse website funded by the Canadian Institute of Health Research (http://ktclearinghouse.ca/cebm/resources/web). Assuming one is drawing from a trustworthy source, the value of this type of evidence is that the work of appraisal has been done and the practitioner can move directly to examining applicability to the context and congruency with patient preference.

In the absence of information from sites that have preappraised the research, searches using individual bibliographic databases are the next action. To begin, start at the top of the evidence hierarchy, searching for systematic reviews and evidence-based guidelines—both preprocessed evidence making it easier for practitioners to use. Clinical guidelines generally promulgated by professional groups, government agencies, and local practices gather, appraise, and combine evidence of varying levels. They include practice recommendations designed to assist the practitioner in making patient decisions. Sources for evidence-based clinical guidelines include the National Guideline Clearinghouse (http://www.guideline.gov), the Agency for Healthcare Research and Quality (http://www.ahrq.gov), and the U.S. Preventive Services Task Force Recommendations (http://www.uspreventiveservicestaskforce .org/recommendations.htm).

Systematic reviews are searched for first because they provide a summary of research findings available on a particular topic or clinical question. Using an explicit, rigorous process to comprehensively identify, critically appraise, and synthesize relevant studies, findings from a systematic review have greater validity than a single research study. The search for systematic reviews should initially focus on sites that focus on this type of evidence. This includes the Cochrane Collaboration (http:// www.cochrane.org), the Campbell Collaboration (http://www.campbellcollaboration .org), and the Joanna Briggs Institute (http://www.joannabriggs.edu.au). One can also search for systematic reviews on PubMed by using the search feature PubMed Clinical Queries or Special Queries.

If systematic reviews are not present on the topic of interest/clinical question, retrieval of individual studies is the next source. Both systematic reviews and individual studies will need to be critically appraised by the practitioner. In searching, the components of the PICO question can be used as search terms. One can further limit the search by stipulating the preferred research design for the question being asked. Knowing the preferred research design (and thus, the strongest evidence), one can begin the search by stipulating the research approach, thus narrowing to "best" available evidence.

Appraise

Once relevant evidence has been acquired, the next step in ensuring that best evidence informs practice is to subject each study to scrutiny, to *appraise* the retrieved systematic reviews or individual studies for quality and confidence in the trustworthiness of the data and its clinical usefulness. The new paradigm of EBP requires developing the skill set to examine a research study for its fit to clinical practice. The appraisal process differs depending on the type of research design used. Both primary studies and secondary reviews must be appraised for their quality. More information about critical appraisal is presented in Chapter 7 as well as in the specific chapters on systematic review of observational, experimental, qualitative, and economic evidence.

Apply

After high-quality studies have been selected from the appraisal process, the next step is to determine whether there is applicability to one's own context and patient population. The decision to *apply* that results in real-time clinical practice is based on the magnitude of the findings, its applicability to different populations, and the strength of the evidence.

In considering the magnitude of the findings or the clinical significance, the practitioner must ask, "Is the size of the benefit (effect size) likely to help my patient?" This requires agreement between the patient and practitioner on the outcome that is important to the patient. The practitioner can provide the evidence to the patient about the likelihood of benefit or harm specific to the intervention, comparison interventions, and the desired outcome in plain language so that the patient can make an informed decision.

In research that examines whether interventions work, such as randomized controlled trials (RCTs), the intervention is often tested in a carefully defined population under tightly controlled situations that do not simulate real-world settings. The practitioners must determine whether the settings and patient populations from the studies or systematic review are similar to their own routine practice, and whether the interventions used can be duplicated and are acceptable to patients. Thus, in the application stage, one is questioning the ability to apply the findings to one's own context and one's own patient population. It is important to recognize that although the data may be objective, the meanings have intrinsically subjective value depending on the audience, and may differ among nurses, physicians, patients, and administrators (Manchikanti, Boswell, & Giordano, 2007).

A final factor to consider in examining applicability is the strength of the evidence. It is not unusual for studies to be of poor quality and, frequently, the recommendations of systematic reviews emphasize the need for more high-quality trials. One only has to consider the progression of recommendations for bed rest in the presence of low back pain. Recommendations from "experience" called for bed rest in episodes of acute back pain and sciatica. Early recommendations from lower levels and lower quality of evidence found bed rest to be effective in alleviating low back pain. Subsequent higher quality clinical trials found different results. In a 2010 systematic review on whether to advise patients to rest in bed versus to stay active for acute low back pain and sciatica, the moderate-quality evidence showed that patients with acute low back pain may experience small benefits in pain relief and functional improvement when advised to stay active, as compared to recommendations for bed rest. There was little or no difference between the two approaches in patients with sciatica (Dahm, Brurberg, Jamtvedt, & Hagen, 2010). In other words, activity was recommended. However, it must be pointed out that hierarchy of evidence is not absolute. It may be that observational studies with sufficiently large and consistent treatment effects may be more compelling than small RCTs (Manchikanti et al., 2007).

Act and Assess

If the practitioner identifies that the evidence can be applied to practice, the final steps are to *act* (put it into practice) and to *assess* whether the expected outcomes are achieved. This ongoing monitoring and review provides ongoing practice-based data on efficacy and effectiveness.

SUMMARY

This chapter has highlighted the new skills that nurses need in light of the paradigm shift to EBP. The components of EBP require best evidence to be integrated with patient values, the clinical context, and with clinical judgment/expertise. The process for incorporating the new paradigm requires an ongoing sense of inquiry in which the practitioner *asks* or challenges the way things are and whether practice is based on best practice, has the skills to *acquire* and *appraise* the evidence, makes decisions about whether to *apply* the evidence, and then *acts* by implementing the new practice and assessing the outcomes of the change.

EXERCISES

Review some of the policies and procedures in your place of employment. Can you tell what evidence was used to write these policies or procedures?

REFERENCES

Akobeng, A. K. (2005). Principles of evidence based medicine. *Archives of Disease in Childhood, 90*(8), 837–840.

Cook, D. J., Mulrow, C. D., & Haynes, R. B. (1997). Systematic reviews: Synthesis of best evidence for clinical decisions. *Annals of Internal Medicine, 126*(5), 389–391.

Dahm, K. T., Brurberg, K. G., Jamtvedt, G., & Hagen, K. B. (2010). Advice to rest in bed versus advice to stay active for acute low-back pain and sciatica. *Cochrane Database of Systematic Reviews, 2010*(6), CD007612. doi:10.1002/14651858.CD007612.pub2.

Dieppe, P., Rafferty, A., & Kitson, A. (2002). The clinical encounter: The focal point of patient-centered care. *Health Expectations, 5*(4), 279–281.

Kitson, A. (2002). Recognizing relationships: Reflections on evidence-based practice. *Nursing Inquiry, 9*(3), 179–186.

Manchikanti, L., Boswell, M. V., & Giordano, J. (2007). Evidence-based interventional pain management: Principles, problems, potential, and applications. *Pain Physician, 10*(2), 329–356.

Melnyk, B. M., Fineout-Overholt, E., Stillwell, S. B., & Williamson, K. M. (2009). Igniting a spirit of inquiry: An essential foundation for evidence-based practice. *American Journal of Nursing, 109*(11), 49–52.

Rycroft-Malone, J., Seers, K., Titchen, A., Harvey, G., Kitson, A., & McCormack, B. (2004). What counts as evidence in evidence-based practice? *Journal of Advanced Nursing, 47*(1), 81–90.

Sackett, D. L. (1998). Evidence-based medicine. *Spine, 23*(10), 1085–1086.

Sackett, D. L., Rosenberg, W. M., Gray, J. A., Haynes, R. B., & Richardson, W. S. (1996). Evidence based medicine: What it is and what it isn't. *British Medical Journal, 312*(7023), 71–72.

Sackett, D. L., Straus, S. E., Richardson, W. S., Rosenberg, W., & Haynes, R. B. (2000). *Evidence based medicine: How to practice and teach EBM* (2nd ed.). Edinburgh, Scotland: Churchill Livingstone.

Salmond, S. (2007). Advancing evidence-based practice: A primer. *Orthopaedic Nursing, 26*(2), 114–123.

Shah, H. M., & Chung, K. C. (2009). Archie Cochrane and his vision for evidence-based medicine. *Plastic and Reconstructive Surgery, 124*(3), 982–988.

Stillwell, S. B., Fineout-Overholt, E., Melnyk, B. M., & Williamson, K. M. (2010). Evidence-based practice, step by step: Asking the clinical question: A key step in evidence-based practice. *American Journal of Nursing, 110*(3), 58–61.

Swanson, J. A., Schmitz, D., & Chung, K. C. (2010). How to practice evidence-based medicine. *Plastic & Reconstructive Surgery, 126*(1), 286–294.

SUGGESTED READINGS

Evans, D., & Pearson, A. (2001). Systematic reviews: Gatekeepers of nursing knowledge. *Journal of Clinical Nursing, 10*(5), 593–599.

Furlan, A. D., van Tulder, M., Cherkin, D., Tsukayama, H., Lao, L., Koes, B., & Berman, B. (2005). Acupuncture and dry-needling for low back pain: An updated systematic review within the framework of the Cochrane Collaboration. *Spine, 30*(8), 944–963.

McCormack, B., Kitson, A., Harvey, G., Rycroft-Malone, J., Titchen, A., & Seers, K. (2001). Getting evidence into practice: The meaning of "context." *Journal of Advanced Nursing, 38*(1), 94–104.

Salmond, S. (2007). Advancing evidence-based practice: A primer. *Orthopaedic Nursing, 26*(2), 114–123.

Stevens, K. R. (2001). Systematic reviews: The heart of evidence-based practice. *AACN Clinical Issues: Advanced Practice in Acute and Critical Care, 12*(1), 529–538.

CHAPTER TWO

Steps in the Systematic Review Process

Susan W. Salmond

OBJECTIVES

Upon completion of Chapter 2, you will be able to:

- Review the definition for systematic review and importance of systematic reviews in clinical practice
- Outline steps involved in conducting a systematic review or steps in the systematic review process

IMPORTANT POINTS

- Systematic reviews provide reliable evidential summaries of completed research.
- A systematic review is a research method undertaken to provide an in-depth answer to a clinical question and to guide best practice.
- Systematic reviews may be quantitative or qualitative in nature or use mixed methods for a more comprehensive review.

INTRODUCTION

How can a practitioner stay current with the exponential expansion of health care literature? Should a clinician be relying on the results of a single study for making decisions in clinical practice? How does a practitioner make sense of the variable quality of published literature and the variable results of quality research? Systematic reviews are an efficient answer to some of these concerns because they provide reliable evidential summaries of past research for the busy practitioner. By pooling results from multiple studies, findings are based on multiple populations, conditions, and circumstances. The pooled results of many small studies can have more precise, more powerful, and more convincing conclusions (Cook, Mulrow, & Haynes, 1997). Table 2.1 captures benefits of systematic reviews over single studies.

TABLE 2.1

Benefits of Systematic Reviews

- Has a clear clinical question guiding the review
- Collapses large amounts of information that has been critically appraised to be rigorous into a manageable, usable form
- Provides clearer and less biased understanding because of the systematic process and the checks and balances of two researchers
- Increases the strength and generalizability/transferability of the findings, because they are derived from a broader range of populations, settings, circumstances, treatment variations, and study designs
- Minimizes bias from random and systematic error
- Pools and synthesizes existing information for decisions about clinical care, economic decisions, future research design, and policy formation
- Assesses consistencies and provides explanations for inconsistencies of relationships across studies
- Increases power in suggesting cause-and-effect relationships
- Increases confidence in conclusions
- Increases the likelihood of results being used in clinical practice
- Provides format for ongoing updates of new evidence
- Helps practitioners keep up-to-date with overwhelming quantity of medical literature

The synthesis is brought forward in a single statement, which is extremely valuable for the busy practitioner, and is likely to reduce the time lag for getting new evidence into practice, which is currently estimated to be about 17 years. For administrators, review articles help generate clinical policies that optimize outcomes using available resources. For researchers, systematic reviews help to summarize and clarify existing data and avoid unnecessary duplication of prior work (Margaliot & Chung, 2007). Systematic review allows new research to be designed and conducted from the most well-informed (and therefore well-armed) standpoint. By critically examining primary studies, it is possible to see the inconsistencies among diverse pieces of research evidence (Cook et al., 1997), and this helps researchers to refine hypotheses, more accurately estimate sample sizes, and define future research agendas.

A systematic review applies the same level of scientific rigor to the review process as used when conducting original research. It uses methods that are transparent, reproducible, and objective, thereby reducing the likelihood of bias and random error in the summarization process. Systematic reviews that follow this process and are appraised to have validity (the extent to which its design and conduct are likely to have been protected from bias) are a quality source of evidence to the practitioner and policy maker, and are replacing primary research as the source of evidence on which decisions are based (Evans & Pearson, 2001). This chapter will describe in depth the purpose of a systematic review and the steps in performing a systematic review.

SYSTEMATIC REVIEW

The word *systematic* refers to order and planning. In a systematic review, there is a set of transparent, orderly, structurally interrelated steps, carried out in a way that avoids bias and allows for peer review and independent verification. The systematic review addresses a clearly defined question. It uses a systematic and explicit methodology to identify, select, and critically appraise relevant studies. As an outcome of the critical appraisal process, decisions are made to include or exclude a study from the review so that the final data extraction and analyses use only data from high-quality, trustworthy studies. After data extraction, data from the primary studies are evaluated; however, it may or may not be possible to combine the data from the different studies. Quantitative aggregation, or meta-analysis, is the statistical pooling of the results from two or more separate studies that generates summary (pooled) estimates of effect. Qualitative aggregation, or metasynthesis, is an interpretive process that provides a framework for the synthesis/summary of findings from multiple qualitative studies relating to a phenomenon of interest (Evans & Pearson, 2001). Integrative review is often used when statistical analysis is not possible (Fineout-Overholt, O'Mathúna, & Kent, 2008).

Systematic reviews are often compared with traditional narrative review articles. However, narrative articles typically do not use explicit, systematic approaches in the review process and are more subjective. In narrative reviews, search strategies are not described, reasons for inclusion and exclusion of studies are not specified, critical appraisal is not done, and methods for synthesizing evidence are not clearly defined. Transparency is missing. Consequently, narrative reviews are more biased with a higher likelihood for inaccurate or unsubstantiated conclusions.

Systematic reviews, on the other hand, are a form of research that aims to identify, evaluate, and summarize the findings of all quality, relevant, individual studies on a topic systematically (Centre for Reviews and Dissemination, 2009), thereby relieving the end user of this time-consuming task. It requires the reviewers to have expertise in both the subject matter and the review method. Rigorous systematic reviews are completed by at least two reviewers, and key steps such as screening for inclusion criteria, critical appraisal, and data extraction are done independently and compared to minimize potential for bias. With methods training, expert practitioners are assuming the critical task of performing systematic reviews.

STEPS IN THE SYSTEMATIC REVIEW PROCESS

Systematic reviews are retrospective, observational research studies (Cook et al., 1997). Like primary research, they have preplanned methods, and the "subjects" in the research are original studies. By following the review steps described in the succeeding texts, it protects against unintended bias in the identification, selection, and use of published work in these reviews, and yields more trustworthy conclusions.

Systematic reviews are undertaken to answer specific, often narrow, clinical questions in depth. Although originally, the review process was focused on experimental studies, most commonly the randomized controlled trial, review methods have evolved for descriptive, observational, and interpretive research. Reviews may be quantitative or qualitative in nature, or a mixed review may be done. The steps in the process are the same; however, the technique used for each step will vary based on the type of question, type of research design, and approach to synthesis.

Step 1: Formulating a Question

Systematic reviews seek answers to specific, often narrow, clinical questions (Cook et al., 1997). The question should be clinically relevant, and often, it stems from unanswered questions in clinical practice. The question serves as the framework for the search, selection, and synthesis of studies (Evans, 2001a). If the question is too narrow, the number of included studies and patients may be small, and the precision of the review will be low. In contrast, if the question is left very broad, it will capture many more studies and patients but may fail to detect important relationships between subgroups of patients and the outcomes of interest (Margaliot & Chung, 2007). The question guides many of the review steps, including establishing eligibility criteria, performing the search for studies, collecting data from included studies, and presenting findings (Higgins & Green, 2008).

The PICO acronym is frequently used as a guide to specify the population or patient groups being studied, the intervention of interest, any comparators, and the outcomes of interest. Dans, Dans, and Silvestre (2008) use the acronym PEO, standing for populations, exposures, and outcomes.

P refers to the *population of interest* and is generally characterized by demographics (older adults, middle-aged women) and disease or condition (older adults at risk for a fall, middle-aged women with menopausal symptoms). *I* or *E* refers to the *intervention* or *exposure* being evaluated, and may include a treatment, diagnostic test, harmful exposure, or a prognostic factor. *C* refers to the *comparison exposure/intervention* and may or may not be included in the question. *O* refers to the *outcome* expected and could include a disease, complication, or a measure of health (Dans et al., 2008), and may be accompanied by a specification of time. For studies of appropriateness and meaning, an adaptation of the PICO (PICo) may be used, where *P* stands for the *population of interest*, *I* for the *phenomena of interest*, and *Co* for the *context* (The Joanna Briggs Institute [JBI], 2010). Criteria for and examples of questions of effectiveness, diagnosis, etiology or harm, prognosis, and meaning are given in Table 2.2. A more in-depth look at question type and development is provided in Chapter 4.

The PICO can be written as a question: "In children and adolescents, do cognitive-behavioral psychological interventions decrease needle-related procedural pain and distress?" or as an objective "to assess the efficacy of cognitive-behavioral psychological interventions for needle-related procedural pain and distress in children and adolescents." Generally, the objective or question is written as a single sentence. Secondary objectives targeting different participant groups, subgroups, and different comparisons of interventions or different outcome measures may also be developed.

TABLE 2.2

Asking Focused Questions

Type of Question	Element of the Clinical Question			
	P Patient	**I** Intervention (or Cause, Prognosis) or Phenomenon of Interest	**C** Comparison (Optional)	**O** Outcome
			Co: In qualitative studies (meaning questions), combine the C and O for context. The context may or may not have a time horizon	
	Describe as accurately as possible the patient or group of patients of interest (e.g., target clinical condition, coexisting condition, ethnicity, age group)	*What is the main intervention or therapy you wish to consider? This can be a form of a treatment, a diagnostic test, type of service delivery, and may also include any exposures to disease, or factors influencing prognosis*	*Describe if there is an alternative/ comparative treatment to the main intervention, including an actual intervention, treatment as usual, no disease, placebo, a different prognostic factor, absence of risk factors*	*Describe the clinical outcome of interest or effects relating to the intervention, such as prevention of side effects, morbidity, quality of life, and cost-effectiveness. Include a time frame if relevant.*
Intervention or therapy	In patients with chronic back pain	does keeping a pain diary	—	reduce pain and increase functional ability?
Intervention or therapy	In patients with sacral pressure ulcers	does the use of hydrocolloid dressings	compared to gauze dressings	provide greater patient comfort?
Intervention or therapy	In acute care hospitals	how does having a rapid response team	compared with not having a rapid response team	affect the number of cardiac arrests during a 3-month period?
Etiology	Are school-aged children	who have been exposed to in-home second-hand smoke	compared with children not exposed to in-home second-hand smoke	at greater risk for asthma and frequent respiratory infections?
Diagnosis or diagnostic test	In patients with suspected deep vein thrombosis	is an ultrasound scan	compared with a venogram	more accurate in diagnosing deep vein thrombosis?

(Continued)

TABLE 2.2
Asking Focused Questions (Continued)

Type of Question	Element of the Clinical Question			
Prognosis or prediction	In older women with osteoarthritis	does the use of a Cox-2 inhibitor	compared with other NSAIDs	decrease the risk of GI bleeding?
Meaning	How do family members	who witness an unsuccess-ful in-hospital resuscitation	perceive the helpfulness or harmfulness of the experience in the first month of grieving?	

Source: Adapted from Salmond, 2007; Melnyk, Fineout-Overholt, Stillwell, & Wiliamson, 2010; and Stillwell, Fineout-Overholt, Melnyk, & Williamson, 2010.

Step 2: Establishing the Inclusion Criteria

The inclusion and exclusion criteria set boundaries on the articles that will be selected for the study. Inclusion/exclusion criteria should address the types of studies, the types of people, the interventions or exposures, and the types of outcomes that are of interest (Farquhar & Vail, 2006; Higgins & Green, 2008; JBI, 2008). Too restrictive a list will yield few studies, small number of patients, and reduced precision, whereas broad criteria may result in an unmanageable number of studies and invalid conclusions. Inclusion and exclusion criteria are established a priori (Margaliot & Chung, 2007). It should be possible to explain the criteria based on a sound rationale from the perspective of the nursing, medical, or social sciences literature, rather than on unsubstantiated clinical, theoretical, or personal reasoning (JBI, 2008).

Inclusion Criteria for Studies

When setting inclusion criteria for studies, the acceptable study designs as well as any threshold criteria within the design need to be identified. Systematic reviews for the Cochrane Collaboration are primarily reviews of effectiveness and set inclusion criteria to include only randomized controlled trials and clinical controlled trials (types of study designs). One could set further criteria by indicating "all randomized controlled comparisons," thus specifying there must be a comparator group or "all randomized controlled trials with allocation concealment" that would restrict the retrieved studies to studies where the treatment to be allocated is not known before the patient entered into the study, or "attrition rate of less than 10%," which would eliminate the bias of mortality.

Unlike the Cochrane Collaboration, the philosophy of the JBI adopts a pluralistic approach to study designs and provides procedures for the review of evidence on feasibility, appropriateness, meaningfulness, and effectiveness. To this end, they do not restrict study designs to randomized controlled trials or clinical controlled trials, but rather, the designs flow from the type of review being conducted. The language used highlights the importance of searching for the "best available" evidence, not simply the preferred design. In many JBI reviews, there will be a hierarchy of studies that specify a range of studies to be used if the primary study type is not found. Thus, for a study of effectiveness, one would specify that randomized controlled trials would be sought but, in the absence of quality RCTs, other experimental study designs would be included. The hierarchy of evidence in an effectiveness study is generally well accepted to begin with RCTs, followed by quasi-experimental studies, cohort (with control) designs, case-controlled designs, observational studies, and finally, expert opinion in the absence of higher levels of evidence. The hierarchical wording for a review of effectiveness could read:

> The review will consider randomized controlled trials; in the absence of RCTs other research designs, such as non-randomized controlled trials and before-and-after studies, will be considered for inclusion in a narrative summary to enable the identification of current best evidence . . . (JBI, 2008, p. 20).

For studies of meaning, the selection of study design stems from whether one is restricting the design to interpretive or critical designs or is inclusive of both. To this end, the inclusion criteria may include interpretive studies with designs such as phenomenology, grounded theory, and ethnography; critical studies with designs such as action research and feminist research; or a combination of both. The wording for inclusion criteria in a study of meaning could read:

> This review will consider studies that focus on qualitative data including, but not limited to, designs such as phenomenology, ground theory, ethnography, action research and feminist research. In the absence of research studies, other text such as opinion papers and reports will be considered in a narrative summary. (JBI, 2008, p. 31).

One must also specify inclusion criteria for dates during which studies should be retrieved (i.e., 2005–2010), and the accepted languages that can be included. Many systematic reviews limit the language to English, which does create a language bias and may call into question the trustworthiness of the findings. For example, if a review topic was "to assess the efficacy of acupuncture in alleviating pain and increasing functional ability in adults with chronic low back pain," restriction to English may exclude many studies published in Chinese that could bias the findings.

Inclusion Criteria for Participants

Inclusion criteria specify the demographic characteristics of the population, the diseases or conditions of interest, and the setting. Characteristics of the population include factors such as gender, age, race, or educational status. These characteristics are used if they have relevancy to the review question. Disease or conditions of interest may include presence of a condition such as hot flashes or stress incontinence or the designation of a disease according to set diagnostic criteria. Settings may include hospitalized patients, residents of nursing facilities, or community-dwelling or residents of specific communities. Exclusion criteria can be used to restrict studies that deal with types of people who may react to the intervention in a different way (Higgins & Green, 2008). The participant inclusion criteria may be written as a narrative, such as "The review included studies where the participants were adult intensive care patients, family members of adult intensive care patients, intensive care nurses caring for the adult critically ill patient, and ward/unit nurses receiving transfer patients from the intensive care unit. Studies examining the transfer experience for infants, children, or psychiatric patients were excluded from this review."

In qualitative studies, the population is frequently combined with the context. Context may include cultural factors, geographic locations, specific gender-based or racial interests, and setting of care because they relate to the meanings that the population ascribes to the phenomenon of interest.

Inclusion Criteria for Interventions/Phenomena of Interest

The interventions of interest and the comparator interventions (if any) must be delineated. Depending on the question, the intervention may be broad such as "anti-inflammatory drugs," or can be narrow such as nonsteroidal anti-inflammatory drugs, or even narrower to a specific drug such as naproxen. According to Higgins and Green (2008), comparators may include inactive control intervention (no treatment, placebo, standard care) or active control intervention (a different option or approach of the same intervention, a different drug or a different kind of therapy). When possible, describe the intervention and comparator in detail. It is not enough to identify a drug or a treatment or exposure. There needs to be further detail of the definition, intensity, timing, duration, and method of delivery (Forbes, 2003). Furthermore, it is necessary to determine how to handle trials that included only part of intervention, or trials that included the intervention of interest combined with another intervention.

In a qualitative systematic review, the phenomenon of interest may vary based on the complexity of the topic. For example, the phenomenon of interest may be transition into the workforce. This could be further delineated as the experience of new graduates in the first 6 months of transition or the experience of second-career new graduates. The phenomenon of interest may be expanded or revised as the protocol develops (JBI, 2008).

Inclusion Criteria for Outcomes

Inclusion criteria for outcomes attempt to delineate the outcomes of interest for the review that are clinically relevant. According to Higgins and Green (2008), outcomes for studies may include survival (mortality), clinical events (need for intubation, resuscitation, strokes), knowledge levels, patient-reported outcomes (pain, suffering, anxiety, functional ability, quality of life, satisfaction), potential and actual adverse events (hospital-acquired pressure ulcers, ventilator-associated pneumonia), burdens (demands on caregivers, frequency of tests restrictions on lifestyle), and economic outcomes (costs and resource use). A review may consider a single outcome or a range of outcomes.

Further consideration is given to whether there are specific methodological approaches required for measuring the outcome and the timing of the outcome (short term, medium term, and long term). Sources to assist the investigator in determining relevant outcomes include clinical experiences, feedback from advisory groups and consumers, and evidence from the literature. Outcomes are established in advance, although others may be added as the review progresses. The Cochrane Handbook for Systematic Reviews suggests no more than seven main outcomes, and defines main outcomes as those that are essential for decision making with a focus on patient-important outcomes (Higgins & Green, 2008).

Step 3: Developing a Search Strategy/Performing the Search

A comprehensive, unbiased search of the literature is the hallmark of a systematic review. The search is meant to be exhaustive, and errors, or lapses, in the search process potentially result in a biased or otherwise incomplete evidence base (McGowan & Sampson, 2005). It is critical to have an expert librarian familiar with searches for systematic reviews as part of the team. It is a time-consuming process and cannot be rushed because the quality of the final product depends on the effectiveness of the search. Chapters 5 and 6 provide more comprehensive information on searching.

The search process used in systematic review science is unlike searches for any other scholarly work in its comprehensiveness and iterative approach. Essential components of the search include keyword identification, search strategies for multiple databases, hand-searching journals, footnote chasing, gray literature (e.g., unpublished research and theses) searching, and author contact (Magarey, 2001). The search strategy is clearly documented, making it transparent so the search can be evaluated for quality as well as facilitating replication of and consistency in the search approach used when the systematic review is updated (Yoshii, Plaut, McGraw, Anderson, & Wellik, 2009).

Planning for the Search

An appointment should be made early in the process with a librarian to discuss end goals for the review. The librarian will need to know the objective of the review, such as "My SR will inform a local community project," or "We are thinking of starting with interventions aimed at teenagers and obesity." Discussion about preliminary searches that the reviewer has already tried and the resources/databases that have already been searched will allow the librarian to provide more direct advice. Bring to the meeting example articles or citations that typify the kind of research being considered to inform the systematic review.

The librarian will work closely with the investigators to understand the systematic review question, refine the questions, and characterize them in terms of their elements within the PICO format. The PICO along with the inclusion and exclusion criteria assist in the formulating of key terms. Concept mapping and synonym identification are important components of key term mapping. The librarian will further assist in expanding the complete set of terms and Boolean logic combinations to use in the search, and will adapt the search to match the structure of the different databases that will be used in the search.

Components of the Search

The search strategy requires identification of the databases to be used. In nursing, there are four major bibliographic databases that are generally searched first—Ovid, MEDLINE, Cumulative Index to Nursing and Allied Health Literature (CINAHL), and Embase. Although there will be redundancy in paper identification because of the differences in indexing across databases, a paper may be in one database and not the other, making a search of each database essential. In addition to bibliographic databases, comprehensive searches may include a search of trial registries and special subject bibliographies (lists of materials that relate to a particular discipline or subject). Registers of clinical trials, available through the CENTRAL database of the Cochrane Collaboration, are an important resource to systematic reviewers.

Searching goes beyond traditional databases to protect against potential publication bias and database bias (McGowan & Sampson, 2005). There is likely valuable information in the gray literature. Timely gray literature captures documents that are not indexed by commercial publishers and cannot be found easily through conventional channels. Scientific gray literature comprises newsletters, reports, working papers, theses, government documents, bulletins, fact sheets, conference proceedings, and other publications distributed free, available by subscription, or for sale. A website called GreyNet (http://www.greynet.org) assists investigators and librarians with the use and production of gray literature. The search should also include strategies to identify unpublished dissertations and theses (Dissertation Abstracts, ProQuest Dissertations & Theses Database, Theses Canada, Index to Theses in Great Britain and Ireland), because it may identify studies that were not accepted for publication. Conference proceedings are a good source of identifying other unpublished studies. Investigators may correspond with authors who have published on the topic of interest or other colleagues expert in the field to also identify any unpublished manuscripts and other gray literature. The Virginia Henderson International Nursing Library of Sigma Theta Tau International (STTI) is a gray literature site holding all of the STTI conference abstracts and author contact information.

Hand searching and footnote chasing are two other approaches to study identification. The investigators should identify the journals that commonly publish on the topic area. These journals should be hand searched for possible articles. Consideration needs to be given to how extensive hand searching should be. Footnote chasing involves reviewing the references of published studies for the primary studies cited. These approaches are especially important in areas where the science is not well established and for qualitative studies where titles may be metaphorical and studies are not always coded by research design. Finally, an author search should be conducted using the names of authors who have published more than two papers on the review topic.

Managing the Citations

Bibliography citation management tools will allow for citations or references to be placed in an online space that the research team can access, organize, and add to. Examples of fee-based bibliography citation management tools or software include

TABLE 2.3

Advantages to Using a Citation Management System

■ Permanent storage of citations, making it easy to keep track of them and use them for this and related projects
■ Sharing of citations among research partners
■ Sorting of citations by author, title, year, or other fields. The citation tool should also allow for organization of references in groups or categories such as "Group 1: Citations for SR Results section."
■ Deletion of duplicate citations. This is especially useful because duplicate references will occur when searching multiple databases.
■ Customization of the look of each reference adding information, such as personal research notes or comments for a reference
■ Ability to attach files near citations or references stored in the manager, such as PDF full-text article files for references
■ Ability to import citations or references of web pages
■ Placement of citations into your systematic review paper in specific formatting styles such as Journal of the American Medical Association (JAMA) or American Psychological Association (APA)

EndNote, Reference Manager, and RefWorks. Some free citation management tools accessible via the Internet include BibDesk (citation manager that works with Macintosh [Apple, Inc.] computers), Carmun, Citavi, CiteULike, Connotea, JabRef, Mendeley, WizCite, and Zotero.

Organization is paramount throughout the systematic review research process. Search strategies should be written down on paper and search steps saved via database save options. Relevant citations should be imported into citation management software or tools. The advantages of this process are reported in Table 2.3.

Citation management software such as EndNote may work with systematic review article analysis tools, such as the JBI's Comprehensive Review Management System (CReMS). Ask a librarian about available fee-based citation management tools that the library may offer. Librarians may provide instructions or workshops on how to use specific managers. They can also alert you to new tools available in online databases to manage citations such as "My Workspace," a feature from Ovid Technologies as of summer 2010, available on all databases you search on the OvidSP search retrieval system. Citations saved in "My Workspace" can be exported into a new Microsoft Word (Microsoft Corporation) document or bibliography management tools such as Citavi, EndNote, or Reference Manager. Microsoft Word 2007 includes a References tab that can be used to format citations in select styles such as APA, MLA (Modern Language Association), and Chicago.

Keeping the Search Current and Documenting the Search

Setting up RSS (Really Simple Syndication) feeds for notification about new manuscripts aids in keeping the search current while the work of appraisal, extraction, and synthesis occurs. Referral to Current Contents, a web-based current awareness database, can inform investigators of new material because it provides daily updates of complete tables of contents, abstracts, and bibliographic information from leading scholarly journals and evaluated websites. Information in this source is usually more up-to-date than traditional databases. Many reviewers will rerun the search (with new date limits) prior to final data extraction and synthesis.

Throughout the search, the strategies used, databases searched, number of items downloaded from each database, and number of duplicate items removed must be recorded for final reporting. This information is often reported both in a narrative and in an algorithm/flow chart describing the total number of records identified through search, total number found in hand searching, author contacting and footnote chasing, and number of duplicates removed. Guidelines for reporting can be found by referring to Consolidated Standards of Reporting Trials (CONSORT), Quality of Reporting of Meta-analyses (QUOROM), Meta-analysis of Observational Studies in Epidemiology (MOOSE), and Strengthening the Reporting of Observational Studies in Epidemiology (STROBE) statements. In essence, these guidelines tell investigators and authors what information is required to ensure that readers (and reviewers) can properly evaluate the study (Brand, 2009).

Step 4: Selection of Articles to Be Included in the Systematic Review

Although conduct of a systematic review is usually a team effort, there are steps that mandate at least two individuals independently perform the function. This enhances the reliability of the study. Selection of articles to be included in the systematic review requires this two-person approach.

Screening of Titles and Abstracts

Once the search has been conducted, the first step in study selection is to screen the titles and/or abstracts for its fit with the PICO question and inclusion/exclusion criteria. Generally, the initial search retrieves a large number of potentially useful articles; however, only a small percentage of these articles end up in the final review article. The first round of elimination occurs as the titles or abstracts are reviewed against the inclusion/exclusion criteria. The article is rejected if its title or abstract is sufficient to provide the information that the publication is not relevant. Oftentimes, it is because the publication is not a research study, there is a population other than specified in the inclusion criteria, the article is anecdotal, or the intervention varied in a meaningful way. Once titles and abstracts have been reviewed by two independent investigators, their findings are reviewed. Any differences are discussed and the articles re-reviewed for a decision whether to exclude or move on to the next step in selection, which is critical appraisal of the full text. If necessary, a third party can be used to resolve any dispute. At this stage, it is better to err on the side of overinclusion (Ryś, Władysiuk, Skrzekowska-Baran, & Małecki, 2009) and the full text article can be retrieved and critically appraised.

Critical Appraisal of Retrieved Studies

The usefulness of the findings from systematic reviews depends on the quality of the individual studies within the review. All studies that met the relevant inclusion criteria are next subject to a quality assessment, a process that ensures that studies included in the final review had adequate internal validity—that their design and conduct are likely to prevent systematic errors or bias. Consequently, the process enhances the credibility of the conclusions drawn (Thomas, Ciliska, Dobbins, & Micucci, 2004; Ryś, et al., 2009). The appraisal is usually based on structured scales or questionnaires that vary according to the type of research (quantitative or qualitative) and the study design used. Most items are scored as *yes, no,* or *can't tell*; or *met, unmet,* or *unclear.*

Reviews are performed independently by two investigators. After independent reviews are completed, the investigators compare the independent appraisals and dialog about any differences—returning to the original study to confirm rationale for their opinion. A third party is used in the event that the two reviewers cannot reach agreement. The final decision in the appraisal process is to include or exclude the study. Exclusion may be based on a proportion of the criteria rated as *no/unmet* or *can't tell/unclear,* or by differentially weighting certain items and needing to obtain a preset score. Excluded studies and the rationale for exclusion are recorded in a table of excluded studies.

Chapter 7 provides more information on critical appraisal, and Chapters 8, 9, 10, and 11 provide specific information related to appraisal of observational, experimental, qualitative, and economic evidence.

Step 5: Data Extraction

In a systematic review, the subject is the primary (original) research article. Data extraction involves sourcing and recording relevant information from the original article. Using a standardized approach by two reviewers ensures accuracy of this process. Data are extracted about the study design components, and these data are summarized in a table of included studies that provides information for each included study. Data extraction tools are available through the Cochrane Collaboration and the JBI and can be individualized to the study. Data collection tools serve as the record of the data collected and help to ensure that all relevant data are collected and that the chances of transcription error are minimized. It also allows for the accuracy of data to be checked (Evans, 2001b). Data extraction tools are part of the research proposal and should be piloted with a representative sample of the studies, and then adapted based on this review (Forbes, 2003; Magarey, 2001).

Although individual chapters will provide more information on data extraction for that particular study design, common design factors are identified as follows and in Table 2.4. These factors are generally included in a "study characteristics table."

- *Methods* information refers to the type of design, and if the study is quantitative, approaches to minimize bias should be described. Information on methodology, methods, and the phenomena of interest should be reported for qualitative studies.

TABLE 2.4

Potential Information for Characteristics of Included Studies

Methodology/ Methods	Participants and Setting	Interventions	Outcome Measures/ Adverse Outcomes	Results	Conclusions
What was the: Study design? Study purpose/aims? Study duration? Specific methods used? For Quantitative Designs: Sequence generation? Allocation sequence concealment? Blinding?	■ Sample Size ■ Relevant demographic characteristics of sample ■ Criteria for diagnosis/condition identification ■ Relevant comorbidities ■ Contextual factors: setting, culture, geography	■ Number of intervention groups ■ Details of specific intervention for each group and integrity of intervention ■ Qualitative studies generally have no interventions but are exploring a phenomena of interest	Quantitative ■ Outcomes and time points when outcome measures are collected ■ Outcome definition ■ Unit of measurement and interpretation of measurement Qualitative ■ Experience of participants	Quantitative ■ Number of participants allocated to each intervention group ■ Number for which outcome is being reported on ■ Missing participants ■ Statistical data ■ Estimate of effect ■ Subgroup analysis Qualitative ■ Findings with descriptive illustrations	Authors key conclusions

- *Participant data* provide not only sample size information, but also any demographic or disease factors that could influence the direction and strength of an intervention effect (quantitative) or the meaning of the experience (qualitative), as well as those characteristics that would assist the readers in determining applicability to their own patient population. The setting is usually indicated for quantitative studies. In qualitative work, establishing the context is quite important, and information regarding setting, geographical location, culture, and participant information is important in establishing the context. Disease characteristics such as staging, diagnostic parameters, or certain symptoms could be relevant data.
- For quantitative studies, details of *interventions* should be provided for the experimental group(s) and control group. This should include enough detail to allow replication. For studies examining drugs or physical interventions, provide detail on route of delivery/surgical technique, dose, frequency, timing, and length of treatment. For educational and psychobehavioral intervention studies, report on the contents of the intervention, who delivered it, and the format and timing of the delivery (Higgins & Green, 2008). Additionally, it is important to report on the integrity of the intervention—did it go as planned?
- *Outcomes* of interest are specified a priori in the research protocol and in data extraction; only those outcomes that were identified in advance are extracted. Outcome measures should be defined (to also include explanation of scoring) along with when the measure will be taken. *Adverse outcomes* are collected when the study is examining harmful effects of interventions and similar to reporting interventions; the definition of the adverse outcome must be clearly described to allow for comparison. In randomized controlled trials, a tool extracting data related to bias is also completed. For qualitative studies, the *method of data analysis* used in the primary study is identified.
- The *results* extracted are based on the research design, and the quantitative research proposal will specify which outcome measures, time points, and summary statistics are to be extracted. When using JBI or Cochrane Collaboration software for quantitative reviews, there are required fields that must be completed inclusive of the sample sizes per group and the intervention or exposure per group. For outcomes that are dichotomous, the number with the exposure and the total sample for both control and treatment groups are entered. For continuous data, the mean and standard deviation plus sample size are extracted for each outcome specified in the protocol for both the control and intervention (exposure) group. If the publication does not provide all of the results data with needed clarity for the different groups, attempts should be made to contact the author. For qualitative studies, the results extracted include the findings or the conclusion reached by the investigator, presented in the form of themes or metaphors with accompanying text, which illustrates these findings (JBI, 2008). The reviewer reads and rereads the paper to identify the findings and the appropriate illustrations that capture the different concepts within the theme. Each finding/illustration is assessed for congruency, and the reviewer grades the credibility of the researcher's interpretation.
- *Author conclusions* are generally reported. Conclusions should be examined for congruency with the findings.
- *Funding sources/conflict of interest* is now considered important information to collect.

Step 6: Data Synthesis

The inherent purpose of a systematic review is not only to provide data about the included studies, but also to summarize the findings of the included studies. This can be accomplished through a statistical analysis, a qualitative synthesis, or a narrative descriptive synthesis. A meta-analysis is a statistical approach that calculates a pooled estimate of effect and its confidence interval, and provides a combined estimate of effectiveness of a particular treatment (Forbes, 2003; Lipp, 2003; Magarey, 2001). Meta-analysis can only be used when the studies have similar questions, use the same population, administer the intervention in a similar perspective, and focus on the same interventions. This is especially valuable when the primary literature consists of small, underpowered studies. Pooling allows for a more precise estimate of the true effect of the intervention (Margaliot & Chung, 2007). Meta-analysis reports odds ratios for dichotomous data and mean and standard deviation for continuous data (Magarey, 2001). Data that are conflicting (i.e., measured with different outcome measures and that are widely variable) cannot be pooled in a meta-analysis; rather, they are reported through a descriptive synthesis. A descriptive synthesis provides a tabular summary of all studies related to each key piece of information identified as important and facilitates analysis of comparison across studies. Both approaches allow for identification of underlying causes of heterogeneity, leading to suggestions for future research.

Metasynthesis is used for qualitative studies pool and seeks to generate new interpretations from the findings of individual studies (Evans, 2001a). Qualitative metasynthesis involves a synthesis of findings across studies using qualitative comparative analysis. The aim of qualitative metasynthesis is to capture similarities and differences in language, concepts, images, and other ideas around a target experience (Sandelowski, Docherty, & Emden, 1997). The goal in quantitative meta-analysis is to reduce findings to a "common metric"; however, the aims for qualitative metasynthesis are quite different—they are to "enlarge the interpretive possibilities of findings and deconstruct larger narrative and general theories" (Sandelowski et al., 1997, p. 369). The approach to metasynthesis is to determine how studies are related, or dissonant, through a compare and contrast analysis (Walsh & Downe, 2004). Common themes/concepts are identified and discordance and dissonance are noted. Cross-study analysis then occurs with findings interpreted using metaphors and concepts applicable across studies, and finally, synthesis statements that capture the essence of the interpreted findings are set forth (Walsh & Downe, 2004).

Step 7: Recommendations for Practice and Future Research and Writing the Review

The purpose of systematic reviews is to guide practice and provide the data on which to base plans for future research. To this end, the goal of the systematic review is to draw conclusions from the data, recognizing that some studies may be more highly rated because of their level of evidence. As one attempts to reach conclusions, it is important to speak of limitations of the primary studies.

Whether this be the fact that reviews were lower levels of evidence, limited to the English language, or not able to perform meta-analysis because of heterogeneity, addressing limitations increases the confidence in the recommendations (Pai et al., 2004). Recommendations for practice and future research should flow from the data synthesis.

There is a growing movement to obtain consistency in the write-up of systematic reviews, and several guidelines are available to standardize the writing process. Guidelines, such as the Preferred Reporting Items for Systematic Reviews and Meta-Analyses (PRISMA; http://www.prisma-statement.org) and Consolidated Standards of Reporting Trials (CONSORT; http://www.consort-statement.org), not only assist with appraising studies, but also help to identify best practices for conducting and writing up a systematic review (Liberati et al., 2009; Turpin, 2005). For writing up studies of controlled trials, the QUOROM guidelines should be used (Moher et al., 1999), and for observational studies, the MOOSE guidelines should be followed (Stroup et al., 2000).

Step 8: Updating the Systematic Review

As science evolves with the accumulation of new knowledge, what was at one point considered to be effective and safe may in the future be shown to be ineffective or harmful or vice versa (Chalmers & Haynes, 1994). Updating systematic reviews aims to incorporate new evidence into a previously completed review (Moher & Tsertsvadze, 2006). Systematic reviews registered with either Cochrane or the JBI require that review authors keep the review up-to-date. The question regarding when a review needs to be updated depends on the rapidity and scope of scientific and technological developments, nature of the health condition, and its public health importance (Moher et al., 2008). As a rule of thumb, the literature should be reviewed every 2 years to determine the advancement of knowledge and need for an updated review.

SUMMARY

This chapter has highlighted the benefits of systematic reviews as compared with traditional narrative reviews. The steps in the systematic review process have been presented to provide an overview of the comprehensiveness and rigor in the process. Systematic reviews that are retrieved to answer clinical questions should be reviewed for their adherence to the steps in this process.

EXERCISES

Read the systematic review: Reisenberg, L. A., Leisch, J., Cunningham, J. M. (2010). Nursing handoffs: A systematic review of the literature. *American Journal of Nursing, 110*(4), 24–34. doi: 10.1097/01.NAJ.0000370154.79857.09

Can you determine the steps the reviewers took in constructing this systematic review? Are they clear enough for you to be able to use this same method?

REFERENCES

Brand, R. A. (2009). Standards for reporting: The CONSORT, QUORUM, and STROBE guidelines. *Clinical Orthopedics and Related Research, 467*(6), 1393–1394.

Centre for Reviews and Dissemination. (2009). Systematic reviews: CRD's guidance for undertaking reviews in health care. University of York: Author. Retrieved from http://www.york.ac.uk/inst/crd/systematic_reviews_book.htm

Chalmers, I., & Haynes, B. (1994). Reporting, updating, and correcting systematic reviews of the effects of health care. *British Medical Journal, 30*(6958), 862–865.

Cook, D. J., Mulrow, C. D., & Haynes, R. B. (1997). Systematic reviews: Synthesis of best evidence for clinical decisions. *Annals of Internal Medicine, 126*(5), 376–380.

Dans, A. L., Dans, L. F., & Silvestre, M. A., Eds (2008). *Painless evidence-based medicine.* West Sussex, England: Wiley-Blackwell.

Evans, D. (2001a). Systematic reviews of nursing research. *Intensive and Critical Care Nursing, 17*(1), 51–57.

Evans, D. (2001b). An introduction to systematic reviews. *Evidence Based Practice Information Sheets for Health Professionals.* September 1, p. 1–6, Joanna Briggs Institute.

Evans, D., & Pearson, A. (2001). Systematic reviews: Gatekeepers of nursing knowledge. *Journal of Clinical Nursing, 10*(5), 593–599.

Farquhar, C., & Vail, A. (2006). Pitfalls in systematic reviews. *Current Opinions in Obstetrics and Gynecology, 18*(4), 433–439.

Fineout-Overholt, E., O'Mathúna, D. P., & Kent, B. (2008). How systematic reviews can foster evidence-based clinical decisions. *Worldviews on Evidence-Based Nursing, 5*(1), 45–48.

Forbes, D. A. (2003). An example of the use of systematic reviews to answer an effectiveness question. *Western Journal of Nursing Research, 25*(2), 179–192.

Higgins, J. P. T., & Green, S. (2008). *Cochrane handbook for systematic reviews of interventions.* West Sussex, England: Wiley-Blackwell.

The Joanna Briggs Institute. (2008). *The Joanna Briggs Institute reviewer's manual: 2008 Ed.* Adelaide, Australia: Author.

Liberati, A., Altman, D. G., Tetzlaff, J., Mulrow, C., Gøtzsche, P. C., Ioannidis, J. P., . . . Moher, D. (2009). The PRISMA statement for reporting systematic reviews and meta-analyses of studies that evaluate health care interventions: Explanation and elaboration. *Journal of Clinical Epidemiology, 62*(10), e1–e34. doi: 10.1016/j.jclinepi.2009.06.006; pii:S0895-4356(09)00180-2.

Lipp, A. (2003). A guide to developing a systematic review. *Association of Perioperative Registered Nurses Journal, 78*(1), 97–107.

Magarey, J. M. (2001). Elements of a systematic review. *International Journal of Nursing Practice, 7*(6), 376–382.

Margaliot, Z., & Chung, K. C. (2007). Systematic reviews: A primer for plastic surgery research. *Plastic and Reconstructive Surgery, 120*(7), 1834–1841.

McGowan, J., & Sampson, M. (2005). Systematic reviews need systematic searchers. *Journal of the Medical Library Association, 93*(1), 74–80.

Melnyk, B. M., Fineout-Overholt, E., Stillwell, S., & Williamson, K. (2010). Igniting a spirit of inquiry: An essential foundation for evidence-based practice. *American Journal of Nursing, 109*(11), 49–53.

Moher, D., Cook, D. J., Eastwood, S., Olkin, I., Rennie, D., & Stroup, D. F. (1999). Improving the quality of reports of meta-analysis of randomized controlled trials: The QUOROM statement. Quality of Reporting of Meta-analyses. *The Lancet, 354*(9193), 1896–1900.

Moher, D., & Tsertsvadze, A. (2006). Systematic reviews: When is an update an update? *The Lancet, 367*(9514), 881–883.

Moher, D., Tsertsvadze, A., Tricco, A. C., Eccles, M., Grimshaw, J., Sampson, M., & Barrowman, N. (2008). When and how to update systematic reviews. *The Cochrane of Systematic Reviews,* (1), MR000023.

Pai, M., McCulloch, M., Gorman, J. D., Pai, N., Enanoria, W., Kennedy, G., . . . Colford, J. M. Jr. (2004). Systematic reviews and meta-analyses: An illustrated, step-by-step guide. *National Medical Journal of India, 17*(2), 86–95.

Reisenberg, L. A., Leisch, J., Cunningham, J. M. (2010). Nursing handoffs: A systematic review of the literature. *American Journal of Nursing, 110*(4), 24–34. doi: 10.1097/01. NAJ.0000370154.79857.09

Ryś, P., Władysiuk, M., Skrzekowska-Baran, I., & Małecki, M. T. (2009). Review articles, systematic reviews, and meta-analyses: which can be trusted? *Polskie Archiwum Medycyny Wewnętrznej, 119*(3), 148–156.

Salmond, S. W. (2007). Advancing evidence-based practice: A primer. *Orthopaedic Nursing, 26*(2), 114–123.

Sandelowski, M., Docherty, S., & Emden, C. (1997). Qualitative metasyntheses: Issues and techniques. *Research in Nursing & Health, 20*(4), 365–371.

Stillwell, S., Fineout-Overholt, E., Melnyk, B. M., & Williamson, K. (2010). Searching for the evidence. *American Journal of Nursing, 110*(5), 41–47.

Stroup, D. D., Berlin, J. A., Morton, S. C., Olkin, I., Williamson, G. D., Rennie, D., . . . Thacker, S. B. (2000). Meta-analysis of observational studies in epidemiology: A proposal for reporting Meta-analysis of Observational Studies in Epidemiology (MOOSE) group. *Journal of the American Medical Association, 283*(15), 2008–2012.

Thomas, B. H., Ciliska, D., Dobbins, M., & Micucci, B. A. (2004). A process for systematically reviewing the literature: Providing the research evidence for public health nursing interventions. *Worldviews of Evidence-Based Nursing, 1*(3), 176–184.

Turpin, D. L. (2005). CONSORT and QUOROM guidelines for reporting randomized clinical trials and systematic reviews. *American Journal of Orthodontics and Dentofacial Orthopedics, 128*(6), 681–685.

Walsh, D., & Downe, S. (2004). Meta-synthesis method for qualitative research: A literature review. *Journal of Advanced Nursing, 50*(2), 204–211.

Yoshii, A., Plaut, D. A., McGraw, K. A., Anderson, M. J., & Wellik, K. E. (2009). Analysis of the reporting of search strategies in Cochrane systematic reviews. *Journal of Medical Librarians Association, 97*(1), 21–29.

SUGGESTED READINGS

Cohen, D. J., & Crabtree, B. F. (2008). Evaluative criteria for qualitative research in health care: Controversies and recommendations. *Annals of Family Medicine, 6*(4), 331–339.

Evans D, & Pearson A. (2001). Systematic reviews: Gatekeepers of nursing knowledge. *Journal of Clinical Nursing, 10*(5):593–599.

Feldstein, D. A. (2005). Clinician's guide to systematic reviews and meta-analyses. *Wisconsin Medical Journal, 104*(3), 25–29.

Hannes, K., Lockwood, C., & Pearson, C. (2010). A comparative analysis of three online appraisal instruments' ability to assess validity in qualitative research. *Qualitative Health Research, 20*(12), 1736–1743. Epub 2010 Jul 29. doi:10.1177/1049732310378656

Pearson, A., Wiechula, R., Court, A., & Lockwood, C. (2007). A re-consideration of what constitutes "evidence" in the healthcare professions. *Nursing Science Quarterly, 20*(1), 85–88.

Stevens, K. R. (2001). Systematic reviews: The heart of evidence-based practice. *AACN Clinical Issues, 12*(4), 529–538.

PART II

A Framework for Conducting Systematic Reviews

CHAPTER THREE

Planning and Organizing a Systematic Review

Cheryl Holly

Upon completion of Chapter 3, you will be able to:

- List the necessary components of a systematic review proposal
- Describe the attributes of a good systematic review proposal
- Develop a systematic review proposal

- A systematic review proposal serves as a map for the review.
- The objective in writing a proposal for a systematic review is to clearly and succinctly describe what you want to do, why it is important that the review should be done, what methods will be used to conduct the review, and how the findings of the review might be used.
- A body of the proposal for a systematic review should not be more than 15–20 pages of double-spaced text. The title page, reference lists, and appendices are additional.
- See Exhibit 3.1 at the end of this chapter for an example of a systematic review proposal.

INTRODUCTION

A well-written proposal serves as a blueprint for a systematic review, and importantly, gives it the transparency that is necessary in this type of research. Transparency eliminates ambiguity and allows anyone to pick up the proposal and follow it precisely to be reasonably certain of obtaining the same results. A proposal serves as a statement of purpose and provides a detailed plan for the project. It is important to spend a considerable amount of time when writing the proposal because it is the groundwork for writing the review findings. The key components of a systematic review proposal are listed in Box 3.1. A personal perspective on organizing and conducting a systematic review can be found in Box 3.2. This perspective highlights the skills needed to successfully complete a systematic review.

BOX 3.1
Key Components of a Systematic Review Proposal

Title
Reviewers
Beginning and ending dates
Background
Objectives
Criteria for inclusion of studies in the review
    Types of studies
    Types of intervention/phenomenon of interest
    Types of outcomes
Search strategy
Assessment of methodological quality
    Critical appraisal
    Method to extract data
    Method to synthesize data
References and appendices

TITLE OF SYSTEMATIC REVIEW PROTOCOL

The title of the systematic review protocol should precisely describe the review to be undertaken. It should not be more than 10–20 words. One simple sentence that includes the aims and the outcomes of the study should suffice. The formal title of the review should be written after the aims and the objectives of the review are finalized to ensure congruency.

Examples of the title of the systematic review protocols are as follows:

"A systematic review of the effectiveness of smoking cessation strategies for adolescents in a residential facility"
"A qualitative systematic review of the experiences of families of patients in an intensive care unit"
"A comparison of the cost effectiveness of three different methods of intravenous dressing change"

REVIEWERS

At a minimum, a primary and a secondary reviewer should be identified. Reviewers work independently of each other. The primary reviewer is responsible for the overall conduct of the review and for keeping the other reviewers on track and moving toward the completion of the review. The secondary reviewer is in charge of setting the agenda and timeframe for the review. Both reviewers should have a good understanding of research design and the ability to critique research studies. It is important

BOX 3.2
Conducting a Systematic Review: A Personal Perspective

Having recently completed my first systematic review, I was asked by esteemed colleagues to offer practical guidance for others who were intending to undertake a similar endeavor. My aim, undertaken with great humility, is to offer insight to the procedures that were used that assisted me to make the best use of the time and effort required for the conduct of a quality systematic review.

It should be understood from the outset that approximately 1,000 hours would be required for the completion of a systematic review. That time expenditure is dependent to a great extent on the degree of organization or industry and the ability of the researchers to "juggle elephants and feathers." Because the actual process of conducting a systematic review has been discussed in this text, guidance, henceforth, will be on organizing processes to ensure ready access/prompt retrieval of all the review documentation and timely completion of the research project.

Permit me to briefly digress by underscoring the value of an online bibliographic management program (EndNote, RefWorks, etc.) through all the phases of the systematic review process—from proposal development through final write-up. Use of a bibliographic management program will circumvent countless hours spent formatting and managing citations and references, which may number in hundreds. Additionally, be prepared to spend almost all of the time not spent in your primary work role toiling away on your systematic review. Days off, weekends, holidays, and vacation time will need to be encroached upon to complete the review in approximately one year. This degree of work output requires focus, organization, and diligence in meeting established deadlines. Teamwork and accountability support the process and foster achievement of goals.

At the outset, it is essential that one of the two researchers working on the review assumes a coordinator role within the dyad to organize the review processes and establish a reasonable timetable for the completion of the review. Mutual respect provides the underpinning for negotiation of the coordinator role. Researchers identify their special organizational skills, time availability, and so forth, and a coordinator is identified. The creation of a "master table" of citations was a major contribution to the organization of the retrieved studies, efficiency of review conduct, and transparency of the review process. Selection of table format (Excel file, Word table, etc.) should be predicated based on the researcher's preference—usually based on familiarity and ease of use—and the goal of readily accessible data by each reviewer. Our master table identified the citation by an assigned number and a code identifying the sources of the citation (e.g., electronic database search, footnote chase, author contact, and hand search). Additional tabulated information included the full citation (author, publication date, title, journal, volume, issue, and page numbers), study design, and a comments column indicating study appropriateness for the critical appraisal process. In the case of the retrieval of an abstract only, the status of the full text article (received/awaited) and the source of the retrieval request (interlibrary loan or by study author) was indicated in the comment column. This detail in record keeping was critical in keeping track of the status of the studies as one moved on to the other aspects in the systematic review process. Correspondingly, the master table (also called a Table of Evidence) was continually updated and a "first cut deletion table" (also called a Table of Excluded Studies) was created which listed deleted citations and rationale for deletion.

Concurrently, a table of "author contacts" was also created. This table contained the names and the contact information of all the authors contacted regarding the requested informations, the dates when the requests were made, and the actual

(Continued)

Box 3.2 (*Continued*)

responses received from the contacts. E-mail responses were imported directly into the table and phone conversations were summarized and added into the table. Additional authors to be contacted and both published and unpublished research, identified from the authors' responses, were followed up and added to the master table of citations or to the first cut deletion table. Dates of all the updates were indicated on the tables to ensure transparency in the systematic review process.

An invaluable time saver was the creation of an electronic library of all citations with the attachment, wherever possible, of the full-text article as a PDF file. Having the full-text article available in the bibliographic database made the article readily available for review during write-ups of the report. The full-text articles were also downloaded from the electronic library databases into a folder entitled *PDF files*. Each article was named with the author, the publication date, and the key title words. This permitted expeditious retrieval and e-mail sharing of the articles with my coreviewer. Additionally, when it came time for comparison of critical appraisals of studies, having the full-text articles electronically available afforded ready access to the primary data from any location. In addition, availability of the full-text articles in the electronic library and the PDF files folder eliminated the time-consuming process of electronically scanning printed materials into a data file. Given that systematic reviews require a considerable amount of time for completion, any efficacious and expedient practice is worthy of consideration.

Studies were condensed and organized into "narrative tables" listing study purpose, design/methods, sample/setting, and outcomes. Further intimacy with the data prompted the creation of "study characteristic tables" for our populations of interest. These tables chronicled studies by sample type according to common features of interest relative to the review focus. All study tables, correspondence, drafts of the review, and so forth were stored in a folder entitled *SR FWR/FWIP* for efficient retrieval and sharing.

Despite some full-text articles of eligible abstracts that are not yet obtained, I proceeded with the selection of studies from the master table of citations to create a listing of "studies for critical appraisal" with assigned due dates. This was important in keeping to the timetable established for the completion of the review. The number of articles assigned for each week was arrived at by discussion with my coreviewer to be equitable regarding workloads. The list was e-mailed and the critical appraisals were compared through phone on the assigned dates. Following the critical appraisal of each group of studies, the master table was updated to reflect the appraisal status of each research study. Those studies that did not achieve the designated cut-off scores were entered into a table entitled *Study Exclusion Table–After Critical Appraisal*, with the rationale for exclusion made explicit.

After data extraction had been done, my coreviewer and I used a remote meeting and desktop sharing software program to facilitate and to expedite collaboration on data synthesis and the final write-up of the review. This program enabled us to work together and keep to our timetable when we were physically remote and whenever we were available to be online together. It made collaboration convenient as well as time efficient.

In summary, the key to a successful systematic review is meticulous organization of the data, frequently updating records, backing up files to as many locations as possible, keeping to an established timetable, committing to a concentrated investment of all free time—for a designated period—to the systematic review, and remaining in close contact with your coreviewer to address concerns as they arise and keep on track. The process of systematic review is labor intensive, but the reward is great in terms of optimizing health care outcomes for those we are privileged to serve.

Lisa M. Paplanus, DNP, RN-C, CCRN, ACNP-BC, ANP-BC

to identify a third reviewer at the beginning of the review in the event that there is a disagreement between the primary and the secondary reviewer. The third reviewer will assist in resolving any differences.

BEGINNING AND ENDING DATES

An attempt should be made to identify the dates when the review will begin and the anticipated date of completion. Determining these dates before the review begins can assist in keeping the project on track. Most reviews require 8–12 months for completion.

BACKGROUND

The background should describe the issue under review in sufficient detail so that the necessity for conducting the review is clear and unambiguous. It should lay a broad base for the issue that led to the review. A description of the target population, the interventions or phenomenon to be reviewed, and the potential uses of the findings should be presented. Judicious use of statistics can aid in understanding the significance of the review. The background should indicate why the review is necessary and its contribution to health care. The background provides the foundation for the development of the review's objectives and aims. Questions that need to be addressed in the background include:

- Who will benefit?
- What are the specific issues to be addressed?
- What is the target population?
- What is the context of the investigation?
- Why is it necessary to review and pool studies on this topic? Why is this work important?
- What has already been published?
- How will this build on published literature, inform practice, or formulate policy?

OBJECTIVES

The review objectives are grounded in the review question and provide the basis for the development of the inclusion criteria. The rationale for the objectives should be found in the background. Review objectives are written in measurable terms and need to address the target population, intervention or phenomenon, and outcomes. An overall objective for the review is provided first, followed by subobjectives, as appropriate. For example, in an economic analysis of human cell-derived wound care products for the treatment of leg ulcers, Langer and Rogowski (2009) explained that their study assessed the cost-effectiveness of growth factors and tissue-engineered artificial skin for treating chronic wounds. An example of a review objective for a qualitative review (a meta-synthesis) is provided by Ho, Berggren, and Dahlborg-Lyckhage (2010): "The aim was to contribute to a deeper understanding of what clients perceive as being important in an effective empowerment strategy for diabetes self-management" (p. 260).

Some questions to ask as the proposal objectives are constructed are:

- Does the overall objective clearly describe the review's purpose and direction?
- Are the objectives realistic and feasible in relation to the selected completion date?
- Do the objectives match what is described in the background?
- Are the objectives stated in measurable terms?
- Are there objectives written that describe the anticipated outcomes of the review?

CRITERIA FOR INCLUSION OF STUDIES IN THE REVIEW

Inclusion Criteria

Systematic reviews are distinguished by the transparency with which they are conducted. One of the features that allow this transparency is the prespecification of the review's inclusion and exclusion criteria, that is, those criteria that make a study eligible for inclusion in the review. Eligibility criteria include parts of the review question and the types of studies that will be sought. The types of participants, the types of interventions or phenomenon of interest, and the expected types of outcomes are addressed in the eligibility criteria for the review (The Joanna Briggs Institute [JBI], 2009). For example, in a study on the effect of aromatherapy on hypertension, Hur et al. (2010) stated, "all prospective randomized clinical trials (RCTs) and non-randomized controlled clinical trials (CCTs) were included if the patient population including those with hypertension who received aromatherapy alone or combined with other treatments" (p. 2).

Types of Studies

This section describes the type of studies that will be considered for review. For example, Moola and Lockwood (2010) stated:

> Low-quality RCTs produce exaggerated estimates of intervention effects. RCTs with unclear generation of the allocation sequence, allocation concealment and double blinding overestimate intervention effects. Therefore, this review considered all identified prospective studies that used a clearly described process for randomization, and/or included a control group. (p. 755)

In those instances where the reviewer believes that it might be difficult to find the preferred study, the type of study or other literature that will be used instead can also be described. For example, in a metasynthesis on the nursing handoffs, Poletick and Holly (2010) explained:

> The reviewers considered qualitative studies that drew on the experiences of nurses at the time of inter-shift nursing handoff, and included designs such as phenomenology, grounded theory, narrative analysis, and action research,

ethnographic or cultural studies. In the absence of research studies, other texts such as opinion papers, commentaries, and reports were to be considered in a narrative summary. (p. 124)

Types of Participants

Participants in a systematic review refer to the subjects used in the primary studies that will be included in the review. The criteria for selection of these participants must be very clear and specific, because the key words for searching are developed using these criteria. Participants should be defined in three ways. First, the disease or condition of interest, such as urinary tract infection, breast cancer, or Type 2 diabetes, must be identified. Second, the population of interest must be described in as few words as possible. This step involves deciding on the characteristics or attributes of the population, such as age, race, ethnicity, educational level, or a particular condition. Finally, a prereview decision needs to be made concerning the type of setting, such as acute care hospital, community mental health center, and ambulatory surgery (JBI, 2009). For example, in a systematic review of the effects of warming methods on hypothermia in the perioperative area, Moola and Lockwood (2010) used the following inclusion and exclusion criteria: "Adults ≥18 years of age, who underwent any type of surgery; patients who were subject to deliberate hypothermia such as those for cardiac or neurosurgical interventions were excluded" (p. 755). In this example, the condition of interest is hypothermia, the population of interest is any adult aged 18 years or older, and the setting of interest is surgery.

Types of Interventions/Phenomenon of Interest

Next, a description of the types of interventions or phenomenon of interest is necessary. If the proposal is for a review of interventions, the primary and comparison interventions need to be fully described. Following a description of the primary intervention of interest, a decision needs to be made regarding the comparisons, for example, a placebo, another intervention, nothing, or usual care (JBI, 2009). For example, Ried, Sullivan, Fakler, Frank, and Stocks (2010) investigated the effect of cocoa as food or drink compared with placebo on systolic blood pressure (SBP) and diastolic blood pressure (DBP) for a minimum duration of 2 weeks, whereas Poletick and Holly (2010) decided that their review would consider "only those studies that described the processes associated with nurse-to-nurse inter-shift report, specifically, how information was transferred between or among participants, and what purpose or function the handoff served in order to present analysis pertaining to these experiences" (p. 125).

Types of Outcomes

Explicit criteria for establishing the appropriate outcomes and, if necessary, their combinations must be specified (JBI, 2009). The background should provide enough information to justify the outcomes included and, potentially, those that were not included. For example, Mattar, Chan, and Liaw (2010) were interested in the "level of performance of nurses performing conscious level assessment using the GCS, ACDU, and AVPU scales" (p. 4).

SEARCH STRATEGY FOR IDENTIFICATION OF STUDIES

The search for articles and papers to be included in the review can be compared to enrolling patients into a primary research study. The articles selected as a result of the search process are, in essence, the subjects for the review. Key words and phrases provide the foundation for searching and are derived from the review question.

A concept map is useful in expanding key words. For example, the phrase *critical care* can be mapped to include intensive care, intensive care unit, critical care unit, or ICU, as well as identified by specialty area (e.g., coronary care unit, pediatric intensive care unit, surgical intensive care unit). By mapping each of the key words and phrases, a more comprehensive search can be conducted. The phases of the search strategy should be very detailed, including the initial search and the subsequent expanded search.

The search should be described in stages. Stage 1 is the first attempt in which the reviewers use a limited set of key words to find potentially relevant studies. These studies are reviewed in an effort to expand key words and phrases for a more in-depth search. At a minimum, Academic Search Premiere Medline, Ovid, and the Virginia Henderson International Nursing Library of Sigma Theta Tau International should be searched during the first stage. In addition, the attempts should be made to determine whether a systematic review already exists on the topic of interest. This is accomplished by searching the databases of Cochrane, Campbell, and the Joanna Briggs Institute. If a review is found that matches the one that is under consideration, a decision needs to be made to forego the review or expand on it in some manner. For example, years can be extended, databases can be added, and a new population or setting can be added. Stage 2 expands the databases used and searches these using the full list of key words developed in Stage 1. Stage 3 involves searching the reference lists of identified articles for any relevant references and hand searching appropriate journals.

A list of all databases, grey literature, and the full list of key words used in the search should be provided. The timeframe for searching each database must be included. For example, Ried et al. (2010) stated the following:

> [We] searched the Medline and Cochrane databases for randomized controlled trials of chocolate or cocoa on blood pressure published between 1955 and 2009 using the following search terms: chocolate OR cocoa AND blood pressure. (p. 2)

METHODS OF THE REVIEW

Assessment of Methodologic Quality

A description of how the quality of each paper will be determined is necessary for the proposal. There are several well-developed quality instruments in checklist format that are available for use (see Chapter 7). The checklist used should be described in full, referenced, and included in the appendices.

Data Extraction

A description of how data will be extracted and managed must also be included. The data extraction tool to be used should be included in the appendices. Data extraction tools can be developed by the reviewers to meet the particular criteria of the study, or an already developed data extraction tool can be used.

Data Synthesis

This section should explain in some detail how you will manipulate the data that were collected to get at the information that you will use to answer your review question. Where meta-analysis is proposed, the statistical methods and the software used should be described and, if appropriate, should be justified. For instance, it would be necessary to provide a rationale for using standard mean differences instead of weighted means. If statistical pooling was not possible and a narrative summary was used, this should be stated (JBI, 2009). If the review is qualitative, the method of data synthesis needs to be described. For example, Ho et al. (2010) explained that their study adhered to the metaethnographic framework of Noblit and Hare for metasynthesis. In addition, any analytic tools to be used should be briefly described (e.g., ethnograph; nonnumerical unstructured data indexing, searching, and theorizing [NUDIST] software; software quality understanding through the analysis of design [SQUAD]; statistical analysis system [SAS]; statistical package for the social sciences [SPSS]; Systat software; Rev-Man; qualitative assessment and review instrument [QARI]; MAStARI).

References

The American Psychological Association (APA) referencing is usually required; however, if the intent is to submit the proposal for peer review to an organization that is devoted to the conduct of systematic review, such as the Cochrane Collaboration or the Joanna Briggs Institute, it is necessary to check the style preferred by that group.

Appendices

Appendices include all critical appraisal tools and data extraction tools to be used.

SUMMARY

This chapter has presented the individual components of a good systematic review proposal. All of these elements are necessary to guide the reviewer through the process of conducting a systematic review.

EXERCISES

Read the proposal in Exhibit 3.1 in this chapter and identify the various components of the proposal.

EXHIBIT 3.1

A Comprehensive Systematic Review of Family-Witnessed Resuscitation and Family-Witnessed Invasive Procedures in Adults in Hospital Settings Internationally

Reviewers
Susan W. Salmond, EdD, RN, CNE, CTN and Lisa M. Paplanus, DNP, RN-C, CCRN, ACNP-BC, ANP-BC
University of Medicine and Dentistry of New Jersey, School of Nursing

Review Objective:

The objective of this comprehensive systematic review is to investigate the evidence on family-witnessed resuscitation (FWR) and family-witnessed invasive procedures (FWIP) in the adult population in emergency departments, intensive care units, and general hospital wards internationally. The aim is to explicate the perceptions of patients, family members, physicians, and nurses regarding this phenomenon. Ultimately, through scholarly reconciliation of the evidence, health care policy and practice will be informed regarding this family-centered care option.

Background:

"Burgeoning consumerism"[1] (p. 494), the expansion of palliative and hospice care, the incorporation of family in the pediatrics and midwifery arenas, transparency in health care organizations' reporting on performance and outcomes, layperson/bystander performance of cardiopulmonary resuscitation, and technology-facilitated exposure to previously censored procedures conducted in emergency departments and trauma centers have contributed to a paradigm shift away from the paternalistic orientation of health care to one of respect for patient autonomy and the incorporation of family in collaborative decision making and determination of care options[2-11] Congruent with this family-centered focus in health care is a movement calling for the inclusion of FWR and FWIP.

FWR is not a new practice; it is several decades old. It has its origins in family members being permitted by staff in the Foote Hospital Emergency Department (ED) in Jackson, Michigan, to stay with their loved ones during cardiopulmonary resuscitation (CPR).[12,13] Positive feedback from surveys, obtained from participants in this ED experience, spurred further inquiry into this phenomenon, generating a growing body of evidence worldwide in support of benefits to patients and their families, and the identification of positive attitudes by clinicians. Benefits to patients and families centered around connectedness; closure; facilitation of grieving; reduction in fear, anxiety, and guilt; lower degrees of intrusive imagery; posttraumatic avoidance behavior; and symptoms of grief; feelings of being supportive and useful; knowing that everything possible was being done; receiving comfort; increased spiritual connectedness; and having an advocate to remind staff of [patient's] humanity.[8,13-20]

Clinicians' favorable attitudes, however, have been tempered by concerns raised about safety, the emotional responses of family members, performance anxiety and stress of health care providers, fear of distraction among the CPR team, and medicolegal concerns.[13,14,20-34] Although nurses have more favorable attitudes than physicians, the reality is that most of the nurses who were studied are not supportive of this practice.[5,14,25,27,32,33,35-41]

(Continued)

Exhibit 3.1 (*Continued*)

There is mounting evidence in acute care settings across patient populations (i.e., adults and children) that families want the choice regarding presence. Most families, when asked if they would want to be present, believe they do.[13,18,20,42–47] In those studies where families have actually witnessed resuscitation attempts and invasive procedures, the majority found it positive and would want to do it again. Further evidence supporting the need for FWR and FWIP is found in the endorsement by numerous professional nursing and medical societies (i.e., the Emergency Nurses Association, the American Association of Critical-Care Nurses, the European Federation of Critical Care Nursing Associations, the Canadian Association of Critical Care Nursing, the American Heart Association, the American College of Critical Care Medicine, the Society of Critical Care Medicine, the American Academy of Pediatrics, the European Society of Paediatric and Neonatal Intensive Care, the European Society of Cardiology Council on Cardiovascular Nursing and Allied Professions, the European Resuscitation Council, the Resuscitation Council [UK], the Royal College of Nursing, the British Association for Accident and Emergency Medicine, the Royal College of Paediatrics and Child Health, and the British Medical Association).[48–61] Despite positive benefits to patients, families, and staffs, FWR and FWIP have not been widely or formally adopted in health care facilities.[7,25,40,48,62] An explanation for this may reside in the lack of congruence between the health care provider and the patient/family perceptions regarding the benefits of this care practice.

Family presence has significance in terms of nursing's holistic, caring, family-centered framework, and commitment to evidence-based practice that supports optimal patient/family health outcomes. As a profession, nursing is committed to the caring of patients and their families as inextricable wholes. The medicalization of care has removed the family from life-threatening situations. The priority of technologic intervention for the goal of rescue has overshadowed the significance of the patient and family member, both being alone during this critical event.[63] To isolate patients from family members may run counter to nursing's commitment to patients in their totality.

Therefore, a critical appraisal is needed for the research on FWR and FWIP. Dingeman et al.[62] have conducted a recent systematic review on the pediatric population. At present, no comprehensive systematic review of the evidence on the phenomenon of FWR or FWIP in the adult population has been conducted. This review will focus on factors that impact the formal adoption of this practice internationally in acute settings with adult patient populations.

Objectives:

The overall aim of this research endeavor is to conduct a comprehensive mixed method of systematic review to reconcile the evidence and provide scholarly insight toward informing practice regarding this family-centered care option.

Specifically, the comprehensive systematic review will determine:

- The beliefs of patients, family members, physicians, and nurses relevant to perceived or actual FWR and FWIP in adult acute care settings.
- The meaning of the experience of FWR and FWIP for patients, family members, physicians, and nurses.
- Factors that are associated with acceptance or rejection of FWR and FWIP by patients, families, physicians, and nurses.
- The effect of family presence on efficiency and perceived competence of resuscitation and invasive procedures for adults in acute care settings.

(Continued)

Exhibit 3.1 (*Continued*)

- Strategies found to be effective in facilitating safety in the practice of FWR and FWIP for patients, family members, physicians, and nurses.
- Congruity of the outcomes in studies evaluating witnessed events compared with outcomes of perceptions and beliefs regarding FWR and FWIP.
- Essential points for policy development.

Inclusion Criteria:

Participants

This review will consider studies involving adult patients, their family members, physicians, and nurses in intensive care units, emergency departments, trauma rooms, and general nursing wards.

Studies involving FWR or FWIP conducted in the field or in the home will be excluded.

Types of Interventions/Phenomena of Interest

The qualitative component of this review will consider studies that investigate the meaning of FWR and FWIP for patients, family members, physicians, and nurses in intensive care units, emergency departments, trauma rooms, and general nursing wards.

The quantitative component of this review will:

1. Examine the outcomes that are associated with FWR and FWIP on patients and family members including but not limited to:
   - Stress and anxiety
   - Grief and bereavement
   - Coping
   - Psychological sequelae
2. Examine the physicians' and nurses' actual or perceived responses to FWR and FWIP including but not limited to:
   - Stress and performance anxiety
   - Interference with teaching
   - Competence in resuscitation performance
   - Adequacy in meeting patient or family needs
   - Safety
   - Medicolegal litigation potential
   - Connection with patients
3. Examine the factors affecting the adoption/implementation of FWR and FWIP including but not limited to:
   - Formal policy and guidelines
   - Family facilitator/chaperone role
   - Educational programming
   - Communication approaches
   - Debriefing

The textual component of this review will examine the position statements and guidelines with respect to FWR and FWIP.

(Continued)

Exhibit 3.1 (*Continued*)

Outcomes

The qualitative component of this review will include experiential and perceptual accounts on the meaning of FWR and FWIP of patients, family members, physicians, and nurses. Additionally, it will identify the perceptions of factors facilitating or obstructing FWR or FWIP.

The quantitative component of this review will consider studies that include, but not limited to, the following outcome measures for:

1. Patients and family members: anxiety levels, stress, fear, guilt, depression, avoidance, intrusive images, knowledge, helpfulness, symptoms of grief, bereavement, psychological acceptance, and adaptation

2. Physicians and nurses: performance anxiety, advocacy for patients and families, interference with teaching and/or resuscitation performance, and litigation potential

The textual component of this review will describe the key components for policies on FWR and FWIP.

Types of Studies

This review will consider studies that focus on qualitative data including, but not limited to, designs such as phenomenology, grounded theory, and ethnography. In the absence of research studies, other text such as opinion papers and reports will be considered.

The quantitative component of this review will consider randomized controlled trials, controlled trials, cohort studies, case-control studies, before-and-after studies, and case series that examine the effectiveness of interventions such as staff education programs and family support personnel on outcomes.

The textual component of this review will consider position papers of professional health care organizations and evidence-based guidelines.

Search Strategy

The search strategy aims to locate both published and unpublished studies. A three-step search strategy will be used in each component of this review. An initial limited search of Medline and Cumulative Index to Nursing and Allied Health Literature (CINAHL) will be undertaken followed by the analysis of the text words contained in the title and abstract, and of the index terms used to describe the article. A second search using all identified key words and index terms will then be undertaken across all included databases. Third, the reference list of all identified reports and articles will be searched for additional studies.

Key words to be used are as follows:

Accident and emergency	Cardiopulmonary resuscitation
Arterial line	Central line
Attitudes	Chaperone
Behavior/behaviour	Chaperoned resuscitation
Beliefs	Chest tube
Bereavement	CPR
Cardiac massage	Critical care unit

(Continued)

Exhibit 3.1 (*Continued*)

Decision making

Defibrillation

Emergency breathing

Emergency department

Emergency room

Emergency ward

Endotracheal tube

Experiences

Facilitator

Family attendance

Family-centered care

Family member

Family member presence

Family needs

Family presence

Family presence policy

Family presence protocol

Family relations

Family support

Family support person

Grief

Health care provider

Health care professional

Holistic care

Hospital policy

Hospital ward

Intensive care unit

Intubation

Invasive procedure

Lumbar puncture

Nursing

Palliative care

Pastoral care

Patient-centered care

Patient comfort

Patient needs

Perceptions

Pericardiocentesis

Perspective

Physicians

Posttraumatic stress disorder

Professional-family relations

Qualitative analysis

Qualitative research

Qualitative study

Randomized controlled trial, randomized
   clinical trial

Relative

Rights

Staff

Systematic review

Tracheostomy

Trauma resuscitation

Trauma room

Tube thoracostomy

Urethral catheterization

Venipuncture

Witnessed cardiac arrest

Witnessed resuscitation

Databases

Searches will be conducted on the following databases:

- CINAHL
- MEDLINE (medical literature on-line)
- PapersFirst (conference proceedings)
- PsycINFO (psychology information)
- ISI (Institute for Scientific Information) web of knowledge
- ERIC (Education Resources Information Center database)
- EBMR (Evidence-Based Medicine Reviews)
- EMBASE (Excerpta Medica Database)

(Continued)

Exhibit 3.1 (*Continued*)

The following registries will be searched:

- JBI (Joanna Briggs Institute)
- Cochrane Collection
- Sara Cole Hirsch Institute

Unpublished Studies

The following databases will be searched for unpublished studies:

- Dissertations Abstracts International
- ProQuest Dissertations & Theses

Additional searching for unpublished studies will be accomplished by communication with key organizations and key researchers in the area.

Grey Literature

A grey literature search will be conducted through the New York Academy of Medicine, Research and Development (RAND), Scirus, http://www.health-evidence.ca, and http://www.greynet.org.

Assessment of Methodologic Quality

All retrieved papers will independently be assessed for methodologic quality by two reviewers, using the appropriate JBI critical appraisal assessment tools. Any disagreements that arise between the reviewers will be resolved through discussion or in consultation with a third reviewer.

Data Collection

Relevant JBI data extraction tools will be used to extract data from quantitative studies, qualitative studies, and opinion pieces. This process will be undertaken by two reviewers working independently. The data extracted will include specific details about the phenomena of interest, interventions, populations, study methods, and outcomes of significance to the review question and specific objectives.

Data Synthesis

Quantitative papers will, where possible, be pooled in statistical meta-analysis using the Joanna Briggs Institute Meta-Analysis of Statistics Assessment and Review Instrument. All results will be subject to double data entry. Odds ratios (for categorical data) and weighted mean differences (for continuous data) and their 95% confidence intervals will be calculated for analysis. Heterogeneity will be assessed using the standard chi-square. Where statistical pooling is not possible, the findings will be presented in narrative form.

Qualitative research findings will, where possible, be pooled using the qualitative assessment and review instrument. This will involve the aggregation or synthesis of findings to generate a set of statements that represent that aggregation, through assembling the finding (Level 1 findings) rates according to their quality, and categorizing these findings on the basis of similarity in meaning (Level 2 findings). These categories are then subjected to a metasynthesis to produce a single

(Continued)

Exhibit 3.1 (*Continued*)

comprehensive set of synthesized findings (Level 3 findings) that can be used as a basis for evidence-based practice. Where textual pooling is not possible, the findings will be presented in narrative form.

Textual papers will, where possible, be pooled using the narrative, opinion and text assessment, and review instrument. This will involve the aggregation or synthesis of conclusions to generate a set of statements that represent that aggregation on the basis of similarity in meaning. These categories are then subjected to a metasynthesis to produce a single comprehensive set of synthesized findings that can be used as a basis for evidence-based practice. Where textual pooling is not possible, the conclusions will be presented in narrative form.

Conflicts of Interest

There are no conflicts of interest. The reviewers are employed in education and clinical service.

References

1. Halm, M. A. (2005). Family presence during resuscitation: A critical review of the literature. *American Journal of Critical Care, 14*(6), 494–511.

2. Williams, J. M. (2002). Family presence during resuscitation: To see or not see? *Nursing Clinics of North America, 37*(1), 211–220.

3. Moreland, P. (2005). Family presence during invasive procedures and resuscitation in the emergency department: A review of the literature. *Journal of Emergency Nursing, 31*(1), 58–72.

4. Walker, W. M. (1999). Do relatives have a right to witness resuscitation? *Journal of Clinical Nursing, 8*(6), 625–630.

5. Fulbrook, P., Albarran, J. W., & Latour, J. M. (2005). A European survey of critical care nurses' attitudes and experiences of having family members present during cardiopulmonary resuscitation. *International Journal of Nursing Studies, 42*(5), 557–568.

6. Van der Woning, M. (1997). Should relatives be invited to witness resuscitation attempt? A review of the literature. *Accident and Emergency Nursing, 5*(4), 215–218.

7. Boudreaux, E. D., Francis, J. L., & Loyacano, T. (2002). Family presence during invasive procedures and resuscitations in the emergency department: A critical review and suggestions for future research. *Annals of Emergency Medicine, 40*(2), 193–205.

8. Clark, A. P., Aldridge, M. D., Guzzetta, C. E., Nyquist-Heise, P., Norris, C., Norris, M., Loper, P., . . . Voelmeck, W. (2005). Family presence during cardiopulmonary resuscitation. *Critical Care Nursing Clinics of North America, 17*(1), 23–32.

9. Rattrie, E. (2000). Witnessed resuscitation: Good practice or not? *Nursing Standard, 14*(24), 32–35.

10. Engel, K. G., Barnosky, A. R., Berry-Bovia, M., Desmond, J. S., & Ubel, P. A. (2007). Provider experience and attitudes toward family presence during resuscitation procedures. *Journal of Palliative Medicine, 10*(5), 1007–1009.

11. Rosenczweig, C. (1998). Should relatives witness resuscitation? Ethical issues and practical considerations. *Canadian Medical Association Journal, 158*(5), 617–620.

(Continued)

Exhibit 3.1 (*Continued*)

12. Hanson, C., & Strawser, D. (1992). Family presence during cardiopulmonary resuscitation: Foote Hospital emergency department's nine-year perspective. *Journal of Emergency Nursing, 18*(2), 104–106.

13. Doyle, C. J., Post, H., Burney, R. E., Maino, J., Keefe, M., & Rhee, K. J. (1987). Family participation during resuscitation: An option. *Annals of Emergency Medicine, 16*(6), 673–675.

14. Redley, B., & Hood, K. (1996). Staff attitudes towards family presence during resuscitation. *Accident and Emergency Nursing, 4*(3), 145–151.

15. Critchell, C. D., & Marik, P. E. (2007). Should family members be present during cardiopulmonary resuscitation? A review of the literature. *American Journal of Hospice and Palliative Care, 24*(4), 311–317.

16. Nibert, A. T. (2005). Teaching clinical ethics using a case study family presence during cardiopulmonary resuscitation. *Critical Care Nurse, 25*(1), 38–44.

17. Belanger, M. A., & Reed, S. (1997). A rural community hospital's experience with family-witnessed resuscitation. *Journal of Emergency Nursing, 23*(3), 238–239.

18. Meyers, T. A., Eichhorn, D. J., Guzzetta, C. E., Clark, A. P., Klein, J. D., Taliaferro, E., & Calvin, A. (2000). Family presence during invasive procedures and resuscitation. *American Journal of Nursing, 100*(2), 32–42.

19. Hanson, C., & Strawser, D. (1992). Family presence during cardiopulmonary resuscitation: Foote Hospital emergency department's nine-year perspective. *Journal of Emergency Nursing, 18*(2), 104–106.

20. Robinson, S. M., Mackenzie-Ross, S., Campbell Hewson, G. L., Egleston, C. V., & Prevost, A. T. (1998). Psychological effect of witnessed resuscitation on bereaved relatives. Lancet, *352*(9128), 614–617.

21. Zoltie, N., Sloan, J. P., & Wright, B. (1994). Should relatives watch resuscitation? *British Medical Journal, 309*(6951), 406–407.

22. O'Shea, F., & Dight, A. (1999). Should relatives be allowed into the resuscitation room? *Nursing Times, 95*(17), 30–31.

23. Eichhorn, D. J., Meyers, T. A., Guzzetta, C. E., Clark, A. P., Klein, J. D., Taliaferro, E., & Calcin, A. O. (2001). During invasive procedures and resuscitation: Hearing the voice of the patient. *American Journal of Nursing, 101*(5), 48–55.

24. Grice, A. S., Picton, P., & Deakin, C. D. Study examining attitudes of staff, patients and relatives to witnessed resuscitation in adult intensive care units. *British Journal of Anaesthesia, 91*(6), 820–824.

25. Duran, C. R., Oman, K. S., Abel, J. J., Koziel, V. M., & Szymanski, D. (2007). Attitudes toward and beliefs about family presence: A survey of healthcare providers, patients' families, and patients. *American Journal of Critical Care, 16*(3), 270–279.

26. Schilling, R. J. (1994). Should relatives watch resuscitation? No room for spectators. *British Medical Journal, 309*(6951), 406.

27. Mitchell, M. H., & Lynch, M. B. (1997). Should relatives be allowed in the resuscitation room? *Journal of Accident & Emergency Medicine, 14*(6), 366–369.

28. Stewart, K., Bacon, M., & Criswell, J. (1998). Effect of witnessed resuscitation on bereaved relatives. *Lancet, 352*(9143), 1863.

29. Chalk, A. (1995). Should relatives be present in the resuscitation room? *Accident and Emergency Nursing, 3*(2), 58–61.

(Continued)

Exhibit 3.1 (*Continued*)

30. MacLean, S. L., Guzzetta, C. E., White, C., Fontaine, D., Eichhorn, D. J., Meyers, T. A., & Désy, P. (2003). Family presence during cardiopulmonary resuscitation and invasive procedures: Practices of critical care and emergency nurses. *Journal of Emergency Nursing, 29*(3), 208–221.

31. Bassler, P. C. (1999). The impact of education on nurses' beliefs regarding family presence in a resuscitation room. *Journal for Nurses in Staff Development, 15*(3), 126–131.

32. Helmer, S. D., Smith, R. S., Dort, J. M., Shapiro, W. M., & Katan, B. S. (2000). Family presence during trauma resuscitation: A survey of AAST and ENA members. American Association for the Surgery of Trauma. Emergency Nurses Association. *The Journal of Trauma, 48*(6), 1015–1022.

33. McClenathan, B. M., Torrington, K. G., & Uyehara, C. F. (2002). Family member presence during cardiopulmonary resuscitation: A survey of US and international critical care professionals. *Chest, 122*(6), 2204–2211.

34. Boyd, R., & White, S. (2000). Does witnessed cardiopulmonary resuscitation alter perceived stress in accident and emergency staff? *European Journal of Emergency Medicine, 7*(1), 51–53.

35. Twibell, R. S., Siela, D., Riwitis, C., Wheatley, J., Riegle, T., Bousman, D., . . . Neal, A. (2008). Nurses' perceptions of their self-confidence and the benefits and risks of family presence during resuscitation. *American Journal of Critical Care, 17*(2), 101–111.

36. Ong, M. E., Chan, Y. H., Srither, D. E., & Lim, Y. H. (2004). Asian medical staff attitudes towards witnessed resuscitation. *Resuscitation, 60*(1), 45–50.

37. Ong, M. E., Chung, W. L., & Mei, J. S. (2007). Comparing attitudes of the public and medical staff towards witnessed resuscitation in an Asian population. *Resuscitation, 73*(1), 103–108.

38. Badir, A., & Sepit, D. (2007). Family presence during CPR: A study of the experiences and opinions of Turkish critical care nurses. *International Journal of Nursing Studies, 44*(1), 83–92.

39. Mortelmans, L. J., Cas, W. M., Van Hellemond, P. L., & De Cauwer, H. G.. (2009). Should relatives witness resuscitation in the emergency department? The point of view of the Belgian Emergency Departments staff. *European Journal of Emergency Medicine, 16*(2), 87–91.

40. Mian, P., Warchal, S., Whitney, S., Fitzmaurice, J., & Tancredi, D. (2007). Impact of a multifaceted intervention on nurses' and physicians' attitudes and behaviors toward family presence during resuscitation. *Critical Care Nurse, 27*(1), 52–61.

41. Demir, F. (2008). Presence of patients' families during cardiopulmonary resuscitation: Physicians' and nurses' opinions. *Journal of Advanced Nursing, 63*(4), 409–416.

42. Belanger, M. A., & Reed, S. (1997). A rural community hospital's experience with family-witnessed resuscitation. *Journal of Emergency Nursing, 23*(3), 238–239.

43. Barratt, F., & Wallis, D. N. (1998). Relatives in the resuscitation room: Their point of view. *Journal of Accident & Emergency Medicine, 15*(2), 109–111.

44. Benjamin, M., Holger, J., & Carr, M. (2004). Personal preferences regarding family member presence during resuscitation. *Academy of Emergency Medicine, 11*(7), 750–753.

(Continued)

Exhibit 3.1 (*Continued*)

45. Wagner, J. M. (2004). Lived experience of critically ill patients' family members during cardiopulmonary resuscitation. *American Journal of Critical Care, 13*(5), 416–420.

46. Sacchetti, A., Lichenstein, R., Carraccio, C. A., & Harris, R. H. (1996). Family member presence during pediatric emergency department procedures. *Pediatric Emergency Care, 12*(4), 268–271.

47. Powers, K. S., & Rubenstein, J. S. (1999). Family presence during invasive procedures in the pediatric intensive care unit. *Archives of Pediatrics & Adolescent Medicine, 153*(9), 955–958.

48. Davidson, J. E., Powers, K., Hedayat, K. M., Tieszen, M., Kon, A. A., Shepard, E., . . . Armstrong, D. (2007). Clinical practice guidelines for support of the family in the patient-centered intensive care unit: American College of Critical Care Medicine Task Force 2004–2005. *Critical Care Medicine, 35*(2), 605–622.

49. Baskett, P. J., Steen, P. A., & Bossaert, L. European Resuscitation Council guidelines for resuscitation 2005. Section 8. The ethics of resuscitation and end-of-life decisions. *Resuscitation, 67*(Suppl. 1), S171–S180.

50. Moons, P., & Norekvål, T. M. (2008). European nursing organizations stand up for family presences during cardiopulmonary resuscitation: A joint position statement. *Progress in Cardiovascular Nursing, 23*(3), 136–139.

51. American Association of Critical-Care Nurses. (2004). *Practice alert: Family presence during CPR and invasive procedures* (pp. 1–3). Aliso Viejo, CA: Author.

52. Emergency Nurses Association. (2005). *Family presence at the bedside during invasive procedures and cardiopulmonary resuscitation* (pp. 1–6). Des Plaines, IL: Author.

53. Canadian Association of Critical Care Nurses. (2005). Family presence during resuscitation. *Dynamics, 16*(4), 8–9.

54. Royal College of Nursing. (2002). *Witnessing resuscitation: Guidance for nursing staff* (pp. 1–16). London, UK: Author.

55. Emergency Nurses Association. (1994). *Position Statement: Family presence at the bedside during invasive procedures and cardiopulmonary resuscitation* (pp. 1–8). Des Plaines, IL: Author.

56. Guidelines 2000 for cardiopulmonary resuscitation and emergency cardiovascular care. Part 2: Ethical aspects of CPR and ECC. (2000). *Circulation, 102*(8 Suppl.), I12–I21.

57. Resuscitation Council. (1996). *Should relatives witness resuscitation?* (pp. 1–14). London, UK: Author.

58. American College of Emergency Physicians, American Academy of Pediatrics. (2001). Care of children in the emergency department: Guidelines for preparedness. *Annals of Emergency Medicine, 37*(4), 423–427. Retrieved from http://www.acep.org/practres.aspx?id529134.

59. American College of Emergency Physicians. (2002). Joint statement by the American College of Emergency Physicians and the American Academy of Pediatrics: Death of a child in the emergency department. Retrieved from http://www.acep.org/practres.aspx?id529160

60. British Association for Accident and Emergency Medicine, Royal College of Nursing. (1995). *Bereavement care in A & E departments. Report of the working group.* London, UK: Author.

(Continued)

Exhibit 3.1 (*Continued*)

61. Fulbrook, P., Latour, J., Albarran, J., de Graaf, W., Lynch, F., Devictor, D., & Norekvål, T. (2007). The presence of family members during cardiopulmonary resuscitation: European Federation of Critical Care Nursing Associations, European Society of Paediatric and Neonatal Intensive Care and European Society of Cardiology Council on Cardiovascular Nursing and Allied Professions joint position statement. *Connect: The World of Critical Care Nursing*, *5*(4), 86–88.

62. Dingeman, R. S., Mitchell, E. A., Meyer, E. C., & Curley, M. A. (2007). Parent presence during complex invasive procedures and cardiopulmonary resuscitation: A systematic review of the literature. *Pediatrics*, *120*(4), 842–854.

63. Timmermans, S. (1997). High touch in high tech: The presence of relatives and friends during resuscitative efforts. *Scholarly Inquiry for Nursing Practice*, *11*(2), 153–168.

REFERENCES

Ho, A. Y., Berggren, I., & Dahlborg-Lyckhage, E. (2010). Diabetes empowerment related to Pender's Health Promotion Model: A meta-synthesis. *Nursing and Health Sciences, 12*(2), 259–267.

Hur, M. H., Kim, C., & Ernst, E. (2010). Aromatherapy treatment of hypertension: A systematic review. *Journal of Evaluation in Clinical Practice*, 1–5.

The Joanna Briggs Institute. (2009). Comprehensive systematic review training program: Module 1. Adelaide, Australia: Author.

Langer, A., & Rogowski, W. (2009). Systematic economic evaluation of human cell-derived wound care products for treatment of venous leg and diabetic foot ulcers. *BMC Health Services Research, 10*(9), 115.

Mattar, I., Chan, M. F., & Liaw, S. Y. (2010). A comprehensive systematic review of the factors that impact nurses' performance in conscious level assessment. Joanna Briggs Institute, Protocol #334. Adelaide, Australia: Joanna Briggs Institute.

Moola, S., & Lockwood, C. (2010). The effectiveness of strategies for the management and/or prevention of hypothermia within the adult perioperative environment: Systematic review. *JBI Library of Systematic Review, 8*(19), 752–792.

Poletick, E. P., & Holly. C (2010). A systematic review of nurses' inter-shift handoff reports in acute care hospitals. *JBI Library of Systematic Review, 8*(4), 121–172.

Ried, K., Sullivan, T., Fakler, P., Frank, O. R., & Stocks, N. P. (2010). Does chocolate reduce blood pressure: A meta-analysis. *BMC Medicine, 8*, 39. Retrieved from http://www.biomedcentral.com/1741-7015/8/39

SUGGESTED READING

Pearson, A., Wiechula, R., Court, A., & Lockwood, C. (2007). A re-consideration of what constitutes "evidence" in the healthcare professions. *Nursing Science Quarterly, 20*(1), 85–88.

CHAPTER FOUR

Developing Clinical Questions for Systematic Review

Marie K. Saimbert, Jenny Pierce, and Pam Hargwood

OBJECTIVES

Upon completion of Chapter 4, you will be able to:

- Define the two broad question types involved in systematic reviews
- List domains or subcategories of foreground clinical questions
- List some study designs/methodologies best suited to answer different types of foreground questions
- Apply Cumulative Index to Nursing and Allied Health Literature (CINAHL) database subject headings or Subject Terms to focus or limit search results to specific study designs and methods
- Develop a clinical question suitable for systematic review

IMPORTANT POINTS

- The systematic review process is methodical, beginning with a clinical inquiry question.
- Background and foreground questions guide systematic reviews.
- Foreground questions deal with patient/population/phenomena of interest and their relationship to an intervention (diagnostic, therapeutic, laboratory value) or outcome.
- Common types of foreground questions include diagnosis/screening, etiology/causation/risk factor, therapy, prognosis, harm, economic evaluation, and meaning.
- Some databases such as CINAHL and PubMed add labels or subject headings to articles in the database. Specific study designs and methodologies can be subject headings; use them to limit or focus searches and/or search results.

INTRODUCTION

The critical issue in any systematic review is to ask the right question. According to Kitchenham (2004), the right question is one that:

- Is meaningful and important to practitioners as well as researchers
- Will lead either to changes in current practice or to increased confidence in the value of current practice
- Identifies discrepancies between commonly held beliefs and reality

TYPES OF CLINICAL QUESTIONS

Clinical questions are the basis or underpinning of professional practice. As such, they drive systematic reviews. Development of a clinical question starts with a very specific clinical inquiry related to a patient, family, or group and their condition. Clinicians ask many questions throughout the course of a day, but it can prove challenging to decide which questions to use as the basis of a systematic review. Booth (2006) suggests looking at high-yield questions: those that deal with high volume, high impact, and high risk. To begin, there are two broad questions to consider: background and foreground questions.

Background Questions

Background questions ask for general knowledge. They are basic inquiries about a phenomenon, disease state/condition, therapy, diagnostic test, or laboratory value (Sackett, 2000). Answers to background questions are facts, as currently known, and can usually be found in print and electronic textbooks, as well as reliable Internet resources such as the Centers for Disease Control and Prevention at http://www.cdc.gov; eMedicine, a free resource part of WebMD at http://www.emedicine.com; and MedlinePlus, a resource from the United States National Library of Medicine (U.S. NLM) at http://medlineplus.gov. Answers to background questions may also be found in review articles such as a meta-analysis because these reviews often summarize information on a topic. Although the factual evidence in review articles may be enough to answer background questions, many types of review articles lack inclusion of all possible evidence on a topic, so they possess limited utility for answering foreground questions. For instance, the "complete picture" or evidence may not be reflected in the references used for a meta-analysis. Further, authors of meta-analyses and similar types of articles may provide limited information on how articles were chosen for their review (Booth, 2006). Some examples of background questions appear below and in subsequent paragraphs. See Table 4.1 for additional examples.

- What are some common indications for a transesophageal echocardiogram?
- What are the forces of magnetism?
- What is cystic fibrosis?
- What are the adverse effects of vigabatrin (Sabril)?

- What are common characteristics of patients exhibiting drug-seeking behavior?
- What is the connection between fava beans and G6PD deficiency?

Foreground Questions

Compared with background questions, foreground questions are less broad, more focused, and ask for specific knowledge (Sackett, 2000). Foreground questions explore a relationship between a phenomenon, patient, family, disease state/condition, an exposure (therapy, diagnostic, or laboratory value), or outcome. There is depth and dimension to foreground clinical questions because they are focused on more than generic factual evidence, reviewing and often comparing options for a specific patient or population. For example, the perceptions of women of childbearing age facing a hysterectomy can be complex and the outcomes of research on this topic are not predictable, but can be explored to gather the range of meaning shared by the women, which can inform clinical interventions designed to assist them. In another example, Laurant et al. (2004) wanted to know the impact of doctor–nurse substitution in primary care on patient outcomes, process of care, and resource utilization including cost. The authors noted that patient outcomes included morbidity, mortality, satisfaction, compliance, and preference. Process outcomes included practitioner adherence to clinical guidelines, standards or quality of care, and practitioner health care activity. Resource utilization was measured by frequency and length of consultations, return visits, prescriptions, tests, and referral to other services and direct or indirect cost.

The complexity of foreground clinical questions can pose challenges for reviewers, but these hurdles can be addressed with thoughtful selection of appropriate online search resources or databases to answer the questions. Some examples of foreground questions are below and a comparison of background and foreground questions are presented in Table 4.1.

- What is the best available qualitative evidence pertaining to the nursing handoff report at the time of shift change to "enhance the transfer of information between and among nurses, and by extension, improve patient care" (Poletick & Holly, 2010, p. 121)?
- What is the best available evidence on the effectiveness of using simulated learning experiences in prelicensure health profession education (Laschinger et al., 2008)?
- What is the best available evidence on the optimal dietetic treatment and management of children and adolescents who are overweight or obese (Collins, Warren, Neve, McCoy, & Stokes, 2007)?
- What are the best interventions for increasing the frequency and quality of questions formulated by health care providers in practice and the context of self-directed learning (Horsley et al., 2010)?
- What is the effect of planned early birth compared with expectant management for pregnancies complicated with preterm premature rupture of membranes (PPROM) prior to 37 weeks' gestation (Buchanan, Crowther, Levett, Middleton, & Morris, 2010)?
- What are the most effective interventions used to treat noisy breathing in patients close to death (Wee & Hillier, 2008)?
- How efficacious are probiotics in the treatment of bacterial vaginosis (BV; Senok, Verstraelen, Temmerman, & Botta, 2009)?

TABLE 4.1

Background and Foreground Questions

Background	Foreground
What are leiomyomas? How common are leiomyomas in pre-menopausal women? How does MRI-guided focused ultrasound work to treat leimyomas?	In premenopausal women with abnormal uterine bleeding, what is the accuracy of transvaginal ultrasonography, sonohys-terography, and hysteroscopy in aiding in the diagnostic workup (Farquhar, Ekeroma, Furness, & Arroll, 2003)?
Who are the most likely groups of patients at risk for falls in the community versus in the hospital? What are some healthcare–based inter-ventions for community and acute care to reduce chance of older adults falling?	How effective are "population-based inter-ventions, defined as coordinated, com-munity-wide, multistrategy initiatives, for reducing fall-related injuries among older people" (McClure et al., 2008, p. 1)?
What is Methicillin-resistant Staphylococ-cus aureus (MRSA)?? What types of infection does MRSA cause in the elderly? What percentage of nursing home resi-dents have MRSA originating from living in a nursing home?	What are the "effects of infection control strategies for preventing the transmis-sion of MRSA in nursing homes for older people" (Hughes, Smith, & Tunney, 2008, p. 1)?
What is telehealth and telenursing? What medications are used to manage CHF? What percentage of patients with heart failure (HF) are readmitted into hospitals?	What is the "best available evidence to determine the effectiveness of telephone-based postdischarge nursing care of patient with HF and to quantify the effect on all-cause readmission rates of these patients" (Lee & Park, 2010, p. 1288)?
What are normal and abnormal vital signs for children?	"What educational interventions are effective in influencing parents to pro-vide effective care for their febrile child" (Young, Watts, & Wilson, 2010, p. 826)?
What alternative therapies decrease the chance for nausea? What is involved in an abdominal laparoscopy?	What are the "most effective noninvasive complementary therapies for reducing the incidence and/or severity of postoperative nausea and vomiting in women under-going abdominal laparoscopies" (Hewitt & Watts, 2009, p. 850)?
What clinical prediction rules can assist in determining the risk of stroke after a transient ischemic attack (TIA)?	In patients with a recent TIA, who are dis-charged from the emergency department, which clinical prediction test(s) best iden-tify those at risk for stroke (Shah, Metz, & Edlow, 2009)?
What is drug-induced psychosis?	In people with acute psychosis, how do outcomes differ for those admitted to open medical wards versus conventional psychiatric units (Hickling, Abel, Garner, & Rathbone, 2007)?

(Continued)

TABLE 4.1

Background and Foreground Questions *(Continued)*

Background	Foreground
What is optimized background therapy for HIV? What is the clinical definition of HIV-associated lipodystrophy?	How can HIV-associated lipodystrophy from long term anti-retroviral therapy be mitigated in people with HIV (Wierzbicki, Purdon, Hardman, Kulasegaram, & Peters, 2008)?
What are some devices currently on the market for home blood glucose monitoring? What are the current treatments for Type 2 diabetes? What is the purpose of measuring hemoglobin A1C or glycosylated hemoglobin?	What is the economic evidence supporting Self-monitoring of Blood Glucose Monitoring (SMBG) by patients with Type 2 Diabetes Mellitus (T2DM) to improve glycemic control (de Verteuil & Tan, 2010)?
What is the structure of clinical nursing leadership in a hospital system?	What is the "best available evidence on the feasibility, meaningfulness and effectiveness of nursing leadership attributes that contribute to the development and sustainability of nursing leadership to foster a healthy work environment" (Pearson et al., 2007, p. 279)?
What are the types of stroke? Which stroke type(s) are most common in the elderly? What percentage of older adults are at risk for strokes? What is involved in physical and psychological recovery from stroke?	What is the "best available evidence on the psychosocial spiritual experience of elderly individuals recovering from stroke" (Lamb, Buchanan, Godfrey, Harrison, & Oakley, 2008, p. 432)?

FOREGROUND QUESTION DOMAINS AND BEST STUDY EVIDENCE FOR DOMAINS

Foreground questions are further categorized by question domain. Common domains of foreground questions are diagnosis, etiology, therapy, prognosis, and qualitative. During literature searches in databases, it may be possible to focus a search, retrieving information from specific study domains by adding select key terms, subject headings, or subheadings to an initial search statement or results of a search. This chapter offers some subject headings or Subject Terms from the CINAHL database on EBSCOhost in the upcoming sections discussing diagnosis, etiology, therapy, prognosis, and qualitative question domains. Searches are constructed using subject headings and subheadings (see Table 4.2).

TABLE 4.2

CINAHL Headings for Retrieving Select Question Domains

CINAHL Subject Headings	Question Domain That Can be Retrieved
■ Clinical Assessment Tools ■ Diagnosis, Differential ■ Diagnostic Errors ■ Measurement Issues and Assessments ■ Nursing Assessment ■ Reproducibility of Results	Diagnosis/Screening
■ Analytic Research ■ Case-Control Studies ■ Epidemiological Research ■ Odds Ratio ■ Prospective Studies ■ Risk Assessment ■ Risk Factors	Etiology (Aetiology) or Causation or Risk Factor
■ Clinical Trials (CINAHL heading to retrieve randomized trials and randomized controlled trials) ■ Comparative Studies ■ Crossover Design ■ Patient Selection ■ Random Sample ■ Placebos ■ Placebo Effect ■ Follow-up (Use the CINAHL heading Prospective Studies instead)	Therapy or Therapeutic Intervention
■ Disease Progression ■ Incidence ■ Morbidity ■ Mortality ■ Prevalence ■ Prognosis ■ Prospective Studies ■ Recurrence ■ Survival Analysis ■ Time Factors	Prognosis
■ Concurrent Prospective Studies ■ Cross-Sectional Studies ■ Nonexperimental Studies	Harm

(Continued)

TABLE 4.2

CINAHL Headings for Retrieving Select Question Domains *(Continued)*

CINAHL Subject Headings	Question Domain That Can be Retrieved
■ Economics as a subheading added to a CINAHL Subject Term ■ "Health Care Costs" as a Subject Heading or Term ■ Other subject headings will vary depending on economic outcomes being sought from studies to be retrieved in database searches	**Economic Evaluation**
■ Qualitative Studies ■ Anthropology, Cultural (heading for ethnography pool of CINAHL articles) ■ Grounded Theory ■ Phenomenology	**Meaning**

Diagnosis/Screening

Diagnosis/screening questions discuss prediction rules (validation tests) and the selection and interpretation of diagnostic tests (utility or performance tests). For questions dealing with prediction, randomized controlled trials (RCTs) are the best choice for the review, followed by cohort and then case control study designs. Similar to research comparing at least two therapies, research on diagnostic tests involves comparing one test to an appropriate reference or gold standard. For example, Farquhar et al. (2003) wanted to know the accuracy of transvaginal ultrasonography, sonohysterography, and hysteroscopy in aiding in the diagnostic workup in premenopausal women with abnormal uterine bleeding.

In the CINAHL database, the "Explode feature" broadens and adds depth to the Subject Term—Diagnosis. Exploding will allow retrieval of papers on the general topic of *diagnosis* and papers on *subject headings* under diagnosis like Clinical Assessment Tools and Health Screening to name a few. Other CINAHL headings or Subject Terms that may prove useful in literature searches for questions on diagnosis are Clinical Assessment Tools; Diagnosis, Differential; Diagnostic Errors; Measurement Issues and Assessments; Nursing Assessment; and Reproducibility of Results.

Etiology or Causation

Etiology questions or causation studies seek to identify the root of a disease or phenomena. Commonly used research designs to answer an etiology, risk factor, prevalence, and frequency/rate research question are controlled trials, quasi-experimental studies, cohort, and case control study types. Whereas cohort studies follow people or subjects forward through time, case control studies follow subjects "backward in time." For example, a researcher could compare high-risk pregnancies that ended with good outcomes to high-risk pregnancies that resulted in bad outcomes and see whether the variable of bed rest had an impact on either group of women.

CINAHL headings or Subject Terms that address etiology questions and can be used in searching are Analytic Research, Case Control Studies, Epidemiological Research, Odds Ratio, Prospective Studies, Risk Assessment, and Risk Factors.

Therapy or Therapeutic Interventions

Therapy or therapeutic intervention questions deal with how to select the proper treatment for a condition or disease. Many parameters will be considered, including, at times, the cost of a therapy. For example, an interventional foreground question may seek to understand the influence of changing central venous access device (CVAD) dressings in 3 versus 7 days on bloodstream-related infection risk (Chang, Tsai, Huang, & Shih, 2003; Garland et al., 2001).

In many cases, a randomized controlled trial will be the best evidence study type for answering therapy questions. However, randomized controlled trials do not exist for every research question. In addition, it is not always possible or ethical to conduct randomized controlled trials for some clinical questions. For example, it is not ethical to do a study on toxic gas, exposing people to the hazard. Instead, researchers will identify a population that has already been exposed to the toxin, such as Vietnam War veterans and Agent Orange victims, and study that group alone or in comparison with others who were not exposed to the toxin. In this instance, a reviewer would be limiting search results to cohort studies.

When searching the literature for answers to therapy questions, some CINAHL Subject Terms to add to search statements include Clinical Trials, Comparative Studies, Crossover Design, Patient Selection, Random Sample, and Placebos. Blinding, follow-up, and randomization are not CINAHL headings but can be added to other words in search statements to facilitate retrieving articles dealing with the therapy domain. The CINAHL heading that includes follow-up studies is Prospective Studies.

Prognosis

Questions from the prognosis domain anticipate the effect or impact of a disease and estimate a patient's likely clinical course over time. High-quality prognosis studies are usually prospective cohort studies. Specifically, cohort and case-control studies are useful when reviewing diseases or conditions that are rare or must be followed for a long time. For instance, it may be desirable to follow a group of ex-heroin users who are pregnant and continuing on methadone therapy during pregnancy to see outcomes on their newborns.

Prognostic tests can give information on disease progression and lead to tests on prediction such as screening tests. Examples of questions in the prognosis domain include the following: In people with acute psychosis, how do outcomes differ for those admitted to open medical wards versus conventional psychiatric units? (Hickling, Abel, Garner, & Rathbone, 2007) and In patients with a recent TIA, who are discharged from the emergency department, which clinical prediction test(s) best identify those at risk for stroke? (Shah, Metz, & Edlow, 2009).

CINAHL headings useful for a literature search for prognosis questions are Disease Progression, Morbidity, Mortality, Prognosis, Prospective Studies, Recurrence, Survival Analysis, Time Factors, Incidence, and Prevalence.

Harm

Harm studies can discuss harm introduced either because of interventions of a diagnostic, prognostic, or interventional nature. Common study designs that inform on harm include systematic reviews of many studies, single RCT and non-RCT studies, and observational studies. For example, questions in the Harm domain of interest to community health nurses might involve the benefits of antiretroviral therapy and subsequent risk of HIV-associated lipodystrophy in people with HIV (Wierzbicki, Purdon, Hardman, Kulasegaram, & Peters 2008).

CINAHL headings for retrieving studies to answer questions in the Harm domain include Concurrent Prospective Studies, Cross-Sectional Studies, and Non-experimental Studies.

Economic Evaluation

Studies of Economic Evaluations review the cost burden (monetary and otherwise) for individuals, groups, and society. It can prove difficult to locate such studies in traditional literature sources such as databases until outcomes sought are detailed from one's systematic review question. For example, the reviewer who wanted to know the impact of doctor–nurse substitution in primary care on patient outcomes, process of care, and resource utilization including cost can expand on the term resource utilization revealing key terms or words that may be useful in future database searches, such as frequency and length of consultations, return visits, prescriptions, tests and investigations, referral to other services, and direct or indirect costs (Laurant et al., 2004).

Meaning

Questions on Meaning are concerned with understanding people and situations and with expanding the understanding of a phenomenon. These questions are explored in qualitative studies and involve the collection of data through interviews or observation and detail social phenomena rather than biomedical phenomena (Giacomini & Cook, 2002), exploring the meaning of a situation for patients, families, and other populations, for example, seeking to understand beliefs of African American men on prostate cancer screening (Blocker et al., 2006; Oliver, 2007). Qualitative studies are quite rigorous and serve to generate theories on phenomenon or set of circumstances (Booth, 2006).

Questions in the Meaning domain can be explored through qualitative studies involving different designs and methodologies (Booth, 2006). Examples of qualitative study designs include case studies, ethnographic, ground theory, historical, participatory action research, and phenomenological (see Table 4.2). Selection of a type of study depends on the Meaning foreground question being reviewed.

CINAHL subject headings for retrieving studies to answer questions on Meaning include Qualitative Studies, Grounded Theory, and Phenomenology. The CINAHL heading for ethnography studies is Anthropology, Cultural. Similar Medical Subject Headings (MeSH) are available in PubMed (U.S. NLM). PubMed also includes filters allowing one to limit search results to Qualitative Research Broad and Qualitative Research Narrow.

STUDY DESIGN AND FOREGROUND QUESTIONS

Foreground questions under specific domains can be classified as quantitative and/ or qualitative in nature. Quantitative questions can be answered with experimental or nonexperimental studies. Answers to qualitative questions are in studies exploring meaning of phenomena for a person or group such as observational studies, and they make use of various methodologies such as interviews and focus groups. While performing searches in databases for citations, large numbers of search results or "hits" can be limited to citations using one or more desired study design (see Table 4.3).

WRITING AND ANALYZING FOREGROUND CLINICAL QUESTIONS

Both asking and formulating a question may prove difficult. At least two frameworks— patient, intervention, comparison, outcome (PICO) and setting, perspective, intervention, comparison, evaluation (SPICE)—may be useful for "diagramming" or analyzing components of a foreground clinical question, assessing whether the question is good, feasible, answerable, and highly relevant.

As mentioned previously, PICO is a framework that can be used to help in formulating a comprehensive, yet tailored, researchable foreground clinical question to guide a systematic review. PICO was first described as a way to formalize the process clinicians go through when dissecting a clinical question about a specific patient with a certain circumstance (Richardson, Wilson, Nishikawa, & Hayward, 1995). Coming up with a good, researchable clinical question is one of the first steps in the path toward evidence for interventions for a patient (Richardson et al., 1995). PICO was originally applied to questions in the therapy domain but was later used to formulate and assess other foreground question domains. All components may not apply to other question domains such as some Prognosis questions that may not have a "C" or comparison. For example, what is the usual progression of myasthenia gravis in children diagnosed under the age of 5 years?

The SPICE framework was constructed by Booth (2006) and is used in the information sciences to assist in constructing and analyzing questions for investigation in the literature. This framework may prove useful for questions in the *meaning* domain where PICO may prove an ill-fitting construct to review meaning foreground question elements.

There are several variations of the PICO framework, which can further refine the question. These include PICO*m*, PICO*s*, and PICO*t*. With *"m,"* one can explore what types of studies or methods are best suited to measure variables in a question. With *"s,"* the focus is on study designs that usually are used to answer one's PICO question. With *"t,"* time is the variable of interest in one's PICO*t* question. See Table 4.4 on PICO framework and variations.

TABLE 4.3
Best Study Designs to Answer Foreground Questions for Writing a Systematic Review

Foreground Question Types and Domains

	Study Designs
Type A–Quantitative Questions	
Diagnosis/Screening	■ Randomized controlled trials
	■ Nonrandomized trials
	■ Analytical/observation studies: cross-sectional, cohort, case control (case series/case reports)
Etiology or Causation	■ Controlled trials
Risk Factor	■ Analytical/observation studies: cohort
Prevalence	
Frequency/Rate	
Therapy or Therapeutic Intervention (includes pharmacologic therapies and/or nonpharmacologic treatment)	■ Randomized controlled trials
	■ Nonrandomized trials
	■ Analytical/observation studies: cohort, case control (case series/case reports)
Prognosis	■ Longitudinal survey
	■ Analytical/observation studies: cohort
Harm	■ Randomized controlled trials
	■ Nonrandomized trials
	■ Analytical/observation studies: cohort, case control (case series/case reports)
Type B–Qualitative Questions	
Meaning	■ There are many qualitative study designs. Examples include case studies, ethnographic, ground theory, historical, participatory action research, and phenomenological.
	■ The appropriate choice of study design will depend on the actual descriptive/meaning foreground question.

By placing a foreground question into the PICO framework, the question is refined and inclusion and exclusion criteria for studies to be retrieved for the review become apparent. Important text words or key words and corresponding synonyms from the PICO or SPICE "diagram" can be highlighted, circled, or underlined for use in search statements during searches. Chapter 5 offers more details and tips for consideration in crafting database search strategies or heuristics.

TABLE 4.4

PICO Framework and Variations

PICO or PICO*m* or PICO*s* or PICO*t*	
P =	Patient, family, population, problem/condition, or disease/situation/phenomena of interest
I =	Intervention or exposure or risk factor
C =	Comparison or control
O =	Outcome
*m = or	Measure or method
*s= or	Study design or types of study
*t =	Timeframe for an intervention or treatment, time for when an outcome is reviewed, and so forth.

*There are variations on PICO such as PICO*m*, PICO*s*, and PICO*t*, where *m* is for methods or measure, *s* is for study design, and *t* stands for time.

SEARCH HEURISTICS FROM FOREGROUND QUESTIONS

As mentioned previously, search key terms can be identified from foreground questions, especially those placed in the PICO or SPICE framework. Key terms can be translated to or replaced with appropriate subject headings or subject terms offered by traditional databases such as CINAHL on EBSCOhost and MEDLINE from the U.S. NLM to increase precise retrieval of all relevant database citations on a topic. Key terms or key text words can also be searched "as is" for possible database citations matching that term or its synonyms. All answers to foreground questions are not represented by traditional literature sources such as databases; often, grey literature has to be explored. It may also be useful to elicit expert opinion and/or patients' perceptions (local or global views as appropriate) to get perspectives or answers to a foreground question.

SUMMARY

This chapter reviewed two broad categories of clinical questions that guide systematic review research: background and foreground questions. Two broad foreground question categories were identified—quantitative and qualitative questions—as well as question subcategories or domains (e.g., diagnosis, etiology, therapy, prognosis, harm, meaning). Search filters and subject headings for study designs and question categories in databases allow searchers to control searches and search results toward retrieval of more precise citations of evidence for answering foreground questions. Some databases, such as PubMed, offer the search feature Clinical Queries, allowing searchers to locate evidence-based citations by question domain—results for etiology, diagnosis, therapy, prognosis, and clinical prediction guideline searches (see Figure 4.1).

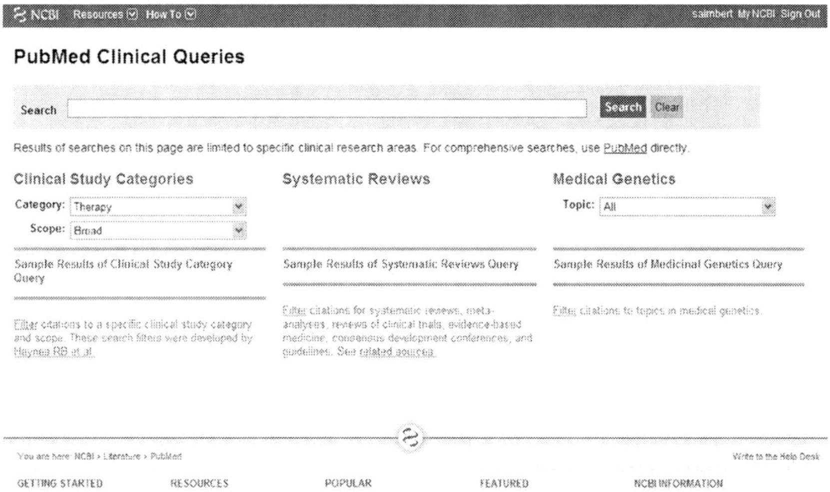

FIGURE 4.1

PubMed Clinical Queries search feature.

For databases not including a special search feature for researching a question by domain or question type, use database filters and subject headings to focus searches as previously noted. For example, a therapy question may be answered by a randomized controlled trial. In this case, limit database search results to include only citations with important terms: controlled trials or randomized controlled trials. Using filters, limits, and subject headings in databases is an art and a science, with each database having some nuances. Explore the "Help" section of *each* database for tips for effective use of filters, limits, and subject headings.

Before conducting literature searches in any online resource, write down the background questions and detail the primary clinical or foreground question in a framework such as PICO or SPICE. Is the foreground question feasible and researchable? Highlight in some way, underline or circle, the important terms from the foreground question. List synonyms for the important terms or key text words. Identify databases likely to include citations on your question and begin searching.

EXERCISES

1. Locating Examples of PICO Questions
   There are many reliable Internet resources from organization (.org) and education (.edu) websites discussing using PICO to formulate and refine foreground questions. Try locating some of these resources on Google; type the search statement *PICO question examples* in the Google search box. Local institution libraries may also have resources on PICO and other frameworks to diagram foreground questions.
2. Placing Foreground Questions in the PICO Framework
   Determine the elements of the PICO question from the foreground question provided and decide what type of systematic review might be done. See answers for Chapter 4, Exercise 2, in Appendix E.

Foreground Research Question #1	PICO #1	Type of Systematic Review
Does the use of nurse practitioners in nursing homes impact the decreasing rate of nursing home patient hospitalizations (Christian & Baker, 2009, p. 1333)?	P = I = C = O =	

Foreground Research Question #2	PICO #2	
What is the best available "evidence related to terminally ill patients' experiences of using music therapy in the palliative setting" (Mabel-Leow, Drury, Poon, & Hong, 2010, p. 344)?	P = I = C = O =	

Foreground Research Question #3	PICO #3	
What is the cost of supporting self-monitoring of blood glucose by Type 2 diabetes mellitus patients to improve glycemic control (Verteuil & Tan, 2010, p. 302)?	P = I = C = O =	

Foreground Research Question #4	PICO #4	
What is the impact of hospital visiting hours on patients and their visitors (Smith, Medves, Harrison, Tranmer, & Waytuck, 2009)?	P = I = C = O =	

Foreground Research Question #5	PICO #5	
What are the spiritual experiences of elderly individuals recovering from stroke (Lamb, Buchanan, Godfrey, Harrison, & Oakley, 2008)?	P = I = C = O =	

3. Fill in the following for Foreground Research Questions into the PICO Framework. See answers for Chapter 4, Exercise 3, in Appendix E.

Foreground Research Question	Question Domain or Category	PICO
What is the effect of open visiting hours on family members of ICU patients?		P = I = C = O =
What is the impact of open versus restricted visiting hours on nurse and patient satisfaction on medical-surgical units?		P = I = C = O =
What is the effect of an ICU residency program for recent (past 6 months) baccalaureate nursing school graduates on ICU nurse retention?		P = I = C = O =
Does discharge teaching on medications decrease congestive heart failure (CHF) patient readmission to the emergency room related to medication noncompliance?		P = I = C = O =
Does bed rounding contribute to a decrease of accidental patient falls in medical-surgical units?		P = I = C = O =

(Continued)

Exercise 3 (*Continued*)

Foreground Research Question	Question Domain or Category	PICO
Does use of advance practice nurses in long-term care facilities decrease patient hospitalizations?		P = I = C = O =
Is there a relationship between nurse–patient ratios and nurse burnout?		P = I = C = O =
Is there any impact or change in bloodstream-related infection when a central vascular access device (CVAD) dressing is changed in 3 days versus 7 days?		P = I = C = O =
Do magnet hospitals experience higher rates of nurse retention compared to nonmagnet hospitals?		P = I = C = O =
What is the occurrence of relocation stress or transfer anxiety in patients and their families upon transfer of the patient from an ICU to a non-ICU?		P = I = C = O =

(Continued)

Exercise 3 (*Continued*)

Foreground Research Question	Question Domain or Category	PICO
What are the most effective strategies for decreasing transfer anxiety in hospital patients?		**P** = **I** = **C** = **O** =
Does education of ICU nurses on oral care and implementation of a *vent bundle* decrease ventilator-associated pneumonia?		**P** = **I** = **C** = **O** =
In children living in an urban environment, does the presence of open spaces, such as parks, lead to positive health outcomes?		**P** = **I** = **C** = **O** =
What is the relationship between patient repositioning and pressure ulcer prevention?		**P** = **I** = **C** = **O** =

REFERENCES

Blocker, D. E., Romocki, L. S., Thomas, K. B., Jones, B. L., Jackson, E. J., Reid, L., & Campbell, M. K. (2006). Knowledge, beliefs and barriers associated with prostate cancer prevention and screening behaviors among African-American men. *Journal of the National Medical Association, 98*(8), 1286–1295.

Booth, A. (2006). Clear and present questions: formulating questions for evidence based practice. *Library Hi Tech, 24*(3), 355–368. doi:10.1108/07378830610692127

Buchanan, S. L., Crowther, C. A., Levett, K. M., Middleton, P., & Morris, J. (2010). Planned early birth versus expectant management for women with preterm prelabour rupture of membranes prior to 37 weeks' gestation for improving pregnancy outcome. *Cochrane Database of Systematic Reviews,* (3). doi:10.1002/14651858.CD004735.pub3

Chang, L., Tsai, J. S., Huang, S. J., & Shih, C. C. (2003). Evaluation of infectious complications of the implantable venous access system in a general oncologic population. *American Journal of Infection Control, 31*(1), 34–39.

Christian, R., & Baker, K. (2009). Effectiveness of nurse practitioners in nursing homes: A systematic review. *JBI Library of Systematic Reviews, 7*(30), 1359–1378. Retrieved from http://connect.jbiconnectplus.org/ViewSourceFile.aspx?0=4838

Collins, C. E., Warren, J. M., Neve, M., McCoy, P., & Stokes, B. (2007). Systematic review of interventions in the management of overweight and obese children which include a dietary component. *JBI Library of Systematic Reviews, 5*(1), 1–70. Retrieved from http://connect.jbiconnectplus.org/ViewSourceFile.aspx?0=4922

Farquhar, C., Ekeroma, A., Furness, S., & Arroll, B. (2003). A systematic review of transvaginal ultrasonography, sonohysterography and hysteroscopy for the investigation of abnormal uterine bleeding in premenopausal women. *Acta Obstetricia et Gynecologica Scandinavia, 82*(6), 493–504.

Garland, J. S., Alex, C. P., Mueller, C. D., Otten, D., Shivpuri, C., Harris, M. C., . . . Maki, D. G. (2001). A randomized trial comparing povidone-iodine to a chlorhexidine gluconate-impregnated dressing for prevention of central venous catheter infections in neonates. *Pediatrics, 107*(6), 1431–1436.

Giacomini, M., & Cook, D. J. (2002). Advanced topics in applying the results of therapy trials. Qualitative research. In G. Guyatt, D. Rennie, M. O. Meade, & D. J. Cook (Eds.), *Users' guides to the medical literature. A manual for evidence-based clinical practice* (2nd ed., pp. 341–360). New York, NY: McGraw Hill Medical.

Hewitt, V., & Watts, R. (2009). The effectiveness of non-invasive complementary therapies in reducing postoperative nausea and vomiting following abdominal laparoscopic surgery in women: A systematic review. *JBI Library of Systematic Reviews, 7*(19), 850–907. Retrieved from http://connect.jbiconnectplus.org/ViewSourceFile.aspx?0=4819

Hickling, F. W., Abel, W., Garner, P., & Rathbone, J. (2007). Open general medical wards versus specialist psychiatric units for acute psychoses. *Cochrane Database of Systematic Reviews,* (4). doi:10.1002/14651858.CD003290.pub2

Horsley, T., O'Neill, J., McGowan, J., Perrier, L., Kane, G., & Campbell, C. (2010). Interventions to improve question formulation in professional practice and self-directed learning. *Cochrane Database of Systematic Reviews,* (5). doi:10.1002/14651858.CD007335.pub2

Hughes, C., Smith, M., & Tunney, M. (2008). Infection control strategies for preventing the transmission of methicillin-resistant *Staphylococcus aureus* (MRSA) in nursing homes for older people. *Cochrane Database of Systematic Reviews,* (1). doi:10.1002/14651858.CD006354.pub2

Kitchenham, B. (2004). *Procedures for Systematic Review. Joint Technical Report.* Retrieved from http://www.mendeley.com/research/procedures-performing-systematic-reviews-joint-technical-report-6/

Lamb, M., Buchanan, D., Godfrey, C. M., Harrison, M. B., & Oakley, P. (2008). The psychosocial spiritual experience of elderly individuals recovering from stroke: A systematic review. *JBI Library of Systematic Reviews, 6*(12), 432–483. Retrieved from http://connect.jbiconnectplus.org/ViewSourceFile.aspx?0=4919

Laschinger, S., Medves, J., Pulling, C., McGraw, R., Waytuck, B., Harrison, M. B., & Gambeta, K. (2008). Effectiveness of simulation on health profession students' knowledge, skills, confidence, and satisfaction. *JBI Library of Systematic Reviews, 6*(7), 265–309. Retrieved from http://connect.jbiconnectplus.org/ViewSourceFile.aspx?0=4914

Laurant, M., Reeves, D., Hermens, R., Braspenning, J., Grol, R., & Sibbald, B. (2004). Substitution of doctors by nurses in primary care. *Cochrane Database of Systematic Reviews, 18*(4). doi:10.1002/14651858.CD001271.pub2

Lee, J., & Park, S. (2010). The effectiveness of telephone-based post-discharge nursing care in decreasing readmission rate in patients with heart failure: A systematic review. *JBI Library of Systematic Reviews, 8*(32), 1288–1303. Retrieved from http://connect.jbiconnectplus.org/ViewSourceFile.aspx?0=4968

Mabel, L. Q. H., Drury, V. B., & Hong, P. W. (2010). The experience and expectations of terminally ill patients receiving music therapy in the palliative setting: A systematic review. *JBI Library of Systematic Reviews, 8*(27), 1088–1111. Retrieved from http://connect.jbiconnectplus.org/ViewSourceFile.aspx?0=4963

Mabel-Leow, Q. H., Drury, V., Poon, W., & Hong, E. (2010) Patient's experiences of music therapy in a Singaporean hospice. *International Journal of Palliative Nursing, 16*(7), 344–350.

McClure, R. J., Turner, C., Peel, N., Spinks, A., Eakin, E., & Hughes, K. (2005). Population-based interventions for the prevention of fall-related injuries in older people. *Cochrane Database of Systematic Reviews,* (1). doi:10.1002/14651858.CD004441.pub2

Oliver, J. S. (2007). Attitudes and beliefs about prostate cancer and screening among rural African American men. *Journal Cultural Diversity, 14*(2), 74–80.

Pearson, A., Laschinger, H., Porritt, K., Jordan, Z., Tucker, D., & Long, L. (2007). Comprehensive systematic review of evidence on developing and sustaining nursing leadership that fosters a healthy work environment in healthcare. *JBI Library of Systematic Reviews, 5*(5), 279–343. Retrieved from http://connect.jbiconnectplus.org/ViewSourceFile.aspx?0=4926

Poletick, E. B., & Holly, C. (2010). A systematic review of nurses' inter-shift handoff reports in acute care hospitals. *JBI Library of Systematic Reviews, 8*(4), 121–172. Retrieved from http://connect.jbiconnectplus.org/ViewSourceFile.aspx?0=4936

Richardson, W. S., Wilson, M. C., Nishikawa, J., & Hayward, R. S. (1995). The well-built clinical question: a key to evidence-based decisions [Editorial]. *ACP Journal Club, 123*(3), A12–A13.

Sackett, D.L. (2000). *Evidence-based medicine: How to practice & teach EBM.* London, UK: Churchill Livingstone.

Senok, A. C., Verstraelen, H., Temmerman, M., & Botta, G. A. (2009). Probiotics for the treatment of bacterial vaginosis. *Cochrane Database of Systematic Reviews,* (4). doi:10.1002/14651858.CD006289.pub2

Shah, K. H., Metz, H. A., & Edlow, J. A. (2009). Clinical prediction rules to stratify short-term risk of stroke among patients diagnosed in the emergency department with a transient ischemic attack. *Ann Emerg Med, 53*(5), 662–673. doi:10.1016/j.annemergmed.2008.08.004

Smith, L., Medves, J., Harrison, M. B., Tranmer, J., & Waytuck, B. (2009). The impact of hospital visiting hour policies on pediatric and adult patients and their visitors. *JBI Library of Systematic Reviews, 7*(2), 38–79. Retrieved from http://connect.jbiconnectplus.org/ViewSourceFile.aspx?0=4802

Verteuil, R. D., & Tan, W. S. (2010). Self-monitoring of blood glucose in type 2 diabetes mellitus: Systematic review of economic evidence. *JBI Library of Systematic Reviews, 8*(7), 302–342. Retrieved from http://connect.jbiconnectplus.org/ViewSourceFile.aspx?0=4939

Wee, B., & Hillier, R. (2008). Interventions for noisy breathing in patients near to death. *Cochrane Database of Systematic Reviews,* (1). doi:10.1002/14651858.CD005177.pub2

Wierzbicki, A., Purdon, S., Hardman, T., Kulasegaram, R., & Peters, B. (2008). Clinical aspects of the management of HIV lipodystrophy. *British Journal of Diabetes & Vascular Disease, 8*(3), 113–119.

Young, M., Watts, R., & Wilson, S. (2010). The effectiveness of educational strategies in improving parental/caregiver management of fever in their child: A systematic review. *JBI Library of Systematic Reviews, 8*(21), 826–868. Retrieved from http://connect.jbiconnectplus.org/ViewSourceFile.aspx?0=4957

SUGGESTED READINGS

Toronto Centre for Evidence-Based Medicine. (2000–2010). *CEBM: Glossary of EBM terms.* Retrieved from http://ktclearinghouse.ca/cebm/glossary/

PART III

Searching and Appraising the Literature

CHAPTER FIVE

Key Principles for Searching Literature

Marie K. Saimbert

OBJECTIVES

Upon completion of Chapter 5, you will be able to:

- Discuss types of searches that can be undertaken to retrieve individual studies for systematic review using primary, secondary, and tertiary literature
- Compare and contrast basic and advanced search features
- Define controlled vocabulary and subject heading/subject term

IMPORTANT POINTS

- Thoughtful, methodical searches for relevant literature to include in systematic reviews are crucial to the systematic review research process. Search details in all resources should be documented and reproducible as needed.
- After preliminary searches of literature, a foreground question, systematic review inclusion and exclusion criteria, important search terms, and/or search statements may need to be revised or expanded.
- Research librarians skilled in the use of advanced search feature in databases, including Medical Subject Headings (MeSH) or subject terms, can help to increase sensitivity (e.g., through use of special search queries or hedges) and precision (e.g., by using applicable subject headings) of obtaining relevant primary studies for systematic reviews.

INTRODUCTION

Performing searches in databases or online search resources to locate relevant, evidence-based literature for foreground clinical questions can be challenging. This chapter reviews common principles on searching that are applicable to researching literature for answering foreground clinical questions, whether for practice or to create a systematic review. Literature can fall under one of three categories: primary, secondary, or tertiary. There is also mention of filtered versus unfiltered literature which can be a way to further describe primary, secondary, and tertiary literature.

TYPES OF LITERATURE

Primary Literature

Primary literature is an original work or first-hand account describing a phenomenon or experiment. Examples of primary literature include quantitative articles on overcooling or therapeutic hypothermia in patients after cardiac arrest (Gillies et al., 2010; Merchant et al., 2006; Prior et al., 2010; Skulec et al., 2008) or qualitative articles on caregivers' burden with a spouse having multiple sclerosis (Akkus, 2010; Knight, Devereux, & Godfrey, 1997; Mutch, 2010; Rivera-Navarro et al., 2009).

Secondary Literature

Secondary literature summarizes and synthesizes primary literature. It also highlights select articles on a topic. Secondary literature, such as meta-analyses or metasyntheses, gathers all information for analysis to promote understanding or illumination of outcomes, either positive or negative from single studies. Metastudy researchers may apply statistical methods, bringing to light effects of primary studies and their overall scientific weight. There is a growing body of literature surrounding metastudies that highlights good and bad metastudies. An example of a good meta-analysis of observational studies according to Andrel, Keith, and Leiby (2009) is on cancer survivors and rate of unemployment compared to the general population (de Boer, Taskila, Ojajarvi, van Dijk, & Verbeek, 2009). Andrel et al. (2009) cite the positive aspects of this meta-analysis as (the researchers) included "inclusion and exclusion criteria, details of databases searched to elicit studies for analysis, methodology quality of individual studies reviewed and detailed, specific calculations using appropriate statistical models and plots of data" (p. 377). The conclusion of the meta-analysis was that survivors of cancer experienced unemployment at rate of 1.37 times more than those who did not have cancer. Andrel et al. (2009) on the other hand, offered a critique of the early meta-analysis finding that rosiglitazone (Avandia) increased the risk of myocardial infarction and cardiac death, noting that the statistical model used in that meta-analysis may have been inappropriate. In fact, a reanalysis using a different statistical model showed insufficient evidence that rosiglitazone increased myocardial infarction risk, but actually had greater impact for rosiglitazone on risk of cardiac death (Andrel et al., 2009).

Meta-analyses should not remain static. Lau et al. (1992) revealed, in a meta-analysis of eight trials before 1973, a significant decrease in mortality for acute myocardial infarction patients taking the thrombolytic agent intravenous streptokinase. Over time, with 25 more trials factored into the meta-analysis, the aforementioned positive effect remained unchanged (Andrel et al., 2009; Lau et al., 1992). Lau et al. postulate that the use of the cumulative metastudy can result in evidence that is constantly updated to give practitioners the best available information for taking care of patients (Lau, Schmid, & Chalmers, 1995). This periodic update is an essential feature of the systematic reviews contained in both the Cochrane Database of Systematic Reviews and the Joanna Briggs Institute Library of Systematic Reviews.

Sometimes, systematic reviewers perform searches and review meta-analyses and metasyntheses related to their foreground question, noting that individual studies cited in the bibliography or reference list of the metastudy may be of value to their research (a technique called footnote or citation chasing). It may be good to remember that citation bias may be introduced into one's systematic review if many original articles are taken from a metastudy, especially because researchers of that metastudy chose to include those articles because it met their inclusion criteria and review objectives, not necessarily the criteria of someone else's systematic review (Shultz, Dell, & Bodan, 2009).

Tertiary Literature

Tertiary literature highlights and/or synthesizes primary and secondary literature, allowing for summaries that reveal information that are otherwise hidden or missed in published literature. This information can facilitate early use of evidence from the literature in clinical practice. An example of tertiary literature is a summary of Type 2 diabetes from online databases such as eMedicine on WebMD and Dynamed on EBSCOhost (Dynamed, 2010; Ligaray & Isley, 2010). The phrase *tertiary source* can also be used to describe an electronic database such as MEDLINE, which is the premier biomedical database from the United States National Library of Medicine (U.S. NLM). MEDLINE includes citations of primary, secondary, and tertiary literature. Another example of tertiary sources are textbooks, because they are often based on or summarize primary or secondary literature.

Filtered Literature

Either primary, secondary or tertiary literature can be filtered, reviewed and pooled to explore common outcomes for patients with similar set of circumstances. Filtered, or synthesized, literature often highlights the latest evidence-based information for a topic or a specific question. Examples of filtered literature include an electronic article or summary on congestive heart failure (CHF) from electronic search resources such as Dynamed or eMedicine, a systematic review, guideline, meta-analysis, and metasynthesis articles. Filtered resources translate evidence from systematic reviews, allowing for quick integration of evidence into practice applicable to specific patients or populations of interest.

Searches in most traditional online or electronic databases and some Internet resources can be manipulated to retrieve filtered or synthesized citations. For example, a search in PubMed using the search box directly located on the Pubmed.gov page will yield both filtered and unfiltered results. Use the *limits* option to narrow down the results pool to filtered information such as *practice guidelines* and *review*. PubMed also offers a unique search box/feature called Clinical Queries, where a searcher can search for both filtered and unfiltered evidence-based studies—systematic reviews and individual studies, respectively.

Examples of unfiltered, or "raw," literature include an original research article on hyperbaric oxygen therapy (HBOT) for chronic nondiabetic wound healing or a report, classified as *grey literature*, on parental control on after-school programs promoting personal and social skills (Durlak & Weissberg, 2007; Hammarlund & Sundberg, 1994; see Chapter 6 section on grey literature). Some unfiltered literature can also be part of search results from Internet search resources such as Google Scholar (scholar.google.com) and searches in traditional databases employing basic search features.

Systematic reviewers are often focused on pooling unfiltered literature to explore answers for their foreground questions, while clinicians at the "bedside" look to filtered literature for assistance in answering their foreground questions, as filtered literature (if one is able to locate it and it matches the patient being considered) can be a powerful tool facilitating evidence-based patient care.

For example, an emergency room nurse practitioner may use a database with filtered evidence such as Best Bets (Best Evidence Topics; http://www.bestbets.org). That resource allows for browsing of emergency medicine scenarios or questions. Examples of BestBETs topics include oral versus nebulized steroids for croup; collar and cuff versus sling for clavicle fractures; eye patches for corneal abrasion; and the Oucher versus Children's Hospital Eastern Ontario Pain Scale (CHEOPS) for pain assessment for children (Carley, 2000; Lyon, 2000; Mackway-Jones, 2000; Maurice, 2000).

Conversely, a researcher conducting a systematic review may need primarily unfiltered evidence, such as primary studies for their review, but may use synthesized literature such as a meta-analysis to answer one aspect of their review question. For example, in the Cochrane review on exercise or exercise plus diet modifications for preventing diabetes, the researchers noted that the included studies for their main analysis were randomized controlled trials lasting at least six months and mentioned incidence of diabetes in people at risk for diabetes. They also sought and analyzed meta-analyses for answers dealing with their review's secondary outcomes. Secondary outcomes included *development of impaired glucose tolerance, cholesterol levels, costs,* and *adverse effects* (e.g., traumatic injuries secondary to leisure physical activity, nutritional deficits; Orozco et al., 2008, p. 8). Similarly, some systematic review researchers performing reviews dealing with education, crime, justice, and social welfare also look at meta-analyses or data in meta-analyses as part of their systematic review work, as in the review *Effects of Cognitive-Behavioral Programs for Criminal Offenders* (Lipsey, Landenberger, & Wilson, 2007).

LITERATURE SEARCHES FOR SYSTEMATIC REVIEW

Being Systematic

Systematic review research involves conscientious retrieval and review of all attainable literature on a research question to decrease bias. There are many types of bias possible that can blemish research and research reporting. Researchers should conduct thorough literature searches, inclusive of worldwide evidence (in all languages) from all sources available to them. This involves searching at least four relevant electronic search resources. Top search resources for a nursing-related systematic review effort include Cumulative Index to Nursing and Allied Health Literature (CINAHL on EBSCOhost), MEDLINE on Ovid or EBSCOhost) or searching MEDLINE within PubMed (U.S. NLM), and EMBASE (Elsevier B.V.). Depending on the foreground search question, other databases, such as PsycINFO (American Psychological Association) or *ProQuest Social Science Journals* (Proquest, LLC), may prove important for locating individual or primary studies for a systematic review. In the literature, there are critiques of systematic review methodologies noting that some reviewers searched too few databases. Some search only one or two databases to answer a foreground clinical question (Petticrew, Wilson, Wright, & Song, 2002). This jeopardizes the applicability of the systematic review outcomes for patients/populations of interest. A systematic review not inclusive of all the possible available evidence in the literature on a question is an incomplete review, and it is therefore biased. Other issues include searching in an imprecise or non-systematic fashion.

Tracking Systematic Review Searches

For searches related to systematic review work, it is not enough to search all the appropriate databases; a researcher must also track the path of searches, so steps could be reproduced by others (see Exhibit 6.1: Comprehensive Systematic Review Search Strategies Worksheet). Information on search resources used to obtain included and excluded studies for a systematic review usually appear in detail in the systematic review Methods section, which also details inclusion and exclusion criteria. At least one example of a search path or a search strategy employed in an online database is presented in the review write-up, but all search steps should be documented in the event that others would like to retrace those search steps, reobtaining the results that a researcher obtained in an online search resources for a selected timeframe. All search strategies employed during systematic review research should be documented. Store searches in a *personal account* provided by most online databases and/or on a search strategies worksheet.

Where to Begin Searching

Preliminary searches should be done in filtered evidence resources, places holding summaries or reviews of already published systematic reviews on the same or similar systematic review question of interest. Most libraries' websites include lists of databases and online research resources. Some offer subject guides, research guides, and toolkits/toolboxes to assist in quick identification of relevant search resources for locating evidence-based information in the literature for foreground clinical questions (see Table 5.1). The guides may highlight which databases are filtered versus unfiltered and other print and electronic resources.

Designing Search Strategies

A search worksheet can be completed to write out search strategies for use in specific databases and other online resources. Important or key text words and phrases

TABLE 5.1

Sample Items in Toolkits/Toolboxes

Toolkit/Toolbox Categories	Example Items in Categories
Electronic Bibliographic Databases	**Biomedical:** ■ CINAHL ■ EMBASE ■ PsycINFO ■ PubMed **Evidence-Based Clinical Care Databases:** BestBETs ■ http://www.bestbets.org/ **Dynamed** ■ http://www.ebscohost.com/dynamed/ **Turning Research Into Practice Database (TRIP)** ■ http://www.tripdatabase.com/ **Social Science:** ■ *ProQuest Social Science Journals* ■ Web of Science
E-books or Select Relevant Books	**Print Book:** *Evidence-based practice in nursing & health-care: A guide to best practice.* Bernadette Mazurek Melnyk, Ellen Fineout-Overholt **E-book:** *Users' Guides to the Medical Literature* http://www.pubs.ama-assn.org/misc/usersguides.dtl
E-journals or Select Relevant Articles on Evidence-Based Practice	**E-journal:** *Worldviews on Evidence-Based Nursing* **Example Article #1:** Dicenso, A., Bayley, L., & Haynes, R. B. (2009). Accessing pre-appraised evidence: Fine-tuning the 5S model into a 6S model. *Evidence-Based Nursing, 12*(4), 99–101. http://www.ebn.bmj.com/content/12/4/99.2.full.pdf **Example Article #2:** McKibbon, K. A., Wilczynski, N. L., & Haynes, R. B. (2004). What do evidence-based secondary journals tell us about the publication of clinically important articles in primary healthcare journals? *BMC Med, 2*, 33. http://www.ncbi.nlm.nih.gov/pmc/articles/PMC518974/?tool=pubmed
Patient/Consumer/ Healthcare Policy-maker Resources	**New York Online Access to Health (NOAH)** ■ http://noah-health.org/ **MedlinePlus** ■ http://www.nlm.nih.gov/medlineplus/

(Continued)

TABLE 5.1

Sample Items in Toolkits/Toolboxes *(Continued)*

Toolkit/Toolbox Categories	Example Items in Categories
Internet Resources with Grey Literature	**Intute—Nursing, Midwifery, and Allied Health** ■ Search or browse a nursing topic under its Medical Subject Heading (MeSH) ■ http://www.intute.ac.uk/nmah/ **AARP Policy and Research for Professionals in Aging** ■ Includes information on many health care topics of interest to seniors ■ Contains reports such as the AARP 2006 Prescription Drug Study With Hispanics and African Americans ■ http://www.aarp.org/research **The Commonwealth Fund** ■ Information for healthcare policy generation related to children, uninsured, minorities and other groups ■ http://www.commonwealthfund.org/ **EDUCATION—Line** ■ Grey literature database from British Education Service in Leeds ■ Contains full-text working papers and conference papers to support education research, policy making, and practice ■ http://www.leeds.ac.uk/bei/index.html **New York Academy of Medicine Grey Literature Report** ■ http://www.nyam.org/library/grey.shtml **OAIster** ■ Contains grey literature–scanned books, audio, images, and statistics datasets on health policy ■ http://oaister.worldcat.org/ **Research and Development (RAND)** ■ Nonprofit, nonpartisan organization around since 1940s; they prepare research reports that can impact health, social, and economic policies. ■ http://www.rand.org/

identified from a foreground systematic review question and synonyms for the text words/phrases should be placed on the worksheet. More can be added as reviewers discover specifics about searching each database.

Search one electronic resource or computerized database at a time. Although it may be offered, avoid searching multiple databases at once because each database will have specific features that will not be the same as another database's, so some article citations may be missed if one uses a federated or *one* search option.

As noted previously, some databases use different terminology in referring to a concept. In addition, some concepts are covered in more detail and/or divided into more subcategories in one database than in another. A database's thesaurus or dictionary reveals controlled vocabulary terms, otherwise known as *subject headings* or subject terms, which are attached to each article citation in a database. How much a database covers a topic (level and depth) may be apparent while reviewing subject headings in the database thesaurus. For example, a search of the CINAHL database controlled vocabulary list or subject terms list for the term *nursing students* reveals articles under a thesaurus term Students, Nursing +. The plus sign in Students, Nursing indicates that thesaurus term "explodes" or expands to deeper subgroups/categories or types of nursing students such as midwifery, baccalaureate, and male nursing students (see Figure 5.1). A similar search of the MEDLINE database-controlled vocabulary list or *Medical Subject Headings* (MeSH) list reveals the heading: students, nursing under the broader heading: students, *health occupations*. In comparing the subject term listing for nursing students in CINAHL and MEDLINE on Ovid, CINAHL offers a more direct route for locating subject headings or subject terms on subcategories of nursing students. In MEDLINE, one will retrieve all articles labeled with the MeSH: students, nursing. To locate articles on select types of nursing students, such as male nursing students or baccalaureate nursing students, one would need to use those specific terms in the MEDLINE on Ovid search box. For instance, to retrieve articles on baccalaureate nursing students, the MEDLINE subject heading *Education, Nursing, Baccalaureate* could be selected during a search.

Search Filters and Hedges

Search hedges and filters have been created to locate information on a topic, and often, those filters have been tested for a balance of precision or accuracy, ability to retrieve all citations in a database on a topic, sensitivity, ability to find and retrieve a certain percentage of citations in a database on a topic, and specificity (i.e., the ability to have a really low number of misses or documents not on a topic). One website that a reviewer can visit to learn more about search hedges and filters is the McMaster University's Health Information Research Unit (HIRU) website at http://hiru.mcmaster.ca/hiru/HIRU_Hedges_home.aspx. Hedges, similar to search statements, may be modified or evolved over time to enhance their accuracy, sensitivity, and/or specificity. There is no all-encompassing search hedge to retrieve qualitative articles; it often comes down to investigators reviewing search results in a database to manually identify qualitative studies. Hedges/filters for quantitative studies may prove more accurate.

Search Resources and their Search Retrieval Systems

Databases are online search resources placed within one or more search retrieval systems. For example, one can search MEDLINE on Ovid or EBSCOhost search systems (depends on what is available at an institution library). Why is attention to a

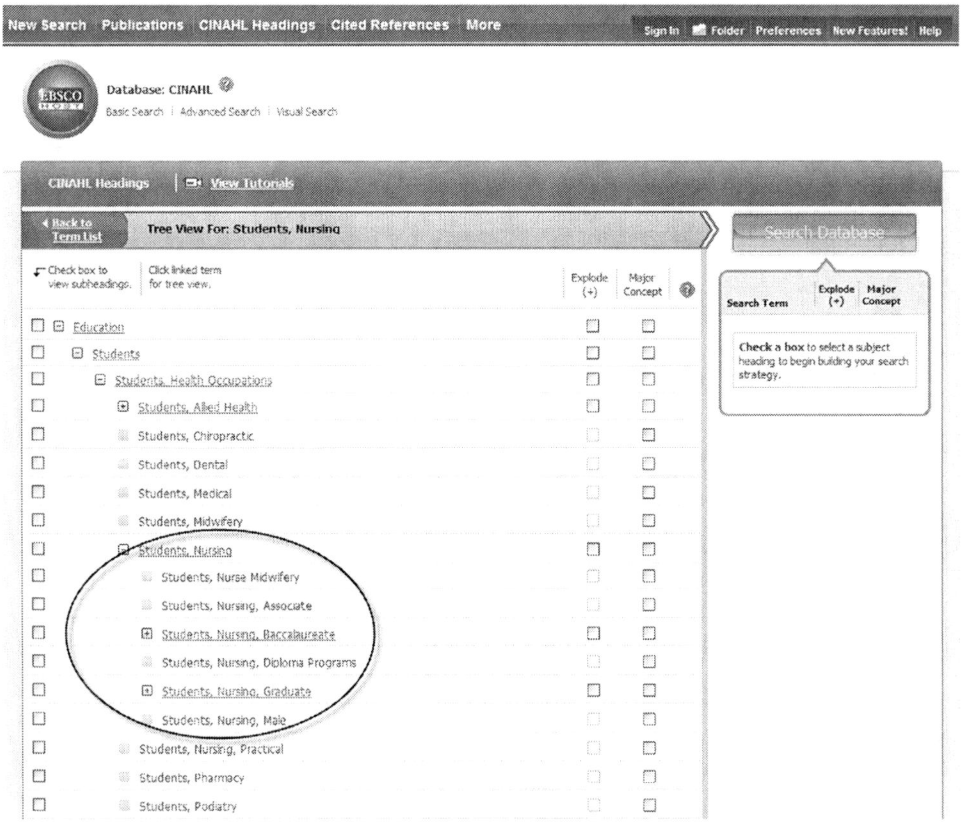

FIGURE 5.1

CINAHL on EBSCOhost: Subject Term: Students, Nursing for keyword: nursing students.

Source: Copyright © EBSCO Industries, Inc.

search retrieval system important? Why not just concentrate on the database being searched? Sometimes a reviewer may find it easier and/or more efficient to search a database on one search system or platform versus another. Depending on the search retrieval system holding a database, a searcher may be able to search and/or manage database citations more easily. Reviewers have searched the same database (e.g., MEDLINE on Ovid versus MEDLINE as part of PubMed), similarly, on more than one system and obtained different results. Reasons may include a time lag between search retrieval systems for entry of citations in a database and differences basic and/or advanced search on one search retrieval platform versus another. Arguably, it is easier to retrieve similar search results from advanced searches of *one* database on *two* different search retrieval systems because, regardless of the search retrieval system, a reviewer could control the search using the controlled vocabulary or thesaurus terms native to the database. Involve a librarian early on in complex search work such as that in systematic review research. A more important thing is to keep track of the full name (such as Ovid MEDLINE) of the resource being used on a search worksheet and be able to share that with librarians or reviewers.

Select Types of Literature Searches

Pearl-Growing Search

A *pearl-growing search* is a search akin to casting a net at sea, only this net is cast in a database to retrieve gems of articles. The phrases "snow-balling" or "going-wide search" are sometimes used in lieu of pearl-growing search. The pearl-growing search can help in the following ways:

■ Gives an idea of what work has been published or is available on a clinical question
■ Assists in identification of other key text words/concepts that can be used during searches
■ Provides clues regarding whether the existing body of literature in a database addresses a research question; it may also verify if a researcher has a detailed enough, answerable foreground question
■ Can be accomplished using text words and the basic search option in a database
■ May make the case for a searcher using the advanced search option in a database and controlled vocabulary or a database thesaurus if available

Preliminary Search

Preliminary searches are initial searches that often are performed for pearl growing. An example of a preliminary search in the systematic review process involves looking for existing systematic reviews on a foreground clinical question.

Comprehensive Search

Comprehensive searches aim to be as thorough as possible; the best strategy to retrieve desired citations is attempted. Usually, the advanced search option and specific database search features are employed to carry out a successful comprehensive search. Part of comprehensive searching is repeating searches in more than one online search resource or database. Attention is placed not only on search accuracy, but also on the sensitivity of databases and search statements employed in them for retrieving relevant citations.

Because the systematic review process will take time, some noting about twelve to eighteen months to complete (Bernard Becker Medical Library, 2009; Holopainen, Hakulinen-Viitanen, & Tossavainen, 2008), some systematic review researchers set up search alerts (for e-mails and RSS feeds) in databases to continue collecting new citations of studies that are potentially relevant for their review. Many databases useful for systematic review work, such as CINAHL, EMBASE, and MEDLINE, include a feature allowing for setup of search alerts, including parameters for when and what type of alerts a searcher wishes to receive. Regardless of when reviewers end searching the literature in a database or other resource, write down the dates searches were performed. This is useful if the original systematic review investigators or future research teams want to go back to duplicate one or more of the searches from a systematic review.

Basic and Advanced Search

The terms *basic search* and *advanced search* do not mean the same things across all databases. For example, what constitutes as basic search in CINAHL may not be the same as basic search in MEDLINE. Also, a basic search of a database on one search retrieval system may not be equivalent to a basic search of the same database on a different search retrieval system. For example, a basic search of EMBASE on Ovid may not produce the same results as searching equivalent EMBASE files on Elsevier's EMBASE.com. Chapter 6 presents some specific basic and advanced search features for select databases.

One thing that often holds true about basic search is that it is equivalent to cooking—where one adds all the ingredients into the pot at once versus adding ingredients one at a time, tasting the dish before adding the next ingredient. For example, in basic search in some databases, searchers are offered one search box to enter important text words from their search statement or research question. Connector words (*AND, OR,* and *NOT*) also called *Boolean logic operators,* can be added between the text words and phrases and then the searcher processes the search, directly obtaining results.

Text words entered into a search box for a basic search are looked for in specific areas of citations and in other places such as internal dictionaries proprietary to a database (Quain, personal communication, July 2010). It would be incorrect to assume that a basic search involves a database looking for text word anywhere it appears in the full text of an article or citation. For example, a basic search in one database may only look for a searcher's text word/phrase in the title, abstract, subject heading, and article picture's captions for an article.

Although advanced search can mean different things in different databases, one thing present in most advanced searches is a way to add text words or phrases in steps—similar to cooking, adding one ingredient at a time and seeing how things *taste* before the next ingredient is added. In the search for information on nurse practitioners and *attitudes* to *clinical information systems,* a researcher can perform a "in one pot–all at once" search (i.e., a basic search) by placing the following in a database's search box: (nurse practitioners OR APNs OR advanced practice nurses) AND attitudes AND (clinical information systems OR CIS OR computerized information systems OR hospital information systems). The alternative search, often an advanced search where a researcher is doing things in steps, is as follows:

1. Type *nurse practitioner* in the database search box and select the appropriate subject heading for nurse practitioner.
2. The next "ingredient" is typing *clinical information systems* in the search box and choosing the appropriate subject heading for that.
3. Then combine the result set for nurse practitioners with the result set for clinical information systems, similar to chopping one ingredient, then another, and then adding them into one pot to make a dish.
4. Lastly, to narrow search results down to articles on *attitudes* of nurse practitioners regarding information systems, the result set from the combining of subject heading: nurse practitioners AND subject heading: information systems was *ANDed*

with the text word attitude. (Text words searched as text words rather than as subject headings are handled by a database in this fashion. The database locates the text word in specific areas of the article such as the abstract and title. It does not look for the text word all throughout an entire article.)

For practice, try the preceding search in MEDLINE on Ovid.

An evidence-based practice workshop or library seminar on searching would be worthwhile to learn more about building advanced searches. The class will cover how to add text words and/or subject headings one by one in a search and then address combining the text words and/or subject headings using Boolean logic operators (*AND, OR,* and *NOT*) to achieve a final result set. See the section Boolean Logic Operators in this chapter for more details about when to use *AND, OR,* and *NOT.* The workshop should also include how to use the limits feature in databases to further narrow search results to relevant citations.

A common advanced search makes use of a database's thesaurus of terms. The database thesaurus or dictionary includes terms or subject headings for topics. All citations in a database are organized by being assigned several subject headings; sometimes, 15 or more thesaurus subject headings are attached to one citation, often by human indexers who read the articles prior to their placement in a database and then "label" or tag each article with the subject headings based on what is the focus of an article. The tagged articles are entered into the database, and retrieval of those articles by an end-user such as a systematic review researcher best takes place by using advanced search strategies to search for the specific subject headings attached to articles in the database. For example, citations on nursing students in CINAHL would be put in the database and labeled or tagged with the thesaurus heading *students, nursing.* When a searcher is looking to retrieve article citations on nursing students in CINAHL, they have a good chance of obtaining search results with more relevant citations on nursing students if their search makes use of the database subject heading: *students, nursing* for the text words: nursing student.

For example, a searcher types the text words *nursing students* in a CINAHL advanced search box and "runs" their search. The database shows the searcher a page listing their text words: nursing students and a list of thesaurus subject headings that may represent their text words. Because the searcher wants this to be an advanced search, they will place a check mark in front of the most appropriate subject heading that represents the original text word they typed. The subject heading: *students, nursing* receives a checkmark, and the searcher will click on *"search database"* to see how many results are in CINAHL for that heading.

More search results may be located using the database subject heading: *students, nursing;* then the keyword: nursing students. For example, in a search performed on December 2, 2010, there were 17,149 citations for the subject heading: students, nursing and 7,443 for the text word/phrase in *quotation marks:* nursing students. In terms of systematic review research, which search move, advanced search using database subject headings, or searching using *key words,* may allow for retrieval of *more relevant* citations? More "on point," not necessarily a greater number of cites should be evident from a search using the subject

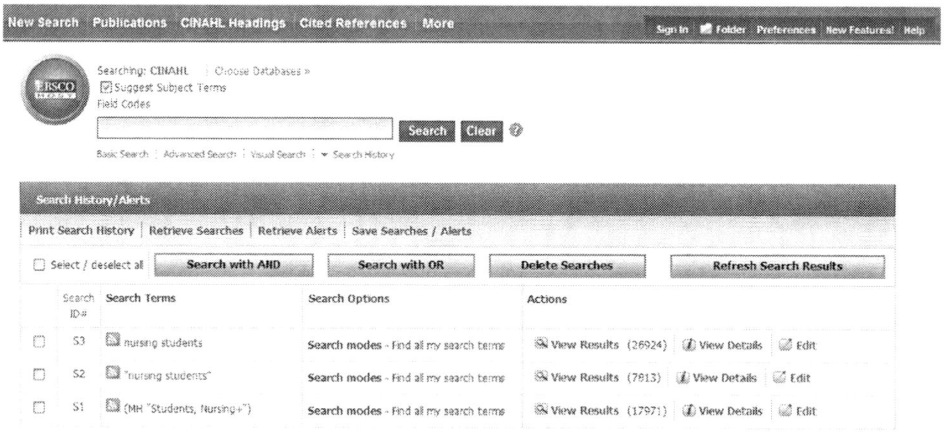

FIGURE 5.2

CINAHL (EBSCOhost) Advanced Search results for Subject Term: Students, Nursing+ (S1) versus the text word: *nursing students* (S2, S3).

Source: Copyright © EBSCO Industries, Inc.

heading: *Students, Nursing* as in set S1 in Figure 5.2. Some relevant citations may also appear from search set S2 representing the search on the text word, nursing students, in quotation marks, but the set of results from the subject heading search may prove more and more useful. A final text word search for nursing students with the words not in quotes was performed, and results are shown in Figure 5.2 under set S3, a yield of 25,721 citations. This was accomplished by removing the check mark on a CINAHL search page for *"suggest subject terms."* Then enter words in the CINAHL search box and that word will be searched as a *"text word"* in select fields or areas of CINAHL citations such as the title or abstract. Although S3 includes more citations than the subject term search in S1, many of the citations in S3 may not be relevant, because the database may have retrieved citations that mention the word nursing, or the word students or citations containing the exact phrase *nursing students*.

Some databases offer more than one search box for searchers to type text words/phrases and/or subject headings, and they refer to this as advanced search (see Figure 5.3). Library database administrators have a hand in controlling how basic and advanced search looks at a searcher's institution and reference librarians are poised to assist researchers with questions related to customization of those databases.

There is a place for both basic and advanced search use in systematic review literature searches. Basic searches are for preliminary searches to gain perspective on what may be in the literature for a systematic review question or to learn more about what way the literature approaches a systematic review topic. Advanced searches are best as reviewers progress in their search, as it offers more control over getting as many relevant citations as possible on a foreground question or topic from a database. Any relevant citations that searchers miss while searching a database may introduce a bias in their systematic review work.

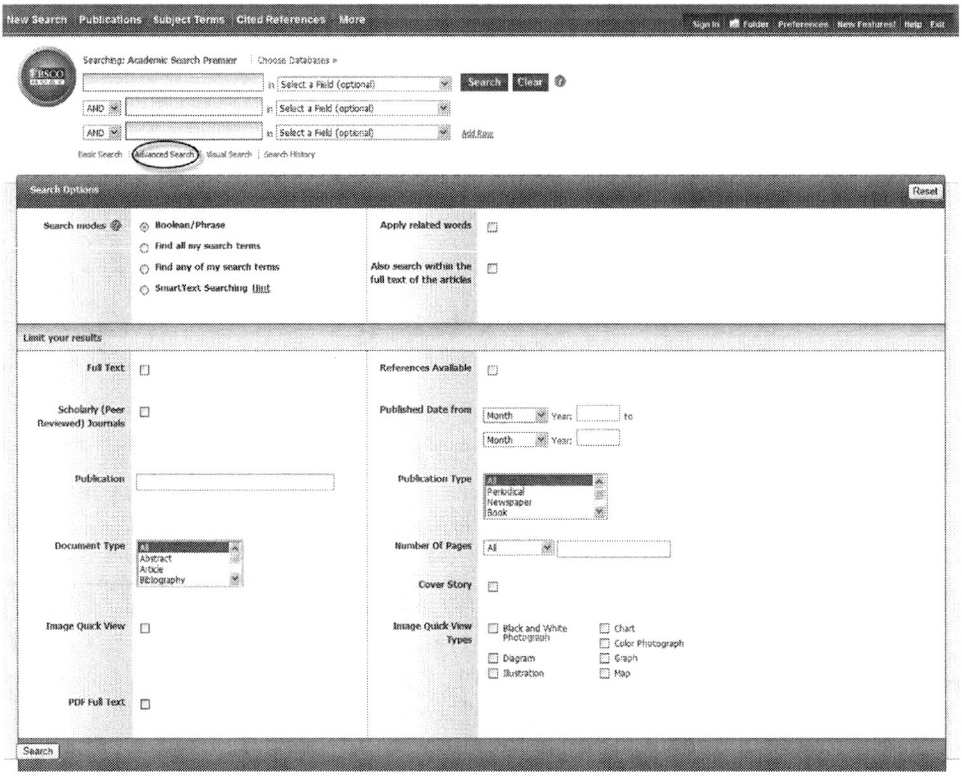

FIGURE 5.3

Advanced Search in Academic Search Premier Database on EBSCOhost.

Source: Copyright © EBSCO Industries, Inc.

SEARCH FEATURES

Controlled Vocabulary

Controlled vocabulary is part of some databases, and it allows searchers a way to manipulate their searches toward a more sensitive and precise search, often with more accurate results than a searcher could obtain when performing a search using only text words/phrases. A database-controlled vocabulary list can be called a *thesaurus* or *dictionary* or a list of *subject headings* or *subject terms*. For example, the name for the controlled vocabulary list in CINAHL is Subject Terms, in EMBASE *Emtree* thesaurus, and in MEDLINE *MeSH*.

Citations of articles in databases with controlled vocabulary are organized under the vocabulary or thesaurus terms (U.S. National Library of Medicine, 2006a). In the MEDLINE database, a citation can have up to 15 controlled vocabulary or MeSH terms attached to it. It becomes easier to locate citations in a database with controlled vocabulary if a researcher makes use of those thesaurus terms in searches rather than try to predict which text words represent a concept or which key words an article author uses for a concept. Ignoring the controlled vocabulary search option in a database often results in searchers performing many searches to locate more important citations, especially in systematic review work because obtaining all accessible, available, relevant evidence is desirable.

For example, a searcher may notice that as they search using different synonyms for congestive heart failure (CHF), new citations continue to surface. The searcher may decide to construct a search strategy with all the possible synonyms for CHF that they can think of. Here is an example of their search statement: *congestive heart failure OR right-sided heart failure OR right heart failure OR leftsided heart failure OR heart failure OR myocardial heart failure OR cardiac failure OR CHF*. This may make searching frustrating, may seem never ending, and may raise doubts as to whether a search is as complete as possible.

Constructing detailed search statements of synonyms for text words/phrases is a long process. It is hard to predict what words that article authors will place in their publication to represent CHF so some synonyms will be missed. Further, as the years go by, the terms that authors use when talking about concepts may change. An example is *Pneumocystis carinii*, which is now called *Pneumocystis jirovecii*. Over the years researchers have renamed the original concept to distinguish the fact that *Pneumocystis jirovecii* is an infection that occurs in humans while *Pneumocystis carinii* occurs in animals. There are many ways to maneuver and adjust search strategies in light of the dynamics of search terminologies in databases, as well as changes in database search systems.

Controlled Vocabulary in Selected Databases

CINAHL's Subject Terms

CINAHL database citations are organized by subject headings or subject terms based on Medical Subject Headings or MeSH from MEDLINE. CINAHL Subject Terms extend to cover nursing and allied health concepts—the focus of CINAHL database. There are more than 12,000 CINAHL subject headings. Similar to MeSH, CINAHL's Subject Terms represent key concepts including some article publication types such as *qualitative studies* and *phenomenological research*. To learn more about CINAHL's subject headings, visit http://www.EBSCOhost.com/cinahl/default.php?id=8.

EMBASE's Emtree

EMBASE's database houses citations on biomedical and drug literature. Its scope is international and proves valuable for obtaining European drug literature. Citations in EMBASE are organized using a subject heading system called *Emtree*; a biomedical and life science controlled vocabulary or thesaurus from Elsevier, the producers of EMBASE. To learn more about the Emtree thesaurus, visit the following links:

- http://www.info.embase.com/about/indexing.shtml
- http://www.embase.com/info/white-paper-registration

MEDLINE's MeSH Terms

The MeSH tree is a way indexers from the United States National Library of Medicine (U.S. NLM) organize citations of articles in PubMed databases such as MEDLINE (U.S. NLM, 2006a). The most extensive database within PubMed is MEDLINE database (U.S. NLM, 2002). MEDLINE database is also available to be searched on its own through other companies such as EBSCO Technologies and Wolters Kluwer Health-Ovid Technologies.

MeSH terms can include a formal name for a concept or phenomena, a drug name or drug class and article publication types such as meta-analysis (U.S. NLM, 2006b). MeSH is not only used to facilitate searching MEDLINE. MeSH terms are part of the thesaurus of other databases as well such as CINAHL, EMBASE, and The Cochrane Library suite of databases.

There is also an NLM product called MeSH Browser and it assists researchers in determining MeSH for search strategies or search statements.

Sensitivity and/or precision of search results retrieved may improve greatly if searchers make use of MeSH terms in searches. In addition, many other database producers such as owners of CINAHL and EMBASE recognize and organize their articles by placing them under MeSH terms, extending the utility of retrieving relevant citations with MeSH search terms, well beyond PubMed and MEDLINE searches.

To summarize, the MeSH Browser (http://www.nlm.nih.gov/mesh/MBrowser.html) is an online tool with many utilities. It can help searchers locate MeSH terms that can be used in searching the MEDLINE database, and sometimes, other databases that include MeSH terms as part of their thesaurus such as EMBASE. The browser can help with constructing complex search statements or search hedges. It can also be used to see subject headings for text words so a searcher can then construct a more powerful search using the located subject headings instead of text words/phrases.

SUBJECT HEADING FEATURES

The next three features (*explode, focus or major heading*, and *subheadings*) explore concepts and database search ideas related directly to subject headings.

Explode

Explode is a feature that can be applied to a selected subject heading in a database's thesaurus. Explode allows a searcher to retrieve all subcategories of citations under or part of a subject heading. For example, if "Fruit" were a subject term in a database, subsets or subcategories of citations on fruit would include citations of articles on apples, bananas, and oranges. Placing a check mark for *explode* for the subject heading Fruit would allow for retrieval of all citations indented under or part of the broad heading Fruit. Using the explode feature in a database is an art; there are times when a searcher will want to explode search results to all subcategories of terms under a subject heading and times when a searcher will deem this inappropriate for their search.

Focus or Major Heading

Similar to explode, the search feature *major heading* is an option in some databases offered next to some subject headings, allowing searchers to retrieve citations of articles where that subject heading is the major focus of an article. For example, a searcher may check mark the subject heading in a database representing CHF and next to that subject heading, also check mark focus or *major heading*, so articles retrieved have the subject CHF as their main focal point. In Ovid databases, the feature major heading is called *Focus*.

Subheadings

During an advanced search, after a searcher places a check or selects a subject heading, a database can offer them a chance to attach one or more subheadings to their subject heading. The purpose of the subheading is to allow the searcher a way to narrow their search. For example, a searcher selects the subject heading: Gout during a search and wants to focus only on diet modification therapy for gout. To achieve this, select the subheading: *diet therapy* on the appropriate database page. Less and more focused articles will be retrieved on Gout > *diet therapy* then if a searcher ran the database search on the subject heading Gout and checked off the option *"include all subheadings."*

Boolean Logic Operators

Boolean logic operators can help focus and narrow search results in a database. The common Boolean operators are *AND, OR,* and *NOT.* Use of *NOT* can be extremely limiting and result in searchers missing important citations; therefore, the use of *NOT* is often not used in search statements. The following are search statements where *NOT* is used as a Boolean operator. One of the examples is from a Google Scholar search where *NOT* is represented by a minus sign.

Antivirals - HIV
- Google Scholar Search example using [−] for *NOT*

Antivirals *NOT* HIV
- PubMed Search where the use of *NOT* in this case is a seemingly good idea because articles are desired on antivirals potentially dealing with other conditions such as shingles, warts, colds, but *not* HIV or AIDS.
- The use of *NOT* is often not recommended because some citations talking about more than one virus such as the HIV and herpes viruses may be eliminated in a search noting antivirals *NOT* HIV. A researcher may not be interested in the portion of an article talking about HIV, but they may have wanted the full article in the end because it talks about other viruses of interest. Unfortunately, the use of *NOT* in their search statement may eliminate that citation and others similar to it from their search results pool.

Role of Boolean Logic Operators in Narrowing Search Results

So, what produces fewer results in a search, is it the use of *AND* or *OR*? The answer, of course, is *AND.* This may seem counterintuitive because in real life, if one walked into a store to shop for hats and potentially bought a black, brown, *AND* a white hat, that shopper would end up with three hats. In the preceding hat example, using *AND* is equal to *MORE* hats in the shopper's closet. The situation resulting in *LESS* hats in the shopper's closet is *OR*. This is where the shopper buys the black *OR* brown *OR* white hat; in effect, they will have one hat in the closet instead of three hats. If the mentioned example is not clear, reread the previous scenario and think of buying different flavors of ice cream in an ice cream shop rather than purchasing hats (Sostack, personal communication, July 29, 2010).

Unlike real life, in the search world—if you will allow the comparison above to play out further—when *AND* is used to connect text words and/or phrases in a search, one ends up with less search results. This is a good thing, because it often means more focused and narrowed results toward answering a research question. See this YouTube video for an interactive example on Boolean logic operators (http://www.youtube.com/watch?v=vube-ZcJFk4). The following are some examples that make use of the Boolean operator *AND*.

- Type 2 diabetes *AND* metabolic syndrome
- Congestive heart failure *AND* noncompliance *AND* emergency room readmission
- Endovascular aneurysm repair *AND* complications

When *OR* is used as a connecting word between text words and/or phrases, one ends up with more search results. This is good for adding two similar result sets—referring to the same concept for text words and/or related subject headings to make one large result set. For example, take a result set for the text word *teens* and a set of results for the phrase *young adults* and then use *OR* (*teens OR young adults*) to create one set. The set created is not as simple as adding all citations for the "ORed" terms because duplicates of some citations will be eliminated from individual set results. See the example below.

- Set 1 = 290 Results for the text word *teens*
- Set 2 = 19,180 Results for the text word *young adults*
- Set 3 = 21,489 Results for combining Set 1 with Set 2 using "OR"—in essence the search statement *teens* OR *young adults* [Straight addition of citations from Set 1 plus Set 2 may have led a searcher to predict Set 3 should = 21,570, but that prediction does not take into account that databases remove duplicate citations when sets are combined using "OR".]

Other examples that make use of the Boolean operator *OR* are:

- Transfer stress *OR* relocation anxiety
- Teens *OR* teenagers *OR* young adults

Default or Implied Boolean Logic Operators

In many databases, when a searcher types more than one text word in a search box, the database interprets the words making use of a default or implied Boolean operator. A

Boolean operator, usually *AND* or *OR* is automatically inserted between a searcher's text words. The *help* or tips section of a database often reveals if an implied operator is used to reinterpret a searcher's text words. Sometimes, librarians at an institution have a hand in choosing default operators for a database, so consult them for more details.

Most of the time, *AND* is the default or implied Boolean operator. This means that typing the concept *brown recluse spider* in a search box will be interpreted as *brown recluse AND spider*. What a searcher hoped that the database saw as a phrase is divided by *AND*, resulting in citations or references that are different from what was expected. The database does not pay attention to the searcher's phrase *brown recluse spider* or processes the three words in the phrase from left to right as one entity. For the searcher's words to be processed as a phrase, quotation marks should be placed around the phrase *brown recluse spider* (Bronson Fitzpatrick, personal communication, July 28, 2010). Another option would be to use the proximity/adjacency search feature, which is available in some databases. Use of proximity/adjacency and quotation marks are covered under the section entitled Proximity or Adjacency Operators in this chapter.

Natural or Plain Language

Many are familiar with searching using "everyday language" in online resources such as Google.com. This can be done by typing a search statement or question in an online resource's search box, as opposed to performing a search where important text words or phrases are typed in a search box and usually connected with Boolean logic operators *AND*, *OR*, or *NOT*. For example, a natural language search may be *what is the occurrence of transfer anxiety*. The database will take the question typed and locate citations that may or may not be on target with what a searcher wants. In some natural language searches, a database will look for alternate words or synonyms from a searcher's statement or question. Regardless, use of natural language is at best a basic search feature that is not sufficient for systematic review search work.

Using Text Words and Phrases

Regardless of whether a search involves basic or advanced search mode, every search begins as a text word or phrase search. Some searches can go beyond the use of text words/phrases when a researcher chooses subject terms or controlled vocabulary to *replace* the text words/phrases typed in a search box.

Use text word/phrase searching to locate information for:

- Cutting edge or new terms—not yet represented in a database by a subject term or subject heading. Examples include clinical nurse leader or EVAR for endovascular aneurysm repair.
- Informatics terms, including names of information systems such as eMAR (electronic medication administration record) or Crib Notes, a documentation system used by neonatal intensive care nurses.
- Hard to locate drug names (consider typing the generic name for a drug), drug categories, or actions of certain medications (e.g., anticholinergics, neuroprotectants)

- A database being searched that does not include much nursing-controlled vocabulary, yet has citations relevant to nursing
- Preliminary searches, when a searcher is trying to get a feel for the literature published on a topic and to see subject terms or headings assigned to citations in results pool from their text word/phrase search

One thing a searcher may note when searching using text words or phrases in either a basic or advanced search is the way the terms or concepts may be interpreted by a database. Searchers realize quickly that they may get different results if, for instance, they searched with text words connected by a Boolean operator versus a search with a phrase. For example, instead of typing *computers AND charts*, consider typing *computerized charts* or *computerized records*. Note that, even with phrase searching, some databases lack precision and/or sensitivity and will still retrieve results that include either the word *charts, computerized*, or the phrase *computerized charts*. A way for searchers to control the way a database processes phrases is to place the phrase in quotation marks.

Quotation Marks

Use double quotation marks (" ") to guide a database toward looking for a certain phrase or concept in a certain order. Consider the phrases *computerized charts* or *computerized records*. A search for those phrases may retrieve results that are more precise; however, even placing text words or phrases in quotes allows some imprecise results—sometimes, almost as if a searcher had not used quotation marks at all.

Parentheses

Use of parentheses also offers a searcher a way to control the way a database processes a search. This is similar to use of parentheses in math. If shown the equation, $1 + (2 + 5)$, one may recall a math principle dictating items in parentheses should be processed first $(2 + 5)$ and the result (7) is processed with what is left outside of the parentheses, yielding an answer of 8 for the equation shown earlier. The *order of operations* using parentheses applies not only with mathematical equations, but also with terms or phrases placed in parentheses in a database search box. If parentheses are omitted from a search, the order of operations is for the database to execute the terms in a searcher's search statement from left to right. For example:

- nurs* *AND* (*computerized charts OR computerized records*)
- (Electronic medical records *OR* EMR *OR* computer*ized* medical records *OR* computer*ised* medical records *OR* automated medical records *OR* computer*ized* patient records *OR* computer*ised* patient records) *AND* medication errors

Alternate Spelling and Language Variation

If a searcher begins by typing a text word or phrase in a search box and then takes the direction of a database by selecting an appropriate, controlled vocabulary term or subject heading, arguably, that searcher will not have to worry about including alternate spellings and language variation for text words/phrases.

Consider the lessons learned in this scenario: A reviewer would like to perform a search for literature on EMR and medication errors. They begin searching a database using its basic search option. Their search statement follows:

Search Statement #1:
 EMRs *AND* medication errors

Before reviewing the search results, the searcher changes their search statement to the following to be more comprehensive, as well as more on point with their research topic.

Search Statement #2:
 (EMR *OR* computer*ized* medical records *OR* computer*ised* medical records *OR* automated medical records *OR* computer*ized* patient records *OR* computer*ised* patient records) *AND* medication errors

The change from Search Statement #1 to Search Statement #2 takes into account other key terms that stand for EMR, such as computerized medical records. In addition, American and British English word variations are used in the second search statement—computerized or computerised, respectively. Other examples of American English terms followed by their British English equivalent are as follows: diaper is nappy, bathroom is loo, gas is petrol, pharmacist is chemist, and stretcher is gurney.

 The biomedical literature also includes verb tense variations. For example, the verb *leap* exists in American English as the past tense form *leaped*, but the British past tense form is *leapt*. Smell is smelled or smelt. Different words can be used to mean the same point in American English, British English, or Canadian English. Consider the American English word hood, it is often referred to as bonnet in British English, and a cookie is known as a biscuit.

Proximity or Adjacency Operators

Sometimes in searching a database, it seems that the desired search results prove hard to find. It may be that a searcher is searching using text words or phrases that are not yet represented by controlled vocabulary or a subject heading in a database. Therefore, a search may have to be tried repeatedly in a database with new text words or phrases and at times make use of synonyms for those text words.

 Another technique is to make use of proximity operators, a letter or series of letters and a number in between text words/phrases. For example, to locate articles in Ovid MEDLINE on computerized prescriber order entry within five words of the word errors, we can type the following search statement *CPOE* adj5 *errors*. This will retrieve citations where CPOE is mentioned, and five words later, the word *errors* appears. Citations where the word *errors* is mentioned and then five words later, citations where the word *CPOE* is mentioned will also appear. It is up to the searcher to choose the number, such as adj5 for the proximity search. Examples of proximity operators used in some databases include *adj*, *N*, and *W*. All databases do not allow for use of proximity operators. PubMed, which includes MEDLINE database, does

TABLE 5.2

Proximity Search Statements from MEDLINE on Ovid and CINAHL on EBSCOhost

Database	Proximity Operator	Proximity Search Statement(s)
CINAHL	*N*—finds words near one another regardless of order of words	"electronic health record" *N4* consumer
	W—finds words next to one another as they were typed	Magnet *W6* librar*
Medline	*adj*—finds words adjacent to another word, in any order, regardless of order of words typed	CPOE *adj5* errors

not allow the use of proximity operators at this time, but searching MEDLINE as a stand-alone database (not as part of PubMed) on the Ovid search retrieval system will allow for use of Ovid's proximity operators. For examples of search statements using proximity operators, see Table 5.2.

Truncation and Wildcard Symbols

A truncation symbol is used to search for a word having variant endings. Depending on the features of a database, a truncation symbol could be allowed before the start of a word or in the middle of a word. The most common truncation symbols are an asterisk (*) or the dollar sign ($). See Table 5.3.

The wildcard symbol is a feature similar to truncation offered by some databases to help searchers control their search results. Common wildcard symbols include the question mark (?) or pound sign (#). Examples showing use of wildcards are shown in Table 5.4.

TABLE 5.3

Truncation Use Examples

Truncation	Citations retrieved include
nurs*	nurse, nurses, nursing . . .
comput*	computer, computers, computerized, computerized, computerization . . .
"computer * records"	computerized records, computer records, computer-assisted records management system, computer-based records, computer-generated records, computer-matched records,
"*order entry"	. . . physician order entry, . . . prescriber order entry, . . . provider order entry, . . . computerized order sets, . . . test *order* entry, . . . consolidated *order* lists

TABLE 5.4
Wildcard Use Examples

Wildcard	Citations retrieved include
an##sthesia	anesthesia, anaesthesia
favo?r	favor, favour
?esophagus	oesophagus

Stop Words

Stop words are terms that are ignored by a database or online search resource even though a searcher includes that term in their search statement. Stop words are extremely common words such as *among, various, these,* and *through.* These words appear in the text of many citations, so a database search using these words would show too many search hits or results. Each database may have a list of different stop words. Examples of stop words for PubMed database can be reviewed at http://www.nlm.nih.gov/bsd/disted/pubmedtutorial/020_170.html.

Depending on the search resource, use of quotation marks can allow a stop word to be included in a search. For example, in searches on Google.com and Google Scholar, a searcher can place a phrase in quotes such as a search for "peanut butter *and* jelly" to have the stop word *and* be included in search results located.

Special Symbols

Truncation and wildcard symbols were discussed in this chapter, but there are more special symbols that databases offer for use in search statements. The number and utility of these symbols will vary from database to database. Consult the help section of a database or online search resource for specific details. For example, a searcher can use the plus sign (+) in Google.com and Google Scholar searches to include the word after the plus sign in search results. The word after the plus sign may be a common word that would have been ignored in a Google product search, or it can be a word that a searcher wants to see in every search result. Google will not expand the search to look for results using synonyms for the word after the plus sign. For example, the Google Scholar search statement: *magnet* + *"shared governance"* will retrieve scholarly articles where the text words *magnet* and phrase in quotes *"shared governance"* are included in every search result (Google Inc., 2000). Note that the use of the quotation marks around the term *shared governance* steers the Google Scholar database to look for that phrase exactly rather than yield search results with the word *shared,* some results with the word *governance,* and some citations with the concept *shared governance.*

Limits

The limits feature in a database can help searchers narrow down or focus in search results, as well as filtering for select types of results. For example, out of a result set with 400 citations, a searcher may apply limits to narrow down the number of results to *clinical trials*, in English, between *2002* and *2010*. Limits can be selected before a search is run or after search results are seen.

Prudent use of limits should include applying one or two limits at a time. A searcher may unwittingly attempt to limit search results—all at once—by language, age range, gender, year range, clinical trials, nursing journals, and full-text only to discover they are left with several results or zero results. In addition, some limits such as English language should not be applied to citations for systematic reviews. If there is no article translation available, then limiting searches to only English language articles is allowed.

A popular limiter allows for restricting search results to full-text articles. This is a tempting option that has its place, such as during preliminary systematic review searches, where one is looking for a few full-text articles on a research question—to get a feel for what is in the literature. Be careful; there may be important articles not available in full text online, but would be best sought because they will impact early research choices in the systematic review process.

Many libraries have placed an icon or an image next to each citation in a database, allowing searchers to quickly navigate to online full-text articles for journals the library subscribes to or put in an order (interlibrary loan request) to have the article located and emailed to them. Therefore, in many cases, full text will be available to a searcher. For more about how to access full-text articles while searching databases, meet a librarian for a one-on-one session at a local institution. They can also talk about the *limits* feature for specific databases that a library subscribes to, because options for *limits* in particular databases are often chosen by librarians at an institution. Examples of limits include the following: English language, inpatient, randomized controlled trial, review article, 0–18 years old, 2002–2012.

Databases may refer to limits using another term, such as in CINAHL where limiters are called *search options*. Explore how to use limits in health science databases: CINAHL, EMBASE, and MEDLINE—databases that are highly useful for most nursing-related systematic reviews.

SUMMARY

Two key principles for searching for literature involve planning (includes general knowledge on searching and use of specific databases on certain systems) and organization (includes managing relevant citations and documenting search information). Searching the literature for citations for a systematic review begins with a researchable question. Carefully, select databases to search for information with the assistance of a librarian involved in reference or literature search activities. On a paper, write down search strategies inclusive of text words and phrases to be entered in databases. Make use of database advanced search features such as controlled vocabulary or thesaurus terms. Own the literature search process; write things down along the way, and keep track of search steps by saving them as allowed in the databases being searched. Manage chosen citations in a bibliographic citation manager such as EndNote or RefWorks. Keep track of the search resources used; dates resources are searched, and consider setting up search alerts as needed to ensure that the review will include the most current evidence-based literature on a foreground question. See more tips in Box 5.1, Getting the Most out of Time for Searching Databases.

A research librarian is a valuable resource in conducting a search as a part of a systematic review. If meeting with a local librarian is not feasible, consider reaching out to virtual librarians on the Internet, who may be part of a state-based Ask-a-Librarian service (Saimbert, 2007). Information science professionals who are *expert searchers* or specifically work with researchers who are writing systematic reviews may also be available for a fee. Lastly, review the *help* section of databases, before searching and as needed, for tips on carrying out basic and advanced searches in those resources.

BOX 5.1
Getting the Most out of Time for Searching Databases

1. Write down a primary foreground clinical question. There may be layers or several themes a researcher hopes to address in answering a systematic review question, but try to stick with one main question to base searches on. If there is more than one foreground question or "smaller" questions that are part of the main foreground question, write them down as well and perform separate searches tailored to answer those questions.

2. Write down any background questions related to the foreground question(s). Literature located in databases may inform those questions, although most often, a textbook or reliable Internet resource will suffice for answering background questions.

3. Use a highlighter to bold key concepts or important text words in a systematic review question to allow for easier recognition of words to use in search statements and for formulation of strategies to facilitate efficient searching in online resources. In addition, list synonyms for the text words, as some database searches may prove more effective at retrieving a larger, more relevant pool of articles if synonyms for important terms are also searched.

4. Underline other words in the systematic review question that may be important in a search but seem to be *common words*—in effect, terminology that would be mentioned in any article. For example, in the question: "What are the most effective strategies for *decreasing* relocation stress or transfer anxiety in patients and their families upon transfer of the patient from an intensive care unit to a non-intensive care unit," *decreasing* is a common word that can be added to a search statement with key text words to retrieve citations. A common word can also be added to a search that made use of controlled vocabulary or thesaurus terms. The results from the controlled vocabulary search can be combined in a new search statement with the common word.

   For example, a searcher using the CINAHL database wants to locate articles on nursing students and stress. The searcher can type *nursing students* in the CINAHL search box and select the controlled vocabulary term for what they typed: *students, nursing*. After viewing the number of results for *students, nursing*, the searcher could type a new search statement, including the common word stress. The search just described is considered an *advanced search*. Work with a librarian to learn about advanced search, because it is not carried out in the same manner across all databases. What constitutes advanced searching in one database may not be equivalent to advance searching in another database. Advanced searching is a challenge that can be rewarding, because it offers more

(Continued)

Box 5.1 (*Continued*)

control in manipulating search steps and may yield more relevant citations for systematic review research. In an advanced search employing *only* controlled vocabulary or subject headings or a search using controlled vocabulary plus common words, often the number of citations retrieved is less but more precise than if one simply performed a search using solely common text words.

5. Write down all inclusion and exclusion criteria for a systematic review. Some of those terms can be used to focus or narrow search results. For example, a searcher may only want articles on *teenagers* with metabolic syndrome or cooling blanket use in *cardiac arrest* patients or only *randomized controlled trials* of chronic asthma patients.

EXERCISES

1. Practice using both CINAHL and MEDLINE. MEDLINE on Ovid is not a free resource, so if an institution does not subscribe to MEDLINE on Ovid or MEDLINE on another search system, try the practice exercise using MEDLINE's MeSH database through PubMed at http://www.ncbi.nlm.nih.gov/mesh. There is no free version of CINAHL. While working on this exercise, take notice of the *scope note* for each subject heading *or* subject term; it will provide definitions for the subject heading and a list of other words that the subject term is *used for.*

Compare answers with the answer key for Chapter 5, Exercise 1, in Appendix E.

Controlled Vocabulary or Subject Headings for Text Words/Phrases

Text Word/Phrase	MEDLINE (Ovid) MeSH Term	CINAHL (EBSCOhost) Subject Term	Comments on Discoveries
AIDS			
Alternative therapy			
Anti-inflammatory			
Aspirin			
Bed rest			
Cardiac catheterization			
Clinical ladder			
Cot death			
CPOE			
Hospital readmission			
Kangaroo care			
Metabolic syndrome			
Nurse burnout			
PT time			
Qualitative			
Swine flu			

2. Alternate Spelling for Terms in Databases
   Fill in the blanks with the alternate spellings. See answer key for Chapter 5, Exercise 2, in Appendix E.

American Spelling	British Spelling
Anesthesia	
	Ageing
Analyze	
Center	
	Favour
Fetal	
Hemorrhage	
	Oesophagus
Pediatrics	

REFERENCES

Akkus, Y. (2011). Multiple sclerosis patient caregivers: The relationship between their psychological and social needs and burden levels. *Disability and Rehabilitation*, *33*(4), 326–333. do i:10.3109/09638288.2010.490866

Andrel, J. A., Keith, S. W., & Leiby, B. E. (2009). Meta-analysis: A brief introduction. *Clinical and Translational Science*, *2*(5), 374–378. doi:10.1111/j.1752-8062.2009.00152.x

Bernard Becker Medical Library. (2009). *Systematic reviews—evidence at Becker—Becker-Guides at Becker Medical Library*. Retrieved from http://beckerguides.wustl.edu/content.php?pid=119750&sid=1031216

Carley, S. (2000). *No evidence for either Collar and cuff or sling after fracture of the clavicle*. Retrieved from http://www.bestbets.org/bets/bet.php?id=13

de Boer, A. G., Taskila, T., Ojajärvi, A., van Dijk, F. J., & Verbeek, J. H. (2009). Cancer survivors and unemployment: a meta-analysis and meta-regression. *Journal of the American Medical Association*, *301*(7), 753–762. doi:10.1001/jama.2009.187

Durlak, J. A., & Weissberg, R. P. (2007). *The impact of after-school programs that promote personal and social skills*. Retrieved from http://casel.org/wp-content/uploads/2011/04/ASP-Exec.pdf

Dynamed. (2010). *Diabetes mellitus type 2*. Retrieved from Ebsco Publishing, http://www.search.ebscohost.com/login.aspx?direct=true&site=dynamed&id=AN+113993

Gillies, M. A., Pratt, R., Whiteley, C., Borg, J., Beale, R. J., & Tibby, S. M. (2010). Therapeutic hypothermia after cardiac arrest: A retrospective comparison of surface and endovascular cooling techniques. *Resuscitation*, *81*(9), 1117–1122. doi:10.1016/j.resuscitation.2010.05.001

Google Inc. (2000). More search help: Google search basics—Web search help. Retrieved from http://www.google.com/support/websearch/bin/answer.py?hl=en&answer=136861

Hammarlund, C., & Sundberg, T. (1994). Hyperbaric oxygen reduced size of chronic leg ulcers: A randomized double-blind study. *Plastic and Reconstructive Surgery*, *93*(4), 829–833.

Holopainen, A., Hakulinen-Viitanen, T., & Tossavainen, K. (2008). Systematic review—A method for nursing research. *Nurse Researcher*, *16*(1), 72–83.

Knight, R. G., Devereux, R. C., & Godfrey, H. P. (1997). Psychosocial consequences of caring for a spouse with multiple sclerosis. *Journal of Clinical Experimental Neuropsychology*, *19*(1), 7–19.

Lau, J., Antman, E. M., Jimenez-Silva, J., Kupelnick, B., Mosteller, F., & Chalmers, T. C. (1992). Cumulative meta-analysis of therapeutic trials for myocardial infarction. *New England of Journal Medicine*, *327*(4), 248–254. doi:10.1056/nejm199207233270406

Lau, J., Schmid, C. H., & Chalmers, T. C. (1995). Cumulative meta-analysis of clinical trials builds evidence for exemplary medical care. *Journal of Clinical Epidemiology, 48*(1), 45–57.

Ligaray, K. P. L., & Isley, W. L. (2010). Diabetes Mellitus, Type 2. *eMedicine*, 91. Retrieved from http://www.emedicine.medscape.com/article/117853-overview

Lipsey, M. W., Landenberger, N. A., & Wilson, S. J. (2007). Effects of cognitive-behavioral programs for criminal offenders. *Campbell Systematic Reviews, 6*, 27. doi:10.4073/csr.2007.6

Lyon, F. (2000). *Oucher or CHEOPS for pain assessment in children.* Retrieved from http://www.bestbets.org/bets/bet.php?id=45

Mackway-Jones, K. (2000). *Eye patches are not indicated for simple corneal abrasions.* Retrieved from http://www.bestbets.org/bets/bet.php?id=42

Maurice, S. (2000). *No difference between oral and nebulised steroids in croup.* Retrieved from http://www.bestbets.org/bets/bet.php?id=7

Merchant, R. M., Abella, B. S., Peberdy, M. A., Soar, J., Ong, M. E., Schmidt, G. A., . . . Vanden Hoek, T. L. (2006). Therapeutic hypothermia after cardiac arrest: unintentional overcooling is common using ice packs and conventional cooling blankets. *Critical Care Medicine, 34*(Suppl 12), S490–S494. doi:10.1097/01.ccm.0000246016.28679.36

Mutch, K. (2010). In sickness and in health: Experience of caring for a spouse with MS. *British Journal of Nursing, 19*(4), 214–219.

Orozco, L. J., Buchleitner, A. M., Gimenez-Perez, G., Roqué I Figuls, M., Richter, B., & Mauricio, D. (2008). Exercise or exercise and diet for preventing type 2 diabetes mellitus. *Cochrane Database of Systematic Reviews,* (3), CD003054. doi:10.1002/14651858.CD003054.pub3

Petticrew, M., Wilson, P., Wright, K., & Song, F. (2002). Quality of Cochrane reviews. Quality of Cochrane reviews is better than that of non-Cochrane reviews. *British Medical Journal, 324*(7336), 545.

Prior, J., Lawhon-Triano, M., Fedor, D., Vanston, V. J., Getts, R., & Smego, R. A., Jr. (2010). Community-based application of mild therapeutic hypothermia for survivors of cardiac arrest. *Southern Medical Journal, 103*(4), 295–300. doi:10.1097/SMJ.0b013e3181d3cedb

Rivera-Navarro, J., Benito-León, J., Oreja-Guevara, C., Pardo, J., Dib, W. B., Orts, E., & Belló, M. (2009). Burden and health-related quality of life of Spanish caregivers of persons with multiple sclerosis. *Multiple Sclerosis, 15*(11), 1347–1355. doi:10.1177/1352458509345917

Saimbert, M. K. (2007). On the right path: Learn how to get the most out of the time you spend searching medical databases. *Nursing Spectrum—New York & New Jersey Edition, 19A*(20), NJ/NY10-NJ/NY10.

Shultz, S. M., Dell, E. Y., & Bodan, C. L. (2009). Are we there yet? When is a literature review complete? *American Journal of Nursing, 109*(9), 78–79. doi:10.1097/01.NAJ.0000360321.92491.ae

Skulec, R., Kovárnik, T., Bělohlávek, J., Dostálová, G., Kolár, J., Linhart, A., & Seblová, J. (2008). Overcooling during mild hypothermia in cardiac arrest survivors—Phenomenon we should keep in mind. [Article in Czech]. *Vnitřní lékařství, 54*(6), 609–614.

United States National Library of Medicine. (2002). *What's the difference between MEDLINE and PubMed? Fact sheet.* Retrieved from http://www.nlm.nih.gov/pubs/factsheets/dif_med_pub.html

United States National Library of Medicine. (Producer). (2006a). *Branching out: The MeSH vocabulary* [Video]. Retrieved from http://www.nlm.nih.gov/bsd/disted/video/

United States National Library of Medicine. (2006b). *Principles of MEDLINE subject indexing.* Retrieved from http://www.nlm.nih.gov/bsd/disted/mesh/indexprinc.html

SUGGESTED READINGS

Benzies, K., Harrison, M. J., & Magill-Evans, J. (2006). Need for comprehensive search words in reviews. *Journal of Nursing Scholarship, 38*(3), 206–207.

Fine, E. V., & Bliss, D. Z. (2006). Searching the literature: Understanding and using structured electronic databases. *Journal of Wound, Ostomy, & Continence Nursing, 33*(6), 594–605.

Muallem, M., Hough, H., & Schmelzer, M. (2008). Searching the literature with professional databases. *Gastroenterology Nursing, 31*(5), 375–376. doi:10.1097/01.SGA.0000338284.70907.a4

CHAPTER SIX

Resources and Techniques to Maximize Search Efforts

Marie K. Saimbert, Jenny Pierce,
Pam Hargwood, and John T. Oliver

OBJECTIVES

Upon completion of Chapter 6, you will be able to:

- Use common health and social sciences online search resources for retrieving citations to answer systematic review questions
- Define point-of-care resources and identify their role for researching practice-based questions
- Define grey literature and explore its role in systematic review research
- Use various search techniques such as *Citation Chasing* and *Hand Searching*

IMPORTANT POINTS

- Searches that make use of a database's controlled vocabulary or subject headings/terms allow investigators a chance for more accuracy and/or sensitivity for retrieval of more relevant citations.
- Reviewers can expand on or tailor their foreground question and text words or key words by performing preliminary searches in filtered resources such as Clinical Evidence by *BMJ Publishing Group* and Dynamed from *EBSCO Publishing.*
- Setting up *search alerts* if available in searched databases can facilitate keeping an ongoing systematic review research project as up-to-date as possible prior to publication.
- All significant results from literature searches should be collected and organized using a bibliographic citation management tool, for example, EndNote from *Thomson Reuters.*

INTRODUCTION

When conducting a systematic review, the search for relevant articles and other pertinent sources should be comprehensive and exhaustive. Literature resources for gathering the evidence for systematic reviews can be divided into two broad categories: filtered and unfiltered. Filtered resources are also known as *synthesized resources* and unfiltered resources may be referred to as *raw resources*.

Filtered or synthesized resources typically offer some interpretation and appraisal. Each piece of filtered literature covers many individual studies or publications. Examples include systematic reviews, meta-analyses, metasyntheses, and guidelines. In contrast, unfiltered literature sources provide access to individual studies or publications. The term *raw* is fitting for this kind of research. Unfiltered resources typically contain large quantities of individual academic articles and many different types of materials, including editorials and commentaries, randomized controlled trials, epidemiologic studies, qualitative studies, basic review articles, and some filtered literature such as systematic reviews. Electronic biomedical databases, such as MEDLINE or Medical Literature Analysis and Retrieval System Online from the *United States Library of Medicine* and CINAHL or Cumulative Index to Nursing and Allied Health Literature from *EBSCO Publishing* are examples of where to find raw literature.

Raw or unfiltered resources form the body of evidence from which filtered resources draw and synthesize research findings. That means that many items found using filtered resources could ultimately be found by directly searching unfiltered resources. Using filtered resources in concert with unfiltered resources carries important benefits. One is that these filtered resources are tremendously valuable discovery tools that can help reviewers quickly find the most important or influential research on a given topic. Finding one very relevant article via a filtered resource can open the gateway to literally hundreds of other related citations. See the diagram in Figure 6.1 for examples of resources with and/or search techniques for locating filtered and unfiltered literature.

FILTERED EVIDENCE RESOURCES

One search strategy when proposing and conducting a systematic review should include a look for existing reviews of filtered evidence on a clinical question. Some of the resource portals include The Campbell Collaboration Library of Systematic Reviews from *The Campbell Collaboration*, Cochrane Database of Systematic Reviews from *The Cochrane Collaboration*, Database of Abstracts of Reviews of Effects available through *The Cochrane Collaboration or Centre for Reviews and Dissemination*, and the Joanna Briggs Library of Systematic Reviews from *The Joanna Briggs Institute*.

American College of Physicians—Physicians' Information and Education Resource

The American College of Physicians—Physicians' Information and Education Resource (ACP PIER) is a searchable database of filtered evidence used by clinicians to answer clinical questions at the point of care. PIER filters evidence from

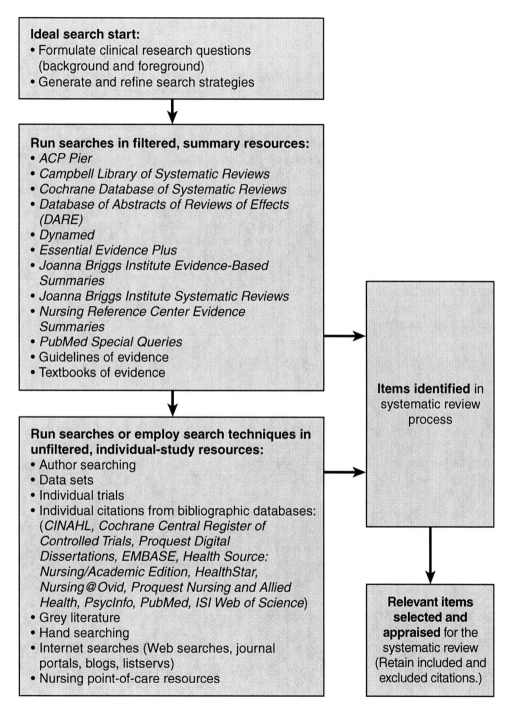

FIGURE 6.1

Searching filtered and unfiltered sources.

the literature and synthesizes it to create clinical summaries that collect synopses, syntheses, and studies to answer clinical questions on disease, screening and prevention, procedures, ethical and legal issues, quality measures, drugs, and alternative therapy topics. Subjects for ACP summary modules are chosen by ACP editors based on the prevalence in clinical practice, and the topics covered lean toward the specialty internal medicine. Once a topic is selected, a search of the literature is performed by editorial consultant staff at McMasters University, one of the three institutions outside of the United States (U.S.) designated by the U.S. Agency for Health Research and Quality (AHRQ) as an evidence-based practice center. Summaries are written by ACP editors, reviewed by a topic expert, and when satisfactory, digitized for inclusion into the PIER database. Currently, there are more than 490 modules with summaries on medical topics in ACP PIER, which are updated quarterly. Like many online search resources, ACP PIER database can be searched through more than one search retrieval system or platform. Become familiar with search systems offered by one's institution library for searching specific resources. Each database has its search features and each search retrieval platform holding a database has features and nuances of its own. So, searchers realize they not only need to know ins and outs of searching a database, but also how to manipulate the search system a database is presented on.

Campbell Collaboration Library of Systematic Reviews

The Campbell Collaboration (C2) is an international research network that produces systematic reviews of the effects of social interventions on policies and services. Started in 2000, C2 covers the subject areas of education, crime and justice, and social welfare. There are less than 200 records in the database (as of December 8, 2010). Records are placed in the Campbell database under vocabulary or thesaurus terms and subject area, as deemed by Campbell producers. All reviews are available for free on the Internet at http://www.campbellcollaboration.org/library.php, and many are coregistered and searchable through The Cochrane Library. For example, a C2 review on children and aggression may also be indexed or found as part of reviews from the Developmental, Psychosocial, and Learning Problems Group within the Cochrane Library database of systematic reviews. Abstracts of many C2 reviews include plain text descriptions of review conclusions. Reviews are updated biannually.

Cochrane Collaboration Products

The Cochrane Library was created by the Cochrane Collaboration and is named after Archie Cochrane, who is considered as the father of evidence-based medicine. Started in 1993, the Cochrane Collaboration is a nonprofit organization based in England with centers all over the world.

The Cochrane Library consists of six medical databases and a database with information about review groups. Databases in the Cochrane Library are predominantly useful for answering foreground clinical questions dealing with the therapy or therapeutic intervention domain. In the past years, Cochrane Database of Systematic Reviews (CDSR) has included some systematic reviews on diagnosis questions. Cochrane reviews are considered the "gold standard" of systematic reviews. As such, their rigor makes them good models for examples of well-constructed systematic reviews. Search techniques are similar for each database in Cochrane, but the content retrieved from each database will be different. In an institution or organization's library, Cochrane Library databases may either be accessible on search retrieval systems from EBSCO, Wiley, or Ovid publishers.

Cochrane Database of Systematic Reviews

CDSR contains all the reviews and protocols prepared by Cochrane review groups. Each Cochrane review is peer-reviewed and supervised by one of the 52 Cochrane review group reviewers working as the editorial team. Written for each review is a protocol for a specific systematic review. Those protocols are also searchable in CDSR. Each review or protocol is prepared according to the methodology set out in the *Cochrane Handbook for Systematic Reviews of Interventions* or *Cochrane Handbook for Diagnostic Test Accuracy Reviews*. As of July 22, 2010, there were 6,244 reviews (around 4,300 completed reviews) and protocols (around 2,000).

The number of reviews and protocols by review group range from four (from the Cochrane Public Health Group) to 316 (from the Cochrane Hepato-Biliary Group). Currently, there are 52 Cochrane review groups and more information on them is located at http://www.cochrane.org/contact/review-groups. Also, consider contacting specific Cochrane review groups for additional guidance on writing a review fitting into that review group category. Some review groups may be more well known than others; reviewers should become familiar with the listing of Cochrane review groups. Reviews relevant to nursing systematic reviews can be found in any Cochrane review group. For example, if one's foreground question is on weight management and blood pressure, browsing the reviews of the Cochrane Hypertension review group may be in order. The Cochrane Effective Practice and Organisation of Care Group (EPOC) includes systematic reviews on reducing hospital admission by having patients be cared for by health professionals in the home, interventions to support shared decision making (SDM) by health professionals, and a review on hand hygiene compliance (Gould, Moralejo, Drey, & Chudleigh, 2010; Légaré et al., 2010; Shepperd et al., 2008). The Cochrane Consumers and Communication review group offers systematic reviews on such topics as family-centered care for children in the hospital and interventions to promote medication compliance and effects of phone calls from peers on persons' health (Dale, Caramlau, Lindenmeyer, & Williams, 2008; Haynes, Ackloo, Sahota, McDonald, & Yao, 2008; Shields, Pratt, Davis, & Hunter, 2007). The following are the links to useful tools for navigating through Cochrane reviews and writing systematic reviews for CDSR:

- **Cochrane Collaboration Glossary of Research Terms**
  http://www.cochrane.org/glossary/5
- **Cochrane Collaboration Handbook for Systematic Reviews of Interventions**
  http://www.cochrane.org/resources/handbook/
- **Cochrane Collaboration—Information for practitioners, providers, and policymakers**
  http://www.cochrane.org/information-practitioners
- **Cochrane Library User Guide, Tutorials and Live Online Workshops**
  http://olabout.wiley.com/WileyCDA/Section/id-390244.html

Database of Abstracts of Reviews of Effectiveness

The Database of Abstracts of Reviews or DARE (http://www.york.ac.uk/inst/crd/) is produced by the Centre for Reviews and Dissemination (CRD) at the University of York, United Kingdom. The CRD is part of the National Institute for Health Research. DARE contains approximately 13,500 abstracts of systematic reviews related to the effects of health interventions. DARE records contain evaluations of the quality of published systematic reviews. Two independent researchers screen and assess identified citations for inclusion on DARE using the following criteria. The reviews chosen must meet criteria 1–3 listed subsequently and at least one more criteria (CRD, 2010) to be included.

1. Were inclusion/exclusion criteria reported?
2. Was the search adequate?
3. Were the included studies synthesized?
4. Was the validity of the included studies assessed?
5. Are sufficient details about the individual included studies presented?

Unlike CDSR, DARE records do not open up to a full-text article, but a page with the citation record information, including the written abstract, with a link to a MEDLINE record for the citation when available and a quality assessment of the systematic review of interest in the DARE record. DARE covers a broader range of health care reviews than CDSR, because it combs through literature from many sources. Although a systematic review is assessed in DARE, that does not imply a recommendation of the quality of that systematic review; however, DARE does alert researchers to important points about a review's methodology and other components—raising questions that can assist in appraisal of systematic reviews. The searches for new systematic reviews for addition to DARE take place monthly (CRD, 2010).

Dynamed

Similar to ACP PIER, Dynamed is a point-of-care resource created by physicians to assist health professionals in answering background and foreground clinical questions. Dynamed is a useful tool for both qualitative and quantitative systematic review research, but it may prove more useful for writing quantitative reviews such as reviews of therapeutic interventions. Dynamed can assist in accumulating background information for context/support of foreground clinical questions, making it useful for writing the background or introduction section of a systematic review. It can also assist in obtaining evidence-based citations of individual studies for possible inclusion or exclusion in a systematic review; discovering information relevant to systematic review research that are not found in journal articles. It can also assist in indexed in MEDLINE, or articles in MEDLINE but not yet assigned subject headings, or articles in MEDLINE indexed under a different topic area or publication type. Dynamed can assist reviewers in finding sources such as reviews, guidelines, or grey literature, as well as aid in retrieving articles that may be excluded from systematic review databases—not because the articles had fatal flaws, but because they did not meet the inclusion criteria for certain systematic reviews.

Dynamed includes over 3,000 evidence-based summaries covering diseases or conditions and drugs. Browsing the resource by category will reveal summaries on *Differential Diagnosis*, *Diagnostic Testing*, and *Quality Improvement* areas for topics such as heart failure. There is also a section including references and guidelines. Dynamed reviewers watch for new literature from about 500 journals and systematic reviews, updating Dynamed content where needed daily. Updating is a process that involves a critical appraisal system to review and rate new evidence. Dynamed producers concentrate on revealing ratings for therapy-based content, although there are ratings of content from question domains such as etiology.

Essential Evidence Plus

Essential Evidence Plus (EE+) was previously known as InfoRetriever and was started in 1994 from a project created by Doctor Mark Ebell. EE+ is a filtered, evidence-based clinical decision support tool, which allows medical providers to find quick answers to clinical questions in the exam room or at the bedside. More than 3,000 Patient-Oriented Evidence that Matters (POEMs) are available in EE+. POEMs are evidence-based summaries of an original article or review. A citation of the article or material that is the focus of the POEM is included. (It is possible to sign up for daily POEMs—delivered to one's e-mail and podcasts for EE+. Essential Evidence Plus also has abstracts of the Cochrane Reviews (>2,500), evidence-based medicine (EBM) guidelines (>1,300), and decision support tools (>3,000) such as interactive diagnostic test calculators.

EE+ consists of 12 databases and/or interactive tools: Essential Evidence Topics, Cochrane Systematic Reviews, Evidence-Based Medical Guidelines (EBMG), National Guideline Clearinghouse (NGC) practice guidelines, Evidence Summaries of guidelines, POEMs Research Summaries, DERM Expert Image Viewer, Decision Support Tools, History and Physical Exam Calculators, Diagnostic Test Calculators, ICD (International Classification of Diseases) Codes, and E/M (Expert, Evaluation and Management) Codes from Medicare. The updates published in EE+ occur one to four times per month.

Joanna Briggs Institute for Nursing and Midwifery

The Joanna Briggs Institute (JBI) for Nursing and Midwifery began in 1996 at the Royal Adelaide Hospital in Australia and is named after the first matron (chief nursing officer) of that hospital. JBI is an international organization with evidence-based health care resources for allied health, medicine, nursing, and midwifery professionals (JBI, 2008). The databases and tools that are currently on the JBI website include review protocols, completed systematic reviews, best practice articles, evidence summaries, evidence-based care "bundles," and tools for assisting in appraisal of literature in writing systematic reviews.

As of 2011, a review of the JBI website revealed the following searchable databases with corresponding number of citations—Evidence Based Recommended

Practices (624), Evidence Summaries (1335), Best Practice Information Sheets (59), JBI Library of Systematic Reviews (174), JBI Systematic Review Protocols (318), Technical Reports (17), and Consumer Information Sheets (115). Many best practice information sheets are freely available to JBI site visitors. Best practice sheets provide the "bottom-line" interventions for clinicians' practice based on systematic review evidence done by JBI reviewers.

The Database of Evidence Summaries is also called JBI COnNECT+ or Clinical Online Network of Evidence for Care and Therapeutics (JBI, 2009a). JBI COnNECT+ leads health care providers, health professionals, and consumers to tools for searching (internal and external websites), appraising, embedding, using, and evaluating evidence. Specifically, searchers can use JBI COnNECT+ to:

- Look for evidence for changing health care practice from several databases in such nodes or areas as acute care, aged care, burns care, infection control, neonatal care, and wound care.
- Search each COnNECT node individually or at once to retrieve "best practice information sheets, evidence summaries, evidence-based recommended practice" documents, "consumer information sheets," and systematic reviews.
- Use tools such as JBI Practical Application to Clinical Evidence System (PACES) for auditing/evaluating the impact of the evidence and JBI Patient Outcomes On Line (POOL) to facilitate collection of prevalence data, both tools assisting in moving and keeping evidence in practice.

The evidence-based care bundles in JBI are the aforementioned JBI COnNECT nodes mentioned in the previous section. Currently, JBI bundles or nodes are in the areas of "Aged Care, Burns Care, Cancer Care, Diagnostic Imaging, Emergency and Trauma, General Medicine, Health Management and Assessment, Infection Control, Mental Health, Midwifery Care, Rehabilitation, Surgical Services, and Wound Healing and Management" (JBI, 2009b). Use the advanced search option in JBI COnNECT+ to search one or more nodes.

From the JBI home page, one can access the evidence-based practice resources under the software System for the Unified Management, Assessment and Review of Information (SUMARI) to assist in assessment, management, and critical appraisal of evidence-based articles. SUMARI includes Comprehensive Review Management System (CReMS), which is a systematic review protocol development and analysis program. CReMS (JBI, 2009c) and the following JBI sponsored programs are available through free registration:

- SUMARI, to assist reviewers in managing and assessment of articles to be included in a systematic review
- Software programs for paper appraisal and data synthesis. Specifically,
  - QARI—Qualitative Assessment and Review Instrument
  - MASTARI—Meta-Analysis of Statistics Assessment and Review Instrument
  - NOTARI—Narrative, Opinion and Text Assessment, and Review Instrument
  - ACTUARI—Analysis of Cost, Technology and Utilization Assessment, and Review Instrument

JBI has an online journal collection where a few articles from first-rate journals are freely accessible and others are available through subscription. As part of a JBI subscription, members may have access to JBI Library of Evaluation Reports, which include articles from the JBI publication: *International Journal of Evidence-Based Healthcare*'s "Evidence Utilisation" section. The journal, available online and in print form, also includes sections on evidence synthesis, which is primary literature and systematic reviews.

UNFILTERED EVIDENCE RESOURCES

CINAHL

CINAHL began in the 1950s as a print index by three librarians in California. In 1983, CINAHL became an electronic search resource or database. It is housed and managed from Glendale Adventist Medical Center, Glendale, California.

Some citations in CINAHL may also be in other biomedical databases such as MEDLINE and the British Nursing Index (BNI), a resource from partner libraries at *Bournemouth University, Poole Hospital NHS Foundation Trust, the Royal College of Nursing, and Salisbury NHS Foundation Trust*, but CINAHL does offer unique content. CINAHL is useful for locating qualitative studies dealing with nursing topics. Citations for articles are placed in CINAHL after review by health professionals who assign each article *subject terms* or *subject headings*. *Major* and *minor headings* and *subheadings* are also assigned to the articles. Searching CINAHL, making use of the *"Suggest Subject Terms"* option is a more powerful way to retrieve citations for a topic.

The CINAHL database includes more than 1 million records from about 3,000 nursing and allied health journals. Biomedical, complementary and alternative medicine, consumer health, and health sciences librarianship literature is also covered. CINAHL includes published literature such as journal articles, book chapters, articles with care plans and critical pathways, research instruments, entries for nursing dissertations, audiovisuals, conference proceedings, and accredited continuing education unit (CEU) articles.

An institution or library may subscribe to a version of CINAHL or CINAHL Plus with or without full text. CINAHL has citations from about 3,000 journals, whereas CINAHL Plus has citations from about 4,000 journals. Citations in CINAHL date back to 1981, and CINAHL Plus citations begin with 1937. All CINAHL database types are updated weekly. Approximately 260,000 new records are added to CINAHL each year.

As with most bibliographic databases, CINAHL offers many search features. For instance, both CINAHL and CINAHL Plus allow for cited reference searches in approximately 1,300 journals. The cited reference feature dates back to the year 2000 for CINAHL and 1994 for CINAHL Plus. There is also a *Save Searches/Alerts* option for keeping searches as temporary or permanent searches. Researchers can also save searches to run as periodic alerts so new search results would be e-mailed or available via an RSS (Really Simple Syndication) feed.

CINAHL database offers both basic and advanced search modes, but regardless of which mode is being used, CINAHL and other traditional electronic databases, such as PubMed, have a list of stop words that, when placed in a search box, will be ignored by the database. The list is periodically updated and currently includes *and, are, as, at, be, because, been, but, by, for, however, if, not, of, on, or, so, the, there, was, were, whatever, whether,* and *would.* Find tips for using basic and advanced search in the succeeding sections.

In the basic search mode, users often type key terms or key concepts and join them with Boolean logic operators, also considered "connector words" such as *AND, OR,* or *NOT.* Additionally, in either basic or advanced search, use the asterisk (*) for truncation.

In advanced search mode, reviewers can choose to search on key terms or make use of CINAHL controlled vocabulary, also called subject headings or Subject Terms. The advanced search feature in CINAHL works best if a searcher can *build their search,* placing *one* key concept in the search box at a time and then use connecting words such as *AND* or *OR* to combine search result sets from the individual key concept searches. Avoid trying to place all possible key terms for a search question in the search box at once. This is the equivalent of placing all ingredients for a stew in a pot at once. The final product may or may not be to one's liking.

Each library may choose a *different look* for CINAHL's basic and advanced search modes. In addition, the library may make decisions on CINAHL *limits'* options or ways database users can narrow down search results, as well decide which other CINAHL features to include or exclude such as the inclusion of a visual search mode in CINAHL. Researchers should consult with a librarian at their institution regarding which version of CINAHL database is available and library changes or customizations to CINAHL that may affect their searches.

As mentioned previously, CINAHL can be searched using controlled vocabulary, also called subject terms, or one can explore CINAHL using plain/natural language. Searching a database such as CINAHL using its subject terms is one of the most powerful ways researchers can control a search and maximize search result yields. Typing a text word or concept into a CINAHL search box and then allowing the CINAHL database to show a listing of subject terms or subject headings that may represent the original text words typed in a CINAHL search box can be a powerful search move.

CINAHL offers several ways for limiting searches or search results by publication type. See the screen captures in Figures 6.2–6.4 for examples on limiting CINAHL search results to publication types such as *systematic review* (Figure 6.2), *meta-analysis* (Figure 6.3), and *qualitative studies* (Figure 6.4A–D). It is possible that qualitative studies may be included in CINAHL, yet may not come up if one follows the steps to locate *qualitative studies.* One or two things may be in play here—the way an investigator is searching and the way a database producer, in the case of CINAHL, EBSCO Publishing, includes citations in its database. In particular, qualitative studies on a topic may be hard to find in one database search. A reviewer may have to search the database a few times, using different terms and/or search strategies and techniques. For example, if a reviewer's inclusion

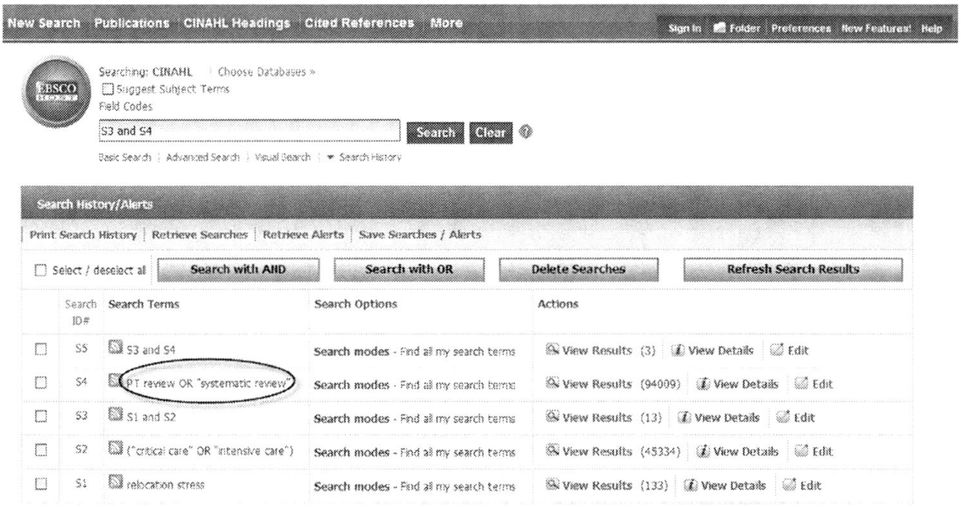

FIGURE 6.2

Search 1—Limit CINAHL results using publication type (PT): *Systematic Review.*

Source: Copyright © EBSCO Industries, Inc.

criteria are for qualitative studies involving interviewing methodology, then the text word *interview* or some variation thereof should be a part of their searches. Similarly, if the reviewer seeks qualitative research involving *phenomenological studies*, that term or equivalent subject heading should be part of their search strategy.

Searchers may already be familiar with a special search feature in PubMed called *Clinical Queries*, which makes use of top-quality search filters based on the type of clinical questions posed by investigators. Question types or domains

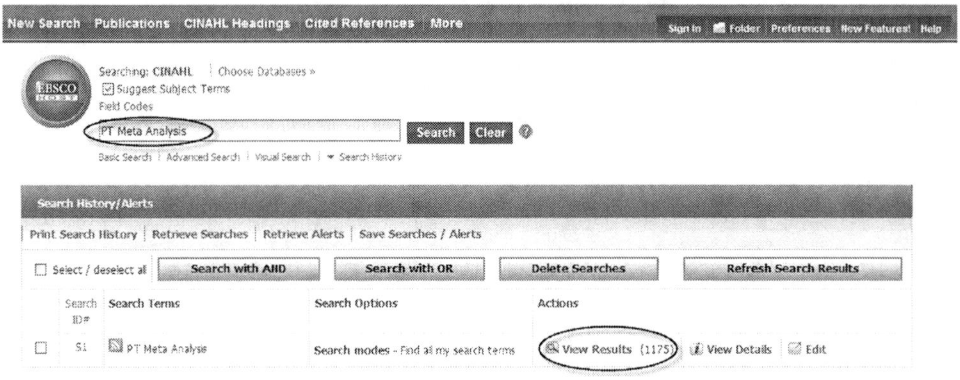

FIGURE 6.3

Search 2—Limit CINAHL results using publication type (PT): *Meta-analysis.*

Source: Copyright © EBSCO Industries, Inc.

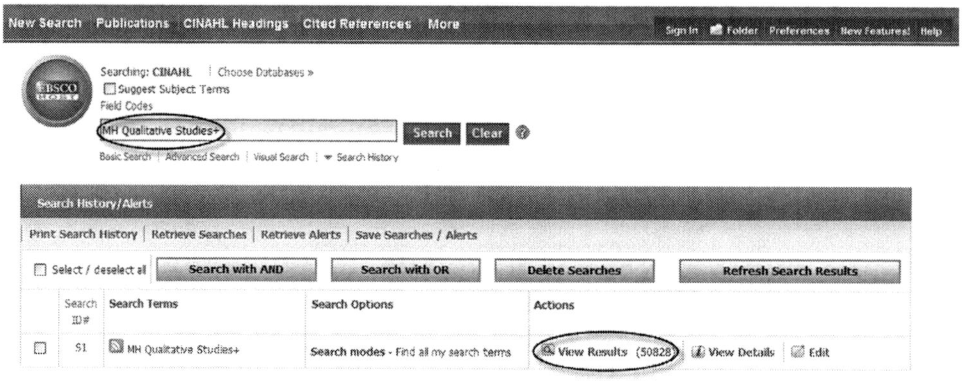

FIGURE 6.4A

Search 3—Step 1: Limit CINAHL citations using the Exact Subject
Heading (code is MH) Qualitative Studies.

Source: Copyright © EBSCO Industries, Inc.

searchable through the clinical queries feature in CINAHL are causation (etiology), qualitative, review, prognosis, and therapy. Select CINAHL clinical query filters at the outset of a search prior to typing text words/phrases in a search box, or apply filters to search results from either basic or advanced searches in CINAHL.

Overall, databases offering the clinical queries option process an investigator's search in a similar way—the user's original search statement is modified often to include the types of articles and/or important terms that would retrieve evidence-based articles from the database on their topic. For example, a user's application of the clinical queries feature to a search for information on a therapy question will be modified by the database to include key terms such as randomized, clinical trials,

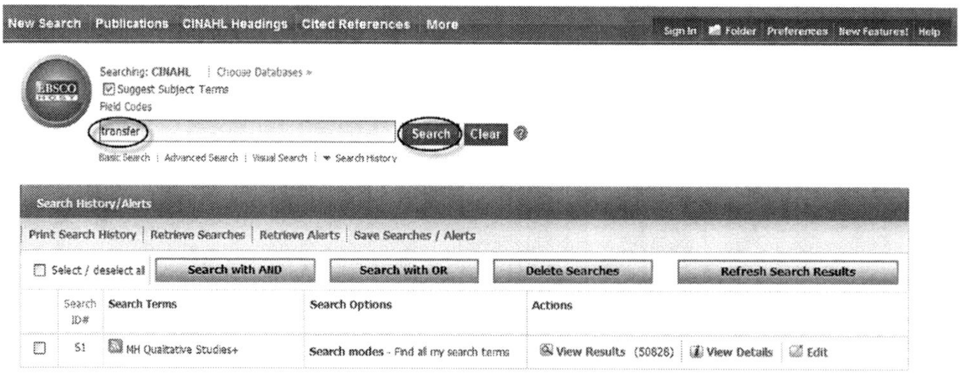

FIGURE 6.4B

Search 3—Step 2: Limit CINAHL citations using the Exact Subject
Heading (code is MH) Qualitative Studies.

Source: Copyright © EBSCO Industries, Inc.

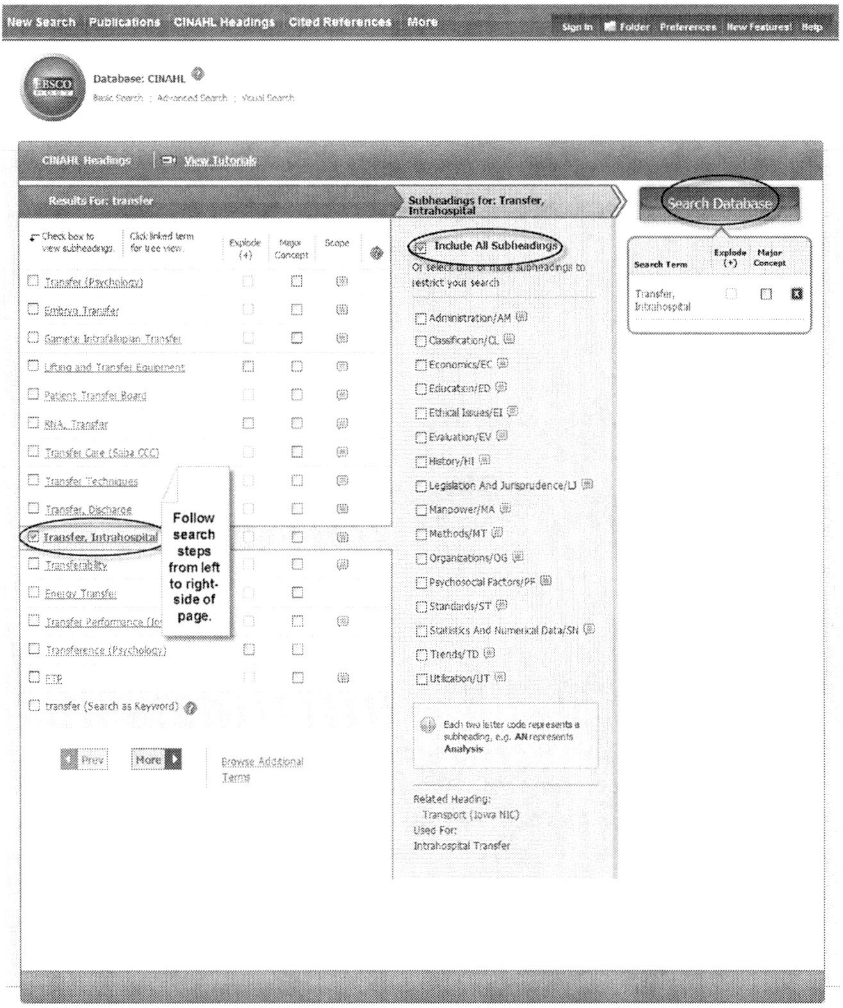

FIGURE 6.4C

Search 3—Step 3: Limit CINAHL citations using the Exact Subject
Heading (code is MH) Qualitative Studies.

Source: Copyright © EBSCO Industries, Inc.

and so on to increase the accuracy and/or sensitivity of relevant citations pulled from the database. An example PubMed Clinical Queries search statement would be:

> *Original search statement placed in PubMed Clinical Queries search box:* ace inhibitors versus calcium channel blockers *AND* African Americans

> *then*

> *PubMed clinical queries filters modified the search strategy as:* (ace inhibitors versus calcium channel blockers *AND* African Americans) *AND* (randomized controlled trial [publication type] *OR* (randomized [title/abstract] *AND* controlled [title/abstract] *AND* trial [title/abstract])

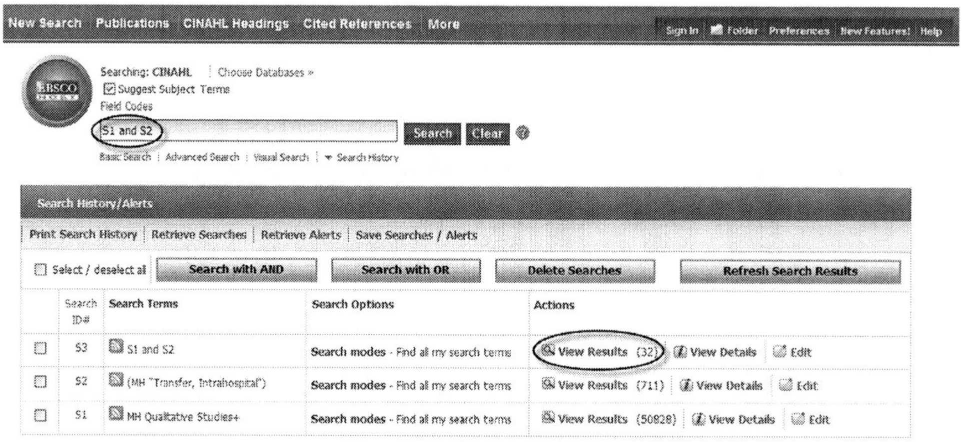

FIGURE 6.4D

Search 3—Step 4: Limit CINAHL citations using the Exact Subject
Heading (code is MH) Qualitative Studies.

Source: Copyright © EBSCO Industries, Inc.

Clinical queries' search filters can be of great help to locate evidence-based cita-tions in a traditional online database such as CINAHL, that normally would retrieve individual "raw" citations, which reviewers would need to assess for quality of evi-dence. The results that reviewers will assess from searches employing the clinical queries option will have a more probability of being relevant for their foreground question research. For each clinical question domain or question type, *any number of study types* may hold evidence that can prove useful. Clinical queries' filters try to include the common study types and/or methodologies, which usually lead to answers for a specific question domain. Put another way, each clinical filter (e.g., eti-ology, diagnosis, therapy, prognosis, clinical prediction guidelines) does not include all the possible study types and methodological qualifier key terms possible, so per-forming a clinical queries search does not guarantee retrieval of all individual, rel-evant evidence-based citations for a systematic review.

Cochrane Central Register of Controlled Trials

Cochrane Central Register of Controlled Trials, also called CENTRAL, is based on regularly run searches for trials from MEDLINE and Embase databases, hand searches by Cochrane centers and Cochrane review groups, and specialized regis-ters created by Cochrane review groups of published and unpublished *randomized controlled trials* (RCT) and *controlled clinical trials* (CCT) that are specific to their area of interest. About three-fifths of the records in CENTRAL are taken from MEDLINE (The Cochrane Collaboration, 2010).

CENTRAL is an indexed collection of approximately 600,000 RCTs with about 350,000 MEDLINE records (1966 onward), 90,000 Embase records (1974 onward), and 160,000 records from hand searches of journals and conference abstracts. CENTRAL searches of specialized registers are created when a Cochrane review group is created. Hand-search resources may be older because searching occurs at centers as well as review groups.

Unlike CDSR, CENTRAL's records are not full text. CENTRAL's records include the title, citation information, and a summary. Because of the nature of CENTRAL, as a resource created for review groups for immediate access to RCT and CCT information, there may be a higher likelihood of duplication and error than in other Cochrane Library databases.

Searches in CENTRAL can be accomplished by looking for a review group or field/network specialized register and hand search codes. See the "Appendix: Review Group or Field/Network Specialised Register and Handsearch Codes" on the CENTRAL help page: http://www.thecochranelibrary.com/view/0/CENTRALHelp. html. Unlike CDSR and DARE, the CENTRAL database is too large to browse and if a researcher selects an option to browse CENTRAL, an advanced search page opens instead for reviewers to enter key words and/or MeSH terms to find trials, rather than listing trials in CENTRAL.

Embase

The database Embase on Elsevier's Embase.com (http://www.embase.com) offers records from Embase classic files, from 1947 to 1973; Embase, from 1974 to present; and MEDLINE, from 1950 to present. Embase covers biomedical, life science (database producers note that the term *life sciences* includes nursing literature), and pharmaceutical literature worldwide, including European literature. Embase includes all MEDLINE citations and about 1,800 unique citations that are not found in MEDLINE from about 2,000 unique journal titles. Citations from more than 7,000 peer-reviewed journals and from 90 countries are in Embase. Citations include books, journal articles, and conferences/meeting abstracts. Near the end of 2010, there were more than 200,000 meeting/conference abstracts from more than 200 journals. Embase is a tool that can assist systematic review researchers in finding clinical studies important for their review that were not part of or indexed in MEDLINE, especially if an answer for a foreground question requires drug information.

Although Embase can be highly useful to locate literature for systematic review work, many libraries may not have a subscription to this resource because of its cost. Embase can be searched on different *search retrieval systems* or platforms such as that provided by Dialog, LLC (Dialog and DataStar platforms), Ovid Technologies (Ovid platform), and Elsevier B.V. (Embase.com). The vendor Dialog also offers Embase ONTAP (online training and practice), an area where reviewers may practice searching Embase before executing final searches in an institution's Embase product on the Dialog platform. The advantages of using Embase ONTAP are that reviewers can practice searching Embase and can think about effective strategies to promote retrieval of relevant results in final searches. When searching Embase ONTAP, the real results will appear as if one were searching a library's Embase database on Dialog, but retrieved results may not reveal all the latest records that a reviewer searching the Embase offered through a library's subscription would see. Visit the following link for information on Dialog ONTAP resources including Embase ONTAP at http://support.dialog.com/ontap/

As mentioned previously, Embase files can be broken down by years. It is important for searchers to realize what years of Embase they are searching. For instance, when searching Embase through Embase.com, the *"Advanced Search"* tab allows for restriction of search results to Embase Classic (1947–1973). There is also a separate database called Embase Alert, available while searching Embase through vendors such as Dialog, Elsevier, and Ovid. Embase Alert is similar to Pre-CINAHL and MEDLINE's *in-process* records, because it allows the most recent 8 weeks of literature or *articles in press* to be accessed as quickly as possible by researchers. The citations are eventually labeled/organized with subject headings or controlled vocabulary and placed in Embase.

Emtree (also known as Embase-controlled vocabulary) is the backbone of how citations are organized in Embase, and it is updated yearly. Updates include addition of new MEDLINE Medical Subject Heading (MeSH) terms, updating Chemical Abstracts Service (CAS) drug registry numbers (See the following link to learn more about CAS registry numbers at http://www.cas.org/expertise/cascontent/registry/regsys.html.). There are more than 55,000 thesaurus terms in Emtree. Depending on which *database provider* or *search retrieval system* one searches Embase on, frequent daily updates to Embase may be apparent.

Emtree includes about 56,000 preferred terms (with a little over 26,300 of those being drug terms) compared to 24,000 terms in MEDLINE's MeSH (with only about 7,000 of those being drug terms). The inclusion of articles on drugs and the specific categorization of those articles under Emtree's thesaurus terms makes Embase a powerful tool for locating drug information. Using the Emtree term for a drug keeps a user from having to know synonyms for drug terms. A drug can have more than 200 synonyms, including laboratory codes; investigational, chemical, and generic drug names; and multiple trade names. In addition, references or names associated with a drug can change over time. Embase's Emtree is a thesaurus including all MeSH vocabulary terms from MEDLINE and unique subject headings on biomedical, life science, and pharmaceutical science topics.

Embase.com is divided into tabs: *Quick, Advanced, Drug, Disease,* and *Article.* The advanced tab allows a searcher to build more precise, complex searches incorporating Emtree thesaurus terms. Retrieving database citations using thesaurus terms assigned to those citations instead of processing searches solely with text words offers a more controlled way to enhance retrieval of relevant search results. It is not necessary to figure out all the text words that represent a concept or know all the possible text words authors would use for a topic. Both the *Drug and Advanced Search* tabs in Embase.com offer the same list of *limits* to help searchers focus in or narrow down search results. Limits include evidence-based medicine, publication type, areas of focus (e.g., cancer, gerontology and geriatrics, internal medicine, public health), and age groups.

In Embase.com *Quick Search,* a searcher can type text words/phrases in a search box. There is a check box for *extensive search (mapping, explosion as key word)* that is check marked by default and, if left checked, can assist searchers in having a more powerful search, which can gather more relevant subcategories of citations on a topic. Mapping means that text words typed in the search box will be matched up and replaced with standard Emtree vocabulary or subject terms. This increases the likelihood that a greater number of articles on a topic can be located with greater precision, because all articles, regardless of what text words a searcher or article authors use for a concept, will be located because they are pooled under one or more Emtree vocabulary or topic terms. Explosion allows *Quick Search* to retrieve citations of articles categorized under the main Emtree vocabulary term. The *extensive quick search* also retrieves citations containing the exact text words/phrases a searcher typed. Quick search also allows for use of Boolean logic and proximity operators and wildcards.

With the *Advanced Search* tab in Embase.com, there is a page with options allowing for searching text words as is, mapping them to Emtree terms and more. Other options offered under both the *Advanced and Drug Search* tabs are as follows. There are *advanced limits*: evidence-based medicine, publication types, areas of focus, article languages, gender, age groups, and animal study types. Specifically, the evidence-based medicine limit allows for Cochrane review, controlled clinical trial, and meta-analysis, and Embase citations tagged with the Emtree term *Systematic Review*.

As noted previously, the *Drug Search* tab offers all the same limits options found under *Advanced Search*. There are a couple of added options: *drug subheadings* such as adverse drug reactions, clinical trial, drug therapy; and *routes of drug administration* such as buccal, epidural, and intratympanic. (Articles dedicated to reviewing routes of administration are something that sets apart Embase from MEDLINE; this proves useful to research a nursing systematic review question such as: "In post-operative patients, is administration of morphine by subcutaneous injection as effective as morphine by intramuscular route.") Allow Embase to search for drugs using an Emtree term because a drug could be mentioned under more than one name in articles, or a searcher may only refer to a drug by one or two synonyms, but there may be others. For instance, in a search for articles on Valium, would a searcher realize that the drug is also called diazepam, Seduxen, Relanium, and Psychopax? When searching for an article on Valium, the Emtree term diazepam would *round up* all the citations on valium, regardless of what article authors call it. Some drugs have more than 50 synonyms. Would a searcher know or want to type all the text words representing a drug in a search box?

In *Disease Search*, one can search for diseases and conditions. The same quick and advanced limits under the *Advanced and Drug Search* are present. There is the added limits option: *disease subheadings* such as complication, congenital disorder, and diagnosis.

The *Article* tab can facilitate the technique, author searching, looking for more articles by one author on a topic.

It is possible to search Embase's thesaurus classification of articles directly using the Emtree tab. A searcher would type a text word or phrase and select the most appropriate Emtree term that represents the text word(s). The searcher can apply features such as explode and focus to the Emtree term selected and add the term to a search box called *query builder*. Repeat the preceding steps to add additional Emtree terms in the search box and run the search.

Emtree includes types of articles or studies (21,825,311 records) and can assist a reviewer in retrieving citations referencing specific study design and methodologies. Examples of items under types of studies include action research, controlled study, experimental study, quasi-experimental study, and prevention study. Examples of methodologies or types of articles include systematic review (35,214 records), cohort analysis, grounded theory, pretest–posttest design, qualitative research, and quantitative study. Embase includes features for managing search results such as save search, e-mail alerts, RSS feeds, and a way to export citations into bibliography citation managers. For instance, direct export of Embase.com records into RefWorks can occur.

Embase.com also offers a link to another Elsevier B.V. product called Scirus. This product is a free Internet search resource for scientific inquiries. A search in Scirus retrieves literature not only from traditional resources such as databases, but also from grey literature sources such as websites. For more on Scirus, see the links mentioned in Appendix C regarding this product.

HealthSTAR

HealthSTAR (Health Services, Technology, Administration, and Research), originally called HSTAR, was a separate database available from the National Library of Medicine (NLM) from February 1994 to December 2000. Materials with a focus on health services research including clinical (emphasizing the evaluation of patient outcomes and the effectiveness of procedures, programs, products, services, and processes) and nonclinical (emphasizing health care administration, economics, planning, and policy) aspects of health care delivery were especially chosen for inclusion in HealthSTAR. Since 2000, the company Wolters Kluwer Health–Ovid Technologies has offered Ovid HealthSTAR as a continuation of the original NLM HealthSTAR database.

HealthSTAR on Ovid retains all existing HealthSTAR citations' back files and is updated with new journal citations culled from MEDLINE using the NLM's HealthSTAR search strategy. The database contains citations and abstracts to journal articles, monographs, technical reports, meeting abstracts and papers, book chapters, government documents, and newspaper articles from 1975 to present. Citations are indexed with the NLM's MeSH to ensure compatibility with other NLM databases. Information in HealthSTAR on Ovid is derived from MEDLINE, the hospital literature index, and selected journals. Ovid HealthSTAR is updated monthly.

Similar to other databases on the Ovid search retrieval system, HealthSTAR can be searched via Ovid basic or advanced search options. The Ovid search system includes similar search features that are also available in other traditional bibliographic databases such as save searches/alerts, which allows users to set up a virtual Ovid account to save searches and RSS feeds. Searchers can also directly export citations to reference management software.

A *basic search* in most Ovid databases, such as HealthSTAR, allows searchers to enter key terms, words, or phrases connected by operators such as *AND, OR,* or

NOT. The database system then parses the question into a search strategy and ranks results by relevance. Default fields searched are *abstract, name of substance word, title, subject heading word,* and *original title.* Subject heading word retrieves every MeSH that includes a particular word.

Reviewers using advanced search in Ovid HealthSTAR make use of MeSH if they leave the *"Map Term to Subject Heading"* box checked before processing a search for their key word. Ovid advanced search is best explored through a tutorial, library database workshop, or a visit with a librarian involved in reference work or literature research activities. Besides MeSH, advanced search allows for use of features to narrow—center or focus and/or expand or explode—search terms. Use of the focus feature retrieves citations where one's term is the primary or major focus of an article. Use of the explode feature not only retrieves general articles on a search concept, but also articles in subcategories represented under a concept. (See the section "Subject Heading Features" in Chapter 5 for more details on explode and focus.)

Even though one may search Ovid HealthSTAR in the advanced search mode, it is still possible to incorporate some basic search features in the advanced mode, as well as make use of special search features such as truncation and wildcards (See Chapter 5 for a review on truncation and wildcards.). In general, the former statement is a tip that applies to searching in other databases with basic and advanced search modes, as well.

MEDLINE

MEDLINE is *the* United States National Library of Medicine (U.S. NLM) original database with biomedical journal citations from over 80 countries. It is available through several different *search systems,* including the NLM's National Center for Biotechnology Information (NCBI) *Entrez retrieval system* and Wolters Kluwer Health's *Ovid system.* MEDLINE is also the largest part of the PubMed database. Which system MEDLINE is available on depends on which *search retrieval system* an institution or library subscribes to for MEDLINE. A subscription to MEDLINE on some search retrieval systems is expensive, so if MEDLINE is not available at a local institution or library, consider searching it on PubMed instead because PubMed is a free database that includes all the content of MEDLINE. Visit the following link for more on *"What is the difference between MEDLINE and PubMed"*: http://www.nlm.nih.gov/pubs/factsheets/dif_med_pub.html

In addition to covering everything in MEDLINE, PubMed also includes out-of-scope citations from certain MEDLINE journals, citations that precede the date journal content was chosen for addition into MEDLINE, and some additional life science journals. PubMed on the NLM system is updated throughout the week and thus parts of it such as MEDLINE. (Depending on which other search retrieval system one searches MEDLINE updating can be daily, weekly, and monthly.) PubMed allows citations of articles to be added directly from journal publishers before the article is indexed or labeled with subject headings.

Currently, PubMed contains more than 20 million MEDLINE citations from approximately 5,500 journals (http://www.nlm.nih.gov/bsd/num_titles.html)

dating back to 1948. The subject scope of PubMed is biomedical and health science literature, including medicine, nursing, allied health, dentistry, veterinary medicine, life sciences, behavioral sciences, chemical sciences, bioengineering, and biophysics.

Searching MEDLINE through PubMed

MEDLINE uses Medical Subject Headings (MeSH), a controlled vocabulary. As mentioned previously, controlled vocabulary is used by database producers to place citations in categories or under subject headings to facilitate maximum and comprehensive retrieval of relevant articles by researchers. PubMed automatically *"maps"* or closely matches terms typed in the basic search box to a MeSH term before processing a search.

The default search in PubMed appears as a basic search box on the PubMed home page, but be aware that this is no ordinary simple search, because words/ phrases entered into the text box are processed to include MeSH terms automatically. So then, why even bother learning how to search PubMed via the MeSH Database— even more control of one's search and to build up more specific, focused search queries that capitalize on the way PubMed group's articles—by medical subject headings and focus less on being a searcher striving to enter all possible key terms and/or synonyms into search boxes.

There are many features allowing for executing searches in a variety of ways on PubMed. Beyond searching MEDLINE on PubMed using the *basic search* box, as suggested one can explore searching PubMed using the *MeSH Database*. With this search, one selects the search option *MeSH Database* and proceed to typing an important *text word* in the search box that appears. PubMed reveals a list of controlled vocabulary terms or subject headings for review and the searcher selects the heading (if any) that appropriately describes the original concept they typed in the MeSH Browser box. Then they click on the option *"Send To,"* which places the chosen subject heading or controlled vocabulary term in a search box. The process is repeated as many times as needed with other subject headings being sent to the search box as representatives for concepts the searcher types in the initial MeSH Database search box. Text words can also be added to the final query before the search is processed. A PubMed MeSH Database tutorial (search the Internet to find one from U.S. NLM) or a workshop session with a reference librarian may prove invaluable to learning how to search MEDLINE within PubMed in this powerful way.

Still another way to search PubMed is through the *advanced search* page, a cool way to search, allowing researchers a preview of the number of search results for each query as they continue building their search. In PubMed Advanced Search, it is easy to see options for limiting searches to a certain author, journal, publication date or date range, as well as a host of other options.

One final way reviewers may want to explore searching PubMed is via the feature Topic-Specific Queries, where one specific interface—the *clinical queries* search box—can be a gem. *PubMed's Clinical Queries* include a search for clinical studies by foreground question category; systematic reviews; and citations on medical genetics.

After a reviewer enters his or her search statement in the Clinical Queries search box and selects a question category, along with scope for the citations to be retrieved (broad or narrow), the queries' page processes their search noting the number of primary studies, systematic reviews, and medical genetics citations on the search statement. The search filters developed by Dr. R. B. Haynes are behind the Clinical Queries search algorithms (http://www.ncbi.nlm.nih.gov/entrez/query/static/clinicaltable.html) and ensure that a reviewer will retrieve evidence-based citations on their topic—bypassing non-evidence that would have been part of their result set (Non-evidence is not filtered out of searches performed using the PubMed basic or advanced search box options.).

One tip for managing PubMed search cites is to set up a group account that will be accessible by all reviewers and/or individual accounts using the *My NCBI* account *sign in*. A My NCBI account will facilitate saving original searches and collections of selected search results (from original searches, *related article* searches, and author chasing and results of handsearches of journals indexed on PubMed). Search results can be set up so that reviewers will receive an automatic e-mail when new citations are available for their systematic review topic.

Under one's personal or group My NCBI account; there are some customizations that may facilitate reviewing of citations in a more efficient manner. Use the My NCBI's *preferences* option to choose a highlighting color. This will mean that the next time a search is performed in PubMed and users are logged in to that PubMed NCBI account, search results will show a searcher's original key words in a *highlighting* color as they review citations. My NCBI also allows for search filters to be applied to searches each time a user is signed in to their My NCBI account. Select frequently requested search filters, search for specific filters, or browse for additional filters (maximum filters one can select to date is 15).

Searching MEDLINE on Ovid

When one searches MEDLINE on Ovid, there is a basic search option that allows searchers to type in a research question in *natural language* (everyday speak) or place important text words/phrases connected with Boolean logic operators (*AND, OR,* or *NOT*), but this search will not be expanded for users to include *MeSH terms*. Basic searches in MEDLINE are appropriate early in reviewers' research process, but more detailed and comprehensive searches will be needed for researching and writing systematic reviews. Some search features applicable for searching MEDLINE on Ovid in basic and advanced search mode follow. The symbol for unlimited truncation is the dollar sign ($) or colon (:). If a searcher would like their key word expanded with a single extra character, then consider the use of the question mark (?) for wildcard truncation (e.g., *an?esthesia* or *p?ediatrics*). This may prove useful when one is trying to retrieve documents with both American (e.g., anesthesia, pediatrics) and British spellings (e.g., anaesthesia, paediatrics).

To search MEDLINE on Ovid with MeSH terms, use the Ovid *advanced search* mode, and manually select appropriate MeSH terms as desired for addition into a search. Similar to U.S. NLM, the producer of PubMed, Ovid Technologies offers a variety of tutorials (http://www.ovid.com/site/help/training.jsp) in several formats to help searchers become proficient in searching databases such as MEDLINE on its platform. Here is a scenario with some lessons learned one can contemplate on before doing an advanced search on Ovid MEDLINE.

- A reviewer types in the Ovid MEDLINE *advanced search* box a key word or text word from their foreground question: *diabetes* and clicks the search buttons. A list of MeSH terms appear on a subsequent screen. The researcher picks *one* MeSH term or subject heading that best represents the key word originally entered—so from keyword: *diabetes* to MeSH term: *Diabetes Mellitus, Type 2*.
- The reviewer then selects the option to *include all subheadings* for the to MeSH term: *Diabetes Mellitus, Type 2* and they click the *continue* button.
- The Ovid system goes about processing their MEDLINE search retrieving results tagged in MEDLINE with the subject heading diabetes mellitus, type 2.
- The preceding process is repeated as needed for other text words from the reviewer's foreground question.
- Eventually the reviewer *combines* result sets for specific subject heading words with the Boolean operator *AND*.
- The reviewer then looks for the MEDLINE on Ovid feature allowing them to create a *personal account* for saving searches and setting up *auto-alerts* to receive new citations on their systematic review topic while they continue on with other processes in the systematic review pathway.

ProQuest Dissertations and Theses Database

The ProQuest Dissertations and Theses (PQDT) database is derived from doctoral dissertations and master's theses from graduate schools and universities in North America and internationally. There are other databases that collect and house dissertations. They include Digital Dissertations, Theses Canada Portal, Index to Theses, Networked Digital Library of Theses and Dissertations, and Digitala Vetenskapliga Arkivet (DiVA). For more dissertation collections, see Appendix 6.

PQDT database contains more than 2 million entries dating back to 1637. Full text is available for more than 1.9 million dissertations and theses, depending on the type of subscription a library has with ProQuest. Each year, 60,000 new entries are added to the PQDT database. Similar to other databases, ProQuest records are cataloged or organized using a unique ProQuest vocabulary of terms. Some records are tagged or organized using terms supplied by the author of a dissertation or abstract.

PQDT can be searched through basic and advanced search modes. The database includes a *My Research* tab that provides users with several options after running a search. They can create bibliographies for e-mailing, printing, or saving as a rich text file, to be opened in word processing programs such as Microsoft Word (*Microsoft Corporation*). Citations can be exported to bibliographic citation management software. There is also a way to create web pages with hyperlinks of researchers' articles, searches, and publications. Set up the theses database using the RSS feed link on the *results* page for sending alerts of new dissertations or theses on a preset topic.

PsycINFO

PsycINFO is a database from the American Psychological Association (APA) that provides systematic coverage of the psychological literature from the 1800s to the present. There are also records from the 1600s and 1700s. PsycINFO includes more than 2.7 million records covering more than 2,450 titles. Ninety-nine percent of the records are peer reviewed. The database also includes 30% journal records from the European literature and 12% U.S. dissertations. In addition, book and books' chapters are included if scholarly, professional, or research-based with psychological relevance. PsycINFO database is updated weekly.

Similar to other search databases, PsycINFO can be offered on many search retrieval systems and/or through vendors such as APA PsycNET, DIALOG/DataStar, EBSCOhost, German Institute for Medical Documentation and Information (GIMDI), Hogrefe Publishing Group, Online Computer Library Center (OCLC), Ovid Technologies and ProQuest (Illumina). Search features to be described in subsequent paragraphs are available when one searches PsycINFO on Ovid. For information on searching PsycINFO on other search retrieval systems, see PsycSEARCH—Guides for APA Databases.

These features apply to both basic and advanced search in PsycINFO: phrase searching, truncation with the dollar sign ($), and wildcard truncation with the number sign (#) for retrieving specialized plural forms of a word. For example, searching for the term "wom#n" retrieves results that contain both woman and women. Another wildcard symbol, the question mark (?) is useful for retrieving documents with British and American word variants. For example, the optional wildcard search "colo?r" retrieves results that contain the words color or colour.

PsycINFO's basic search allows searchers to enter a topic in ordinary English including in the form of a question. The database system then parses the question into a search strategy and ranks results by relevance. Default fields searched are the *abstract, heading word, table of contents* (TOC), *key concepts,* and *title.* Key concepts concisely summarizes a document's subject content and is in addition to subject headings. Heading word searches the words and phrases in subject headings, and the TOC searches the table of contents of books.

Advanced search in PsycINFO allows researchers to make use of controlled vocabulary and subject headings for a more effective search. Available features for application to chosen subject headings include explode and focus. (See the section "Subject Heading Features" in Chapter 5 for more details on explode and focus.) PsycINFO has two areas with a controlled vocabulary/classification, *thesaurus of psychological index terms* and *classification categories and codes.* The thesaurus of psychological index terms can be considered as the APA's version of MeSH. During an advanced search in PsycINFO, users can select appropriate thesaurus terms as shared by the database to increase retrieval of desired search results. Another opportunity that researchers have to retrieve article citations that were placed under a thesaurus term in PsycINFO is when performing a search for a term using the subject headings field. PsycINFO offers a cited reference search. It is comprehensive starting from 2001. PsycINFO database producers are currently adding more cited reference records for earlier years as available. For general information on cited reference search, see the section in this chapter entitled "Cited Reference Search or Citation Chasing."

PsycEXTRA and PsycARTICLES

PsycINFO is only one of the databases from the APA. Another APA database that may be of interest is PsycEXTRA, a grey literature database. PsycEXTRA content was written for professionals and disseminated outside of peer-reviewed journals and includes abstracts and citations. To date, there is no coverage overlap between PsycINFO and PsycEXTRA. PsycEXTRA contains more than 159,000 records, of which, 70% are full text. An estimated 30,000 records are added yearly.

PsycARTICLES is a full-text database of publications from APA, the APA Educational Publishing Foundation, the Canadian Psychological Association, and Hogrefe Publishing Group. All full-text records in PsycARTICLES are indexed as citations in PsycINFO. There are 71 journals covered starting from 1894. Articles are entered into PsycARTICLES on average of 2 weeks after the print issue is mailed. More than 142,000 articles are included and with historical files added, the collection stands at 72,699 full-text records. PsycARTICLES in conjunction with PsycINFO and PsycEXTRA is updated monthly.

Scopus

Scopus is a relatively new database, less than 20 years old, including both biomedical and social science literature. It has some features and set-up that includes the following: Locate Embase database records via a search of Scopus. The Embase search via Scopus only allows for searching Embase via a text word search. Another interesting feature of Scopus involves the presentation of search results in clusters. Searchers can review result clusters for citations by specific authors from particular journals or disciplines such as nursing. Many different journal citations are represented in Scopus that may not be in Embase, MEDLINE, or Web of Science (Gavel & Iselid, 2008). Currently, Scopus cannot be searched using the controlled vocabulary feature part of databases such as CINAHL and MEDLINE. Both Scopus and Web of Science are useful for performing cited reference searches. With a cited reference search, one is looking for the names of other authors who cited or included an original author's paper as part of their work. This is actually a form of the search technique citation chasing.

Web of Science

Web of Science (WoS) is available through the Institute for Scientific Information (ISI) Web of Knowledge platform provided by Thomson Reuters. It consists of seven databases. They are Science Citation Index (SCI) Expanded, Social Sciences Citation Index (SSCI), Arts and Humanities Citation Index, Conference Proceedings Citation Index-Science, Conference Proceedings Citation Index-Social Sciences and Humanities, Index Chemicus, and Current Chemical Reactions. The first three databases allow researchers to do cited reference searching. The conference proceedings indexes include published literature of the significant conferences, symposia, seminars, colloquia, workshops, and conventions in various disciplines. Many nursing researchers look for materials for systematic review work in SCI Expanded, SSCI, and the conference proceedings indexes.

WoS indexes more than 10,000 journals covering the years 1900 to the present. SCI Expanded covers the scientific topics from agriculture to zoology including behavioral sciences, biochemistry, biomedical sciences, chemistry, medicine, microbiology, and pharmacology and dates back to 1900.

Some of the disciplines covered in SSCI are psychiatry, psychology, public health, social work, and substance abuse, and this database goes back to 1956.

There are weekly updates for WoS content. WoS's records are not indexed via a searchable list of controlled vocabulary words, so searchers need to search WoS using synonyms for their search terms.

The truncation symbols used in WoS are the asterisk (*), the question mark (?), and the dollar sign ($). The asterisk is used to replace any group of characters. This is useful for truncating journal or publication titles. The question mark represents any single character. If one is unsure of the ending of an author's last name, the question mark would be a useful truncation symbol. The dollar sign can represent a single character such as "a" in the British spelling for p?ediatrics.

WoS users can create a personal ISI Web of Knowledge profile. This personal account allows for saving searches (any search up to 20 sets) and for creating search alerts, including alerts of when an article on a citation alerts list has been cited by a new article. Alerts are active for 1 year, but can be renewed as needed. WoS allows one to perform cited reference searches. Search for a cited reference by searching for the author, the work's source, and the publication year.

Most libraries or institutions have WoS set up to open to its basic search page that includes three search boxes for users to type in search terms. WoS allows for addition of more search boxes as needed. For each search box, there is a corresponding drop-down menu to choose the search field that one wants the search term to be found in (for example, in the *topic, title, document type*). Terms in each search box are under a searcher's control for linkage with either selection of Boolean operators (*AND, OR,* or *NOT*) to connect words from one search box to another. Refine search results by applying limits from one or more of the following categories: subject areas, document types, authors, source titles, publication years, institutions, funding agencies, languages, or countries/territories.

When searching WoS, it is important to remember that capitalization of text words is not necessary, and the use of Boolean operators varies, depending on which search fields one is selecting for a search box entry. For example, use the Boolean operator *AND* when searching a topic but not when searching for a publication name. Use quotation marks when searching for an exact phrase as part of a topic or title.

There is an advanced search option in WoS that allows investigators to search for records using field tags and combinations of result sets. The following link is from WoS producers and includes brief videos on searching WoS products: http://wokinfo.com/training_support/training/recordedtraining/#wos.

GREY (GRAY) LITERATURE

Grey literature was defined in 2004 at the International Conference on Grey Literature as government, academics, business, and industry information in electronic and print formats not controlled by commercial publishing (TextRelease, 2009). Grey literature should be searched as applicable to avoid publication bias in systematic reviews. Elements involved in publication bias may include limiting searches for systematic review articles to "English language," omitting negative studies or studies with less favorable results, or those showing no difference in effect. More successful studies or studies with more positive outcomes may already overwhelm the literature; therefore, when performing searches for studies to include in a systematic review, one should be sure to identify and transfer the full text of all qualified studies for possible inclusion into a systematic review. Include studies with opposing views in systematic reviews if they meet the systematic review inclusion criteria.

For example, after a state-of-the-art analysis of systematic reviews on treatment for schizophrenia, with some reviews including grey literature while others did not, a group of authors noted that the inclusion of certain grey literature in some of the systematic reviews increased bias (Martin, Pérez, Sacristán, & Alvarez, 2005). Thus, the reason a study was not published must be taken into account when reviewing mental health literature and, arguably, literature from other disciplines. Not all grey literature belongs in a systematic review. Consider when it is appropriate to include grey literature in a review. For a closer look at bias and systematic reviews, see Chapter 1.

Government or organization reports, conference proceedings, and trials where the results were not published in a traditional venue, can all show evidence that should be included in a systematic review. Statistical analysis of the research cited in published reviews has shown that the lack of grey literature can lead to overestimation of the impact of an intervention (Hopewell, McDonald, Clarke, & Egger, 2007; McAuley, Pham, Tugwell, & Moher, 2000).

Therapy or treatment is not the only type of review that should include grey literature. There are questions that can be asked when deciding whether to include grey literature in a systematic review (Benzies, Premji, Hayden, & Serrett, 2006).

Finding grey literature in traditional electronic biomedical databases such as PubMed or CINAHL is unlikely. Grey literature is not peer-reviewed and is less likely to reference sources of information. Six ways to locate grey literature have been identified: search CENTRAL, hand searching, review databases of unpublished and ongoing studies, search the Internet, comb through reference lists, and seek and consult subject experts (Blackhall, 2007).

Another source of grey literature in the health sciences field is the Grey Literature Report from the New York Academy of Medicine (NYAM). The report is bimonthly, alerting readers to new grey literature publications in public health and health services research topics (NYAM Library, 2009). All items in the Grey Litera-ture Report are searchable through NYAM's online catalog at http://nyam.waldo.kohalibrary.com/.

Grey literature can also come from websites on laws, drug-regulating body documents such as those from the U.S. Food and Drug Administration (FDA), con-sults with professionals at departments of health and related departments, and nursing centers housing health research and policy data. A useful Internet presen-tation that provides information on grey literature is at http://www.slideshare.net/giustinid/finding-the-hard-to-finds-searching-for-grey-gray-literature-2010 (Gius-tini, 2010). In addition, see Appendix: Social Science and Biomedical Science Grey Literature.

Grey literature can be an important addition in systematic reviews, even though such literature does not usually meet the same strict guidelines or provide high level of evidence similar to randomized control trials (RCTs). Document the form of grey literature used, date/time span of the literature, and other details to keep track of what has been reviewed.

Conference Proceedings

It is a good idea to add conference proceedings, congresses, and meeting abstracts to reviewers' lists of places to search for information related to a systematic review topic. These may be pieces of literature addressing new angles or putting forth new solutions for a foreground question, which may not yet be part of an article indexed in traditional resources. Searching proceedings and the like helps decrease pub-lication bias in a systematic review, as reviewers are making an attempt to get all possible literature on their foreground question. Some traditional search resources or databases may include information on meetings too, such as BioMed Central (BioMed Central Ltd.; free resource), BIOSIS Previews (Thomson Reuters), Embase, MEDLINE, NLM Gateway (free resource), ProceedingsFirst (OCLC), WoS, and WorldCAT (OCLC).

Databases of Ongoing Research

Clinical Trials

Clinical trials may fit in the category of a type of continuing or ongoing research. Trials in this category include those currently enrolling subjects, active trials beyond the subject enrollment phase, and trials where data analysis is in process. For trials where the results are never published, these resources may be the only online record of the work.

In 2000, the NLM created ClinicalTrials.gov (http://www.clinicaltrials.gov/), the first trial registry. In 2007, the FDA Amendments Act was passed requiring Phase II trials and beyond to be registered at ClinicalTrials.gov and, regardless of publication, results of the trial must be listed in the registry, generally within 1 year of the trial's completion. In addition, the International Committee of Medical

Journal Editors (ICMJE) noted that from 2005 onward, there would be a commitment to publish research where a trial had been registered. As a result, trial registration in the United States increased and new registries were created (*The Evolution of Trial Registration*, 2009; Mathieu, Boutron, Moher, Altman, & Ravaud, 2009). The good news is that there are clinical trial registries, and the bad news is there is not just one trial registry in each country or worldwide. This means that searches for information may have to be performed in multiple registry databases. Sometimes, a website such as Current Controlled Trials (http://www.controlled-trials.com/) is available and such a site offers a metaRegister of Controlled Trials (mRCT; http://www.controlled-trials.com/mrct/), allowing one to search multiple registries at once.

The rate of publication of registered trials has been reviewed in the literature, and it has been noted that not all trials are published and that inconclusive and negative results are less likely not to be published. Further, discrepancies are present in some published results noted in some registries (Mathieu et al., 2009; Ross, Mulvey, Hines, Nissen, & Krumholz, 2009). The group Consolidated Standards of Reporting Trials (CONSORT; http://www.consort-statement.org/) advocates for transparent reporting of randomized controlled trials (RCTs).

ClinicalTrials.gov

As mentioned previously, ClinicalTrials.gov is the largest and oldest of all trial registries, and it includes both government and privately funded trials. There are more than 80,000 trials, and trials are from the United States and about 170 other countries. The ClinicalTrials.gov database is updated daily to accommodate newly received trial data.

On the basic search page for ClinicalTrials.gov, enter important text words/phrases to locate specific studies. These may include words describing diseases, interventions, and/or trial locations such as South America. (The ClinicalTrials.gov database does allow for browsing lists of trials by *conditions, drug intervention, sponsor,* and *location.*) A search for two or more terms in ClinicalTrials.gov is processed using *AND* as the default Boolean operator between the terms typed in the search box. Searchers can choose to exercise more control over searches in ClinicalTrials.gov by making use of the following Boolean operators: *AND, OR,* or *NOT.* Consider using quotation marks (" ") for terms the database should interpret as a phrase or to search a Boolean operator as a word (e.g., *peanut butter and jelly*). Parentheses can also be used to control the way the database interprets a search statement. For example, *(heart disease OR heart attack) AND (stroke OR clot).* It is not necessary for users to brainstorm every synonym for a term and include it in parentheses when searching ClinicalTrials.gov. The ClinicalTrials.gov database does try to determine synonyms for search terms when possible. For example, a search for *heart attack* will also find occurrences of *myocardial infarction.*

For more precise results, use the ClinicalTrials.gov advanced search screen and use, when appropriate, the optional additional fields provided. Only fill in the fields appropriate for specific search needs. Boolean logic operators can be used in any field that is free text. Place the logic operators in all capital letters (see Table 6.1).

TABLE 6.1
ClinicalTrials.gov Advanced Search—Tips on Searching Some Fields

ClinicalTrials.gov Advanced Search Field	Search Tip
Recruitment	Use the provided drop-down menu to choose among all studies, open studies, or closed studies.
Study Results	Use provided drop-down menus to choose among all studies, studies with results, or studies without results.
	The study results field is relatively new and not many studies include results.
Study Type	Use provided drop-down menus to choose among all studies, interventional, observational, or expanded access studies.
Conditions, Interventions, Outcomes Measures, Lead Sponsors, Sponsors, and Study IDs	All are fields allowing one to type one's own terms.
Lead Sponsors, Sponsors	Check mark a box for exact match to have the database locate exactly what was typed in either the lead sponsors or sponsors option.
State/Country	State/Country are fields where one can select from a provided drop-down menu.
Location Terms	Location terms is a free text field allowing one to type free text to search a city or facility as in Mayo Clinic. Not all studies include this level of detail, but if they do, this will find them.
Gender	Select from the provided drop-down menu.
Age Group, Study Phase, and Funded By	More than one box can be checked for age group, study phase, and funded by.
Date	Options include first received and last updated

With either basic or advanced search, results will display a list of studies found. Click on the *refine search* option to modify search results using the same fields offered in advanced search.

Registered Trials in PubMed and Ovid MEDLINE

When attempting to locate registered trials in PubMed and MEDLINE on Ovid, type *clinicaltrials.gov [si]* in the PUBMED basic search box. The abbreviation SI stands for secondary source ID. The *SI field* contains information pertaining to the registration of several types of data discussed in MEDLINE articles including, as of summer 2005, clinical trial numbers. The SI field is composed of the *source* (e.g., ClinicalTrials.gov), followed by a slash, and then followed by an ID (e.g., ClinicalTrials.gov trial identifier number). Currently, there were about 6,630 trial results from ClinicalTrials.gov.

Results from the SI field can be combined with text words to limit and focus the number of results.

To locate trials from ClinicalTrials.gov in MEDLINE on Ovid, click on the search fields option in Ovid MEDLINE and follow these steps.

- Step 1, type ClinicalTrials.gov in the search box.
- Step 2, place a check mark in front of the box for SI.
- Step 3, click on the search button near the search box to run the search.

Review the results. Similar to searching PubMed, results from an SI search of MEDLINE on Ovid can be manipulated to retrieve a more focused set of clinical trial citations.

World Health Organization International Clinical Trials Registry Platform

Another ICMJE approved registry, the searchable World Health Organization (WHO) registry focuses on bringing as many international registries together as possible. According to the website, the WHO registry network is composed of WHO primary registries, partner registries, and registries working with the International Clinical Trials Registry Platform (ICTRP) toward becoming WHO primary registries.

Any registry that enters clinical trials into its database prospectively, that is, before the first participant is recruited, and meets the WHO registry criteria or that is working with ICTRP toward becoming a WHO primary registry, can be part of the WHO registry network. Partner registries meet the same criteria as primary registries, except, they do not need be national or regional in scope, have the support of a government, be managed by a not-for-profit agency, or be open to all prospective registrants, as in disease-specific registries. Registry data sets from providers are updated every Tuesday evening.

The standard WHO ICTRP search is very sensitive, finding as many records as possible. The resource looks for terms (words or phrases) in the fields: title, primary sponsor, health condition(s), intervention(s), countries, main source ID(s), and SI(s). Do not enclose a phrase in double quotes; the system is set to consider two or more words as a phrase. The standard search automatically includes synonyms for terms.

Use Boolean logic operators such as *AND, OR,* or *NOT* in searches on WHO ICTRP. Do not use parentheses, the WHO ICTRP database does not process searches according to what is in parentheses first. The resource does process searches by paying attention to terms connected with the Boolean operator *NOT* first, then attends to terms joined by *AND,* and then focuses on terms joined with *OR*. The asterisk (*) can be used as a wildcard for truncation in searches, but realize that this will keep the database from coming up with synonyms for words typed by a searcher. Truncation such as the (*) does not work if placed in the middle of a word or phrase, only when placed at the end of a word or phrase.

Advanced search in WHO ICTRP also allows for use of Boolean logic operators in a similar fashion to that described previously in the basic search section. One can still have more control in combining search terms in advanced search, because one or more fields can be searched and limits can be added at the beginning of a search. Fields that can be searched include title, condition, intervention, recruitment status, primary sponsor, SI, countries of recruitment, and date of trial registration.

It is possible to search for trials registered in certain WHO primary registries in the following languages: Chinese, Dutch, German, Japanese, and Persian. Searches are sensitive to punctuation (anti-depressants vs. antidepressants). Consider searching for both terms using *OR*. Any number of terms can be combined. However, some combinations of *AND, OR*, and *NOT* can lead to ambiguity. Care must be taken when constructing complex searches.

RePORT Expenditures and Results

The Research Portfolio Online Reporting Tool (RePORT) provides access to reports, data, and analyses of National Institutes of Health (NIH) research activities, including information on NIH expenditures and the results of NIH-supported research. To search RePORT, use RePORT Expenditures and Results (RePORTER); this replaced Computer Retrieval of Information on Scientific Projects (CRISP). RePORTER has more information on research, providing links to PubMed Central, PubMed, and the U.S. Patent and Trademark Office Patent Full-Text and Image Database.

RePORTER is limited by the fact that the information provided goes back 25 years; downloading is sort of all or nothing and results go into Microsoft Excel (*Microsoft Corporation*). On the positive side, if articles have been published from the research, they are listed, contact information is easy to find, and it is possible to limit to projects funded by specific agency or center including the National Institute of Nursing Research (NINR).

The results of a search are returned in a project listing that can be downloaded. Information includes project number and title, contact information for the principal investigator and organization, year(s) of funding, funding institutes, and total amount of funding by year. The project number, subproject ID, and the project title are linked to more detailed information on a series of tabs: description, the science being conducted; detail, administrative and budget details on the project; results, the publications and patents associated with the project; history, past years' project information; and subprojects (for multiproject grants only), all of the component subprojects.

RePORT/ER is updated on a weekly basis. Each update includes not only the addition of newly funded projects, but also revisions to prior awards (e.g., change of grantee institution or revised award amounts).

Use one or more term or words to search RePORTER and place quotation marks around terms to be interpreted exactly as typed by the RePORTER database. Use Boolean logic operators *AND* or *OR*, but not both. *AND* is the default Boolean operator in RePORTER. RePORTER returns results (projects) in which the search terms are found within the title, abstract, or scientific terms. There is also a long list of *stop words* (referred by RePORTER as reserved words) that can be found at http://projectreporter.nih.gov/reporter_help.html.

Most fields have strictly controlled vocabulary terminology. Free text fields include terms, principle investigator, organization, and request for applications

(RFA)/program announcement (PA), which comes from RFA, PA, or notice (NOT) and Public Health Relevance. Not all fields are available for all years.

SEARCH TECHNIQUES

Depending on the foreground question, reviewers may also consider search methods or techniques such as the ones discussed in the subsequent sections to decrease bias and increase the number of citations in a systematic review. Many authors have weighed in on this and some have taken a close look at systematic review search methodology and search yields, highlighting search flaws or missteps, as well as reviews omitting or missing relevant articles on a foreground question (Bassler et al., 2007; Goodman, 2008; Honest & Khan, 2002; Lundh & Gøtzsche, 2008; Sterne, Egger, & Smith, 2001; Trowman, Dumville, Torgerson, & Cranny, 2007).

Author Searching

Author searching is useful to find out who the prolific authors are in a topic area. This form of searching can be undertaken in several ways. Before electronic databases, most researchers looked for authors by checking the references at the end of the articles retrieved from a literature search. If an author was mentioned often in a reference list at the end of an article or has written much on a topic, one would use available tools to "chase" or locate more articles from that same author. Most databases today have some sort of author-searching tool. For example, Ovid MEDLINE has a search aid that lets users narrow their search by authors. After performing a search, click on *authors* in this search aid to view a list of the top five authors who have written on a search topic.

Another resource for author searching is the Virginia Henderson International Nursing Library from Sigma Theta Tau. This is a database of nursing research abstracts from research studies, conference presentations, practice innovations, and evidence-based projects. It also provides contact information for the authors of the abstracts.

Cited Reference Search or Citation Chasing

There are many ways to characterize citation chasing. It can be viewed as a search technique that involves taking an article and searching "backward in time," using the references found at the end of that article to see what authors, publications, including journals are covering on a topic of interest (Bates, 1989).

A form of citation chasing is the *cited reference search*. Using this technique, one can see which authors are citing a particular article, as well as how many times an article has been cited in other publications. A cited reference search is available in commercial databases such as WoS, Scopus, and recently, CINAHL and PsycINFO. Google Scholar also allows for cited reference searching. A closer look into a database is needed to see how far back or what year cited references date back to in that database. In addition, it may be good to locate information on the process used by the database to derive cited references.

How Is a Cited Reference Search Performed in Online Search Resources?

A researcher has one article of interest in hand. Usually, they type that article's title and/or the article's author in search boxes in a database. When the search is processed, the researcher sees which authors cited the original article of interest in their article's reference list.

Researchers need some details to maximize their search yield from a cited reference search in specific search resources and databases. For instance, more than one source has suggested that if an article was published after 1995, performing a cited reference search in Scopus is sufficient, because Scopus includes all MEDLINE and Embase database content, making it a resource with more content than WoS. For cited reference searches of articles published before 1995, a search of both WoS and Scopus is recommended (Falagas, Pitsouni, Malietzis, & Pappas, 2008). Google Scholar is a useful source for locating books, journal articles, web pages, and other web ephemera, but the resource has limited quality control, and its producers offer little information or transparency on how search results are processed compared to the information one receives when searching traditional bibliographic databases such as CINAHL and MEDLINE. Google Scholar should not be the sole source used by a researcher for cited reference searching (Jacsó, 2009).

Web of Science Cited Reference Searching

WoS is a search resource consisting of seven databases. Two WoS databases include the feature cited reference search: SCI Expanded and SSCI. SCI Expanded includes content from about 8,060 major journals across 150 disciplines, dating back to 1900, and SSCI covers 697 journals across 50 social science disciplines, as well as items from 3,500 of the world's leading scientific and technical journals, from 1900 to the present.

The WoS' cited reference search feature page includes a link to a brief recorded training tutorial (https://www.brainshark.com/brainshark/vu/view.asp ?pi=34671484) on cited reference searching. It is a good idea to complete that prior to performing a cited reference search in WoS. Use WoS to search for a cited author or cited work (article). When using WoS cited reference searches, look for a cited author, cited work, and/or cited year(s) for a work. Only the first cited author of a publication is indexed and will display with the reference or citation. Secondary authors are not indexed but are searchable. Therefore, if Ben Johnston is the first or primary author for an article, look for cited references to the article by Ben Johnston et al. by typing his last name in the cited author search box in WoS.

Once articles are located by citing an original author's work, search for more information on those articles, and see those articles' reference lists and other works that cite the authors who cited the original author. Sometimes, one discovers a cited reference and it does not offer a clickable hyperlink, just plain black text. In that case, the item a searcher is interested in may be a reference to a book or other document not indexed in WoS, an article that is not a part of their institution's journal subscription, or the item of interest was not cited correctly in a publication.

Scopus Cited Reference Searching

Scopus is a relatively new database that includes citations from biomedical and social sciences literature, as well as quality data from the Internet. Scopus has fully indexed or categorized article citations including their references beginning with citations from 1996. This makes it possible to browse the cited references for Scopus article citations published from 1996 onward. To use the citation capabilities, use the appropriate link within a Scopus record.

Google Scholar's Cited By Number (#)

Google Scholar is an Internet resource from Google that boasts inclusion of articles, theses, books, abstracts, court opinions, repositories, and other scholarly literature from various research areas. One thing searchers may have noticed when searching Google Scholar is the possible inclusion of multiple versions of an article in a search results list. There may be several reasons for this, including the possibility of a different version of an article. Each article that appears in Google Scholar has a link called *cited by* #. Clicking on the link cited by # reveals other articles that Google Scholar has determined to contain some version of the source article information. Choose Google Scholar from the Google toolbar under *more* or type http://www.scholar.google.com directly into the computer browser. Once in Scholar, enter information on an author and/or title of a source article. Use the available option to pick *articles excluding patents* and then click the search button.

If using advanced Scholar search, consider limiting search results by date, journal, and author. When typing search terms in the advanced Scholar search box, keep in mind the way Google processes searches. For instance, if a researcher is used to typing asthma *AND* therapy in a search box, note that Google automatically places *AND* in between words when more than one word is typed in a search box. Therefore, a search for *chronic asthma* is processed by Google search engines as chronic *AND* asthma. Depending on what an investigator is looking for, the way Google processes this search may be either a good or a bad thing. Similar to a search performed in Google.com, Google Scholar searches can be performed using advanced operators or search connector words or symbols such as the following:

- + operator makes sure results include common words, letters, or numbers that Google's search technology generally ignores, as in (+de knuth)
- − operator excludes all results that include this search term, as in (flowers–author: flowers)
- Phrase search only returns results that include this exact phrase, as in ("as you like it");
- *OR* operator returns results that include either of a researcher's search terms, as in (stock call *OR* put);
- intitle: operator, as in intitle:mars, only returns results that include search term in the document's title.

A more comprehensive listing of Google Search features is available at:

- Google Guide Quick Reference: Google Advanced Operators (cheat sheet) http://www.googleguide.com/advanced_operators_reference.html

Google Scholar also has a set of preferences that can be selected before one starts searching it. It covers languages and links about potential local libraries' linking their library journal subscriptions to make it easier for users to access full text and citation management export options.

EvidenceUpdates

EvidenceUpdates is a collaboration of *British Medical Journal* (BMJ) and McMaster University's Health Information Research Unit (HIRU). This resource at http://plus. mcmaster.ca/EvidenceUpdates/ may be useful as part of Pearl-Growing searches or searches aimed at generating ideas for systematic reviews. EvidenceUpdates can also be used at later stages in the systematic review search process to locate specific evidence on a foreground research question. Currently, anyone can complete an online registration to search EvidenceUpdates database for free. EvidenceUpdates citations come from more than 120 clinical journals, and each citation is rated by EvidenceUpdate research staff.

Hand Searching

Hand searching is a method of physically searching the entire contents of a journal or journals considered relevant to one's research topic. This was more common in the predigital age. However, it is still a useful searching technique today because sometimes studies are missed during the electronic searching process. The area where hand searching is most useful is when reviewers are looking at journal supplements and special issues of journals, because these are not always indexed in the databases. The Cochrane Collaboration has a manual for hand searching available at http://us.cochrane. org/sites/us.cochrane.org/files/uploads/pdf/Handsearcher%20Training%20Manual. pdf; see also http://www.cochrane.org/training/handsearchers-tscs.

SUMMARY

In this chapter, we reviewed many search resources, traditional search databases such as MEDLINE and CINAHL, nontraditional resources such as grey literature, and Internet resources such as Scirus. Search tips and search techniques to maximize search time in each resource were explored. One of the best things reviewers can do is to set about conducting systematic review searches—keeping track of all search histories and research notes using a worksheet (in conjunction with saving actual search steps within each database). See Exhibit 6.1 for a comprehensive systematic review search strategy worksheet.

EXHIBIT 6.1

Comprehensive Systematic Review Search Strategies Worksheet

Foreground Search Question (Use the most appropriate question framework (others available besides PICO) to diagram your research question.)

P =   S =

I =   P =

C =   I =

O =   C =

        E =

Harvesting Search Text Words or Key Concepts

_____

_____

_____

_____

Equivalent Database Search Limits

Search Inclusion Criteria (informs keywords and ways to Limit search results after searching)

_____

_____

_____

_____

FILTERED EVIDENCE DATABASES	Search Databases (Checkmark all to be used)	Database Date Limit for Search	Month/Year Search(es) Performed	Search Text Words	Name for Save Searches/ Alerts	My Research Notes
ACP PIER						
The Campbell Collaboration (C2) Library of Systematic Reviews			Search #1 = Search #2 =			

(Continued)

EXHIBIT 6.1

Comprehensive Systematic Review Search Strategies Worksheet (Continued)

	Search Databases (Checkmark all to be used)	Database Date Limit for Search	Date(s) Searches Performed	Search Text Words	Name for Save Searches/ Alerts	My Research Notes
Cochrane Database of Systematic Reviews (CDSR)						
Clinical Evidence Electronic Textbook						
Dynamed						useful for background questions
Essential Evidence Plus (EE+)						
JBI Evidence Summaries						
JBI Systematic Review Library						
EBSCO's Nursing Reference Center Evidence Based Summaries						
PIER						
TRIP Database						
GUIDELINES						
National Guideline Clearinghouse						
National Institute for Health and Clinical Excellence (NICE)						

(Continued)

EXHIBIT 6.1

Comprehensive Systematic Review Search Strategies Worksheet *(Continued)*

UNFILTERED OR RAW ARTICLE DATABASES	Search Databases (Checkmark all to be used)	Database Date Limit for Search	Date(s) Searches Performed	Search Text Words	Name for Save Searches/ Alerts	My Research Notes
CINAHL						Database Retrieval System: EBSCO Host
Cochrane Central Register of Controlled Trials (Central; Clinical Trials)						
Current Contents						
Database of Abstracts of Reviews (DARE)						
Dissertations and Theses						
Embase						
Health Source: Nursing/ Academic Edition						
HealthStar						
MEDLINE						
Mosby's Index						
Nursing@Ovid						
Proquest Nursing and Allied Health Source						
PsycINFO						Includes citations from PsycARTICLES
PubMed						
Scopus						
Web of Science						

(Continued)

EXHIBIT 6.1

Comprehensive Systematic Review Search Strategies Worksheet *(Continued)*

POINT-OF-CARE RESOURCES	Search Databases (Checkmark all to be used)	Database Date Limit for Search	Date(s) Searches Performed	Search Text Words	Name for Save Searches/ Alerts	My Research Notes
EBSCO's Nursing Reference Center (NRC)						
Mosby's Nursing Consult (MNC)						

OTHER SEARCH RESOURCES	Search Databases (Checkmark all to be used)	Database Date Limit for Search	Date(s) Searches Performed	Search Text Words	Name for Save Searches/ Alerts	My Research Notes

143

EXERCISES

1. Try this search in CINAHL *advanced search*.
- Type the text word *nurses* in an advanced search box; be sure to look above the search box to see if the *suggest subject terms* option has a check mark in front of it.
- Next, click the search button.
- On the next page that appears, scroll all the way down the page to see the text word that was originally typed in a highlighting color (usually, pink rectangle bar).
- Now scroll back up, slowly browsing the suggested subject terms for the original text word *nurses*.
- To execute or process a search for citations on nurses, one can either place a check mark in front of the original key word *nurses* and click *search database* button near the top right of the page.
- This will reveal results where the word *nurses* appears in certain areas of a citation. (Do not assume that the database CINAHL or other databases will comb through entire article citations looking for a text word. In addition, do not assume that the database will look for citations including variations or synonyms for the word *nurses*.)
- There is a difference in searching for citations processing a search for nurses, as a text word, versus processing a search with the subject term or subject heading *nurses*.

How many citations are obtained for a search in CINAHL for citations including the text word *nurses*?

How many citations are obtained for a search using the Subject Term: *Nurses*?

2. Visit the link http://hsl.mcmaster.ca/research/tutorials/cinahl.html to review a video detailing one way to search CINAHL making use of subject terms assigned to CINAHL citations.

3. Practice using the *clinical queries* limiter in CINAHL.
- Uncheck the *suggest subject terms* option, usually above CINAHL search boxes in the advanced search mode.
- Type a search statement dealing with bed rest and pregnancy in the search box.
- Use the search options or *limit your results* area (may appear below search boxes in CINAHL depending on how local institutions or libraries have customized the look of CINAHL for their community) to apply the filter *therapy-best balance*.

How many citations were retrieved?

REFERENCES

Bassler, D., Ferreira-Gonzalez, I., Briel, M., Cook, D. J., Devereaux, P. J., Heels-Ansdell, D., . . . Guyatt, G. H. (2007). Systematic reviewers neglect bias that results from trials stopped early for benefit. *Journal of Clinical Epidemiology, 60*(9), 869–873. doi:10.1016/j.jclinepi.2006.12.006

Bates, M. J. (1989). The design of browsing and berrypicking techniques for the online search interface. *Online Review, 13*(5), 407–424. Retrieved from http://www.gseis.ucla.edu/faculty/bates/berrypicking.html

Benzies, K. M., Premji, S., Hayden, K. A., & Serrett, K. (2006). State-of-the-evidence reviews: advantages and challenges of including grey literature. *Worldviews on Evidence Based Nursing, 3*(2), 55–61. doi:10.1111/j.1741-6787.2006.00051.x

Blackhall, K. (2007). Finding studies for inclusion in systematic reviews of interventions for injury prevention the importance of grey and unpublished literature. *Injury Prevention, 13*(5), 359. doi:10.1136/ip.2007.017020

Centre for Reviews and Dissemination. (2010). Help section: About DARE. Retrieved from http://www.crd.york.ac.uk/crdweb/html/helpdoc.htm#item2

The Cochrane Collaboration. (2010). About the Cochrane Library—The Cochrane Library. Retrieved from http://www.thecochranelibrary.com/view/0/AboutTheCochraneLibrary.html.

Dale, J., Caramlau, I. O., Lindenmeyer, A., & Williams, S. M. (2008). Peer support telephone calls for improving health. *Cochrane Database of Systematic Reviews*, (4), CD006903. doi:10.1002/14651858.CD006903.pub2

Falagas, M. E., Pitsouni, E. I., Malietzis, G. A., & Pappas, G. (2008). Comparison of PubMed, Scopus, Web of Science, and Google Scholar: Strengths and weaknesses. *Faseb Journal, 22*(2), 338–342. doi:10.1096/fj.07-9492LSF

Gavel, Y., & Iselid, L. (2008). Web of Science and Scopus: A journal title overlap study. *Online Information Review, 32*(1), 8-21. doi:10.1108/14684520810865958

Giustini, D. (2010). Finding the hard to finds: Searching for grey (gray) literature [online slides]. San Francisco, CA: SlideShare.

Goodman, S. N. (2008). Systematic reviews are not biased by results from trials stopped early for benefit. *Journal of Clinical Epidemiology, 61*(1), 95–96. doi:10.1016/j.jclinepi.2007.06.012

Gould, D. J., Moralejo, D., Drey, N., & Chudleigh, J. H. (2010). Interventions to improve hand hygiene compliance in patient care. *Cochrane Database of Systematic Reviews*, (9), CD005186. doi:10.1002/14651858.CD005186.pub3

Haynes, R. B., Ackloo, E., Sahota, N., McDonald, H. P., & Yao, X. (2008). Interventions for enhancing medication adherence. *Cochrane Database of Systematic Reviews*, (2), CD000011. doi:10.1002/14651858.CD000011.pub3

Honest, H., & Khan, K. S. (2002). Reporting of measures of accuracy in systematic reviews of diagnostic literature. *BMC Health Services Research, 2*(1), 4.

Hopewell, S., McDonald, S., Clarke, M., & Egger, M. (2007). Grey literature in meta-analyses of randomized trials of health care interventions. *Cochrane Database Systematic Reviews* (2), MR000010. doi:10.1002/14651858.MR000010.pub3

Jacsó, P. (2009). The h-index for countries in Web of Science and Scopus. *Online Information Review, 33*(4), 831-837. doi:10.1108/14684520910985756

The Joanna Briggs Institute. (2008). About the Institute. Retrieved from http://www.joannabriggs.edu.au/About%20Us

The Joanna Briggs Institute. (2009a). JBI COnNECT. Acute care. Retrieved from http://www.jbiCOnNECT.org/acutecare/ebhc/summarise/search-form.php

The Joanna Briggs Institute. (2009b). JBI COnNECT+ nodes. Retrieved from http://COnNECT.jbiCOnNECTplus.org/Nodes.aspx

The Joanna Briggs Institute. (2009c). Welcome to the Joanna Briggs Institute—SUMARI software suite. Retrieved from http://www.joannabriggs.edu.au/Appraise%20Evidence/JBI%20SUMARI%20(systematic%20review%20software)%20FREE

Légaré, F., Ratté, S., Stacey, D., Kryworuchko, J., Gravel, K., Graham, I. D., & Turcotte, S. (2010). Interventions for improving the adoption of shared decision making by healthcare professionals. *Cochrane Database of Systematic Reviews*, (5), CD006732. doi:10.1002/14651858.CD006732.pub2

Lundh, A., & Gøtzsche, P. C. (2008). Recommendations by Cochrane Review Groups for assessment of the risk of bias in studies. *BMC Medical Research Methodology, 8*, 22.

Martin, J. L., Pérez, V., Sacristán, M., & Alvarez, E. (2005). Is grey literature essential for a better control of publication bias in psychiatry? An example from three meta-analyses of schizophrenia. *European Psychiatry, 20*(8), 550–553. doi:10.1016/j.eurpsy.2005.03.011

Mathieu, S., Boutron, I., Moher, D., Altman, D. G., & Ravaud, P. (2009). Comparison of registered and published primary outcomes in randomized controlled trials. *Journal of the American Medical Association, 302*(9), 977–984. doi:10.1001/jama.2009.1242

McAuley, L., Pham, B., Tugwell, P., & Moher, D. (2000). Does the inclusion of grey literature influence estimates of intervention effectiveness reported in meta-analyses? *Lancet, 356*(9237), 1228–1231. doi:10.1016/S0140-6736(00)02786-0

New York Academy of Medicine Library. (2009). Grey Literature Report. Retrieved from http://www.nyam.org/library/online-resources/grey-literature-report/

Ross, J. S., Mulvey, G. K., Hines, E. M., Nissen, S. E., & Krumholz, H. M. (2009). Trial publication after registration in ClinicalTrials.Gov: a cross-sectional analysis. *PLoS Medicine*, *6*(9), e1000144. doi:10.1371/journal.pmed.1000144

Shepperd, S., Doll, H., Angus, R. M., Clarke, M. J., Iliffe, S., Kalra, L., . . . Wilson, A. D. (2008). Admission avoidance hospital at home. *Cochrane Database of Systematic Reviews*, (4), CD007491. doi:10.1002/14651858.CD007491

Shields, L., Pratt, J., Davis, L. M., & Hunter, J. (2007). Family-centred care for children in hospital. *Cochrane Database of Systematic Reviews*, (1), CD004811. doi:10.1002/14651858.CD004811.pub2

Sterne, J. A., Egger, M., & Smith, G. D. (2001). Systematic reviews in health care: Investigating and dealing with publication and other biases in meta-analysis. *British Medical Journal*, *323*(7304), 101–105.

TextRelease. (2009). GreyNet International, Grey Literature Network Service. Retrieved from http://www.greynet.org/

Trowman, R., Dumville, J. C., Torgerson, D. J., & Cranny, G. (2007). The impact of trial baseline imbalances should be considered in systematic reviews: A methodological case study. *Journal of Clinical Epidemiology*, *60*(12), 1229–1233. doi:10.1016/j.jclinepi.2007.03.014

SUGGESTED READINGS

Chou, R. (2008). Using evidence in pain practice: Part I: Assessing quality of systematic reviews and clinical practice guidelines. *Pain Medicine*, *9*(5), 518–530.

Egger, M., Juni, P., Bartlett, C., Holenstein, F., & Sterne, J. (2003). How important are comprehensive literature searches and the assessment of trial quality in systematic reviews? Empirical study. *Health Technology Assessment*, *7*(1), 1–76.

Goodfellow, L. M. (2009). Electronic theses and dissertations: A review of this valuable resource for nurse scholars worldwide. *International Nursing Review*, *56*(2), 159–165.

The GRADE Working Group. (2005–2009). GRADE Working Group. Retrieved from http://www.gradeworkinggroup.org/index.htm

Haynes, B. (2007). Of studies, syntheses, synopses, summaries, and systems: The "5S" evolution of information services for evidence-based healthcare decisions. *Evidence-Based Nursing*, *10*(1), 6–7. doi:10.1136/ebn.10.1.6

Haynes, R. B. (2006). Of studies, syntheses, synopses, summaries, and systems: The "5S" evolution of information services for evidence-based health care decisions. *ACP Journal Club*, *145*(3), A8. doi:ACPJC-2006-145-3-A08

Khan, K. S., Daya, S., & Jadad, A. (1996). The importance of quality of primary studies in producing unbiased systematic reviews. *Archives of Internal Medicine*, *156*(6), 661–666.

Laupacis, A. (1997). Methodological studies of systematic reviews: Is there publication bias? *Archives of Internal Medicine*, *157*(3), 357–358.

McGowan, J., & Sampson, M. (2005). Systematic reviews need systematic searchers. *Journal of the Medical Library Association*, *93*(1), 74–80.

McKibbon, A., & Wilczynski, N. (2009). *PDQ: Pretty Darned Quick. Evidence-based principles and practice* (2nd ed.). Shelton, CT: People's Medical Publishing House.

CHAPTER SEVEN

Critical Appraisal

Susan W. Salmond

OBJECTIVES

Upon completion of Chapter 7, you will be able to:

- Explain the importance of critical appraisal to the systematic review process
- Select the appropriate critical appraisal tool based on the design of study
- Critically appraise a primary study or a systematic review

IMPORTANT POINTS

- Critical appraisal is an assessment of the benefits and strengths of research against its flaws and weaknesses.
- There are several different tools available for assessing quality of research studies within the context of a systematic review based on the type of study design used.
- Critical appraisal is essential for the inclusion of only the highest quality studies available for a systematic review

INTRODUCTION

A systematic review is a form of secondary research that gathers primary studies on the clinical question of interest and analyzes the data from these multiple studies to reach a conclusion. The quality of this research is, in part, dependent on the believability of the primary studies that are included in the review. To ensure this quality, critical appraisal is an integral part of the systematic review process (Hammick, Dornan, & Steinert, 2010). Critical appraisal is completed independently by two reviewers to assess for methodologic rigor to determine whether the results of the primary research are sufficiently valid to be considered useful information (Evans, 2001). A detailed log of the rejected articles is kept, and in the final write-up, a table of excluded articles providing the citation and the reason for exclusion is included.

Greenhalgh (2006) reminds us that the goal of critical appraisal is not finding methodologically flawless papers and that, in reality, there are flaws in 99%

147

of research studies. Rather, the aim is to identify papers that are "good enough" (Hoffmann, Bennett, & Del Mar, 2010). The critical appraisal provides a balanced assessment of the benefits and strengths of research against its flaws and weaknesses. The parameters used for evaluating validity vary according to the specific research design.

Three broad questions are addressed with quantitative critical appraisal—are the results valid, what are the results, and will the results help with one's own patient population. Validity refers to one's assessment of how close the study results are to the truth. In studies where the aim is to determine cause and effect, the focus of validity appraisal is on internal validity. Thus, validity questions focus on assignment of participants to treatments, whether participants who entered the study are sufficiently accounted for at its conclusion, whether the groups were similar at the start of the trial, whether blinding was used, and whether groups were treated ethically. Validity of qualitative research follows a different paradigm, and the research is appraised for credibility of the researcher and credibility of methods. Appraisal focusing on quantitative results ensures that there is adequate reporting of data collection methods and that analysis was appropriate, whether key findings and the significance and precision of the results are reported appropriately. In qualitative research, the focus is on confirmability and dependability. Applicability questions examine whether the results can be applied to one's own practice and population. In quantitative research, the focus is whether all important outcomes and the benefits of the intervention versus the harms and the costs were considered. In qualitative research, the aim is not to generalize but to transfer findings to situations that are contextually similar. Questions focus on the contextual similarity.

TOOLS FOR CRITICAL APPRAISAL

There are many different tools available for assessing the quality of research studies within the context of a systematic review. Tools vary based on the type of design used. These generally take the form of scales wherein quality criteria are scored and combined in a summary score or checklists in which specific questions are asked, and the reviewers must determine which questions are critical to quality for inclusion. Checklists are the most commonly used and recommended. No single score is universally accepted, and validity has not been established for many of the appraisal approaches (Margaliot & Chung, 2007). If undertaking a systematic review for Cochrane Collaboration, Campbell Collaboration, or Joanna Briggs Institute, there are requirements for what appraisal tools are used, and the reader should refer to the appropriate website.

Papers need to be read and reread during the appraisal process. For novice appraisers or for novice review researchers, there is a learning curve to understanding and applying the appraisal criteria. For the novice, this can be facilitated by using a mentor for appraisal of a select number of articles until the mentor has deemed the researcher to have the necessary skills and competencies. Because all appraisals are done by two reviewers, with availability of a third for areas of dispute, accuracy is enhanced.

APPRAISAL OF EFFECTIVENESS RESEARCH

Randomized controlled trials (RCT) are considered the gold standard for intervention research. RCTs usually measure short-term effects in select populations under strict (highly controlled) conditions—thus, testing for efficacy. By using randomization or allocation by chance, the intent is that the groups being compared are similar in terms of both measured and unmeasured baseline factors (Rochon et al., 2005), thus increasing the likelihood that differences in the dependent variable are attributable to the treatment variable. Critical appraisal of this type of design examines internal validity or the extent to which the study design, conduct, and analysis has minimized or avoided biases in its comparison of treatments. Bias is a form of systematic or predictable error in which the observed results may in fact be different from the true results. In the presence of significant bias, the results may not be considered valid or trustworthy. Therefore, in considering whether a study should be included in a systematic review of effectiveness, it is important to appraise for sources of bias. With RCTs, one would assess for four types of systematic errors that could result in bias: (a) selection bias, (b) performance bias, (c) attrition bias, and (d) detection bias (Magarey, 2001; The Joanna Briggs Institute, 2008). An explanation of these systematic biases and how to appraise for them is described further in Table 7.1.

There are dozens of scales and checklists that can be found for appraising effectiveness studies. Most of the tools measure beyond internal validity, and capture criteria of quality, precision of the study, and applicability. Questions such as "Did the study ask a clearly focused question?" "Did the study have enough participants to minimize the play of chance?" and "How are the results presented and what is the main result?" are examples that capture quality of the study rather than bias. Questions such as "Are your patients so different from those studied that the results may not apply to them?" target applicability. Questions such as "Were participants appropriately allocated to intervention and control groups?" "Were participants, staff, and study personnel 'blind' to participants' study group?" and "Were all of the participants who entered the trial accounted for at its conclusion?" are examples of questions focusing on potential bias. The Cochrane Collaboration has a separate tool for assessing the risk of bias in RCTs.

The Cochrane group distinguishes bias from quality. Bias addresses the issue of believability of the findings. Quality focuses on whether the study was carried out to the highest possible standards and is larger in scope than bias. It is possible to have a study carried out with the highest possible standards, yet still have an important risk of bias. For example, in a study where participants are not blinded to their group allocation, the study may be carried out with high quality, yet performance bias may still be an issue (Higgins & Green, 2008).

A challenge to the reviewer appraising studies is that review of the published articles often does not clearly report the methodology. This may require contacting the author for clarification on the approaches used. There is an international movement to improve the reporting of an RCT research. The Consolidated Standards of Reporting Trials (CONSORT) Statement calls for better reporting of a trial's design, conduct, analysis and interpretation, and can be used to assess the validity of its results. A 25-item checklist of information to include when reporting a randomized trial is available through the CONSORT website at http://www.consort-statement.org/home.

TABLE 7.1

Appraising for Bias in Effectiveness Studies

Type of Bias	Explanation of Bias	Critical Appraisal for Bias
Selection bias	■ Results from errors in the way that research participants were selected into the study from the target population or because of factors that influence whether research participants remained in a study. ■ The intervention group is therefore different from the control/comparison group in measured or unmeasured baseline characteristics, and this difference may impact prognosis or outcomes ■ Also used to mean that the participants are not representative of the population of all possible participants ■ Greater chance for selection bias with nonrandom samples or when the individual assigning participants to intervention groups has the ability to select which group the individual will be assigned to	Randomization and allocation concealment are key to minimizing selection bias. Evaluate whether: ■ Randomization was used ■ The allocation sequence was appropriate (such as using a random component in the sequence generation, such as a random-number table, coin toss, or throwing dice) ■ Allocation was adequately concealed
Performance bias	■ Systematic differences in care provided to the participants in the intervention and control/comparison group ■ In the presence of differences in the care provided, one cannot confidently conclude that the intervention under investigation caused the effect ■ More likely to occur if the caregiver is aware of whether a patient is in a control or treatment group ■ Blinding is an approach to prevent the subject and/or researcher clinician from knowing the allocated intervention	■ Was there blinding of subject? ■ Was there blinding of researcher/clinician?
Attrition bias	■ Differences between control and treatment groups in terms of patients dropping out of a study, or not being followed up, as thoroughly as others in the groups ■ Attrition of participants from a study can produce bias if the incidence rates in people who drop out differ from those who complete the study ■ Although dropouts will occur, the researchers want to be assured that missing outcome data is balanced in numbers across groups with similar reasons for missing data across groups	■ Was loss to follow-up (dropout, nonresponse, withdrawal, protocol deviators) reported? ■ Did researchers apply the concept of intention to treat?

(Continued)

TABLE 7.1

Appraising for Bias in Effectiveness Studies *(Continued)*

Type of Bias	Explanation of Bias	Critical Appraisal for Bias
Detection (assessor or ascertainment) bias	■ Occurs if outcomes are measured differently for patients depending on whether they are in the control or treatment group ■ A detection bias generally occurs when the assessor (the one determining the outcome results) knows whether the subject is in the control or intervention group	■ Was blinding of the assessor carried out?

APPRAISAL OF OBSERVATIONAL STUDIES

Observational studies include various types of designs (cohort, case-controlled) that compare outcomes in groups that did and did not receive an intervention, but allocation is not through randomization. Evans and Pearson (2001) point out that observational studies are frequently the best choice in cases where ethics does not allow exposing a group to harmful agents, when measuring infrequent adverse outcomes, evaluating interventions designed to prevent rare events, and when examining long-term outcomes. Because observational studies do not use randomization and generally have less restrictive inclusion and exclusion criteria compared with RCTs, they typically are at greater risk for bias but are more reflective of the population at large (external validity). In fact, one of the advantages of a cohort design is that it can determine whether efficacy observed in randomized trials translates into effectiveness in broader populations and in more realistic settings (Rochon et al., 2005).

When randomization is not used or when subjects can select their own treatments, or their environments inflict treatments on them, there is a greater risk that the differences in outcomes are caused by pretreatment differences (confounders) rather than to the effects of the treatment. The CONSORT definition of confounding is a situation in which the estimated intervention effect is biased because of some difference between the comparison groups apart from the planned intervention. This could include baseline characteristics, prognostic factors, or concomitant interventions (http://www.consort-statement.org). Selection of the comparison group should be done so that it is as close to matching the intervention group as possible, and the decision making regarding comparison group selection should be clear.

To minimize this risk, recruitment of subjects should use techniques such as matching to achieve comparability of the covariates of concern across groups. For example, in a case-control study where smoking is deemed as a confounding factor, cases and controls can be matched by smoking status, so that for each case who smokes, a control who smokes is found (Boccia et al., 2007). Information on the distribution of potential confounders within the two comparison groups should be provided to demonstrate comparability. Restriction is another approach to control confounders.

In restriction, one uses more restrictive inclusion/exclusion criteria to limit the potential of a known confounder. However, there may be unknown confounders that would typically be evenly distributed in the randomization, but with matching, there is less protection. Post hoc analysis can also minimize confounding effects. Use of stratification or multivariable modeling can provide estimates of the confounding effect.

Because observational studies do not use randomization, appraisal focuses on the approach to recruitment of cases and controls in order to have matching or comparability of subjects, the accuracy of measurement of exposure and outcome to minimize bias, the identification of potential confounders, careful definition of exposure for case selection, precision of results, and applicability to the local population. Although questions for reporting and applicability are generally similar to effectiveness studies, questions on validity will differ. Typical questions examining validity include whether there is support for the choice of the study method, whether the population studied is appropriate, whether confounding and bias are considered, and whether follow-up was long enough.

APPRAISAL OF QUALITATIVE STUDIES

Critical appraisal of qualitative studies differs significantly from quantitative approaches; in fact, there is even a debate whether critical appraisal should be done for qualitative syntheses (Hannes, Lockwood, & Pearson, 2010). In this chapter, we have adopted the viewpoint that critical appraisal is an integral part of the systematic review process with the goal to synthesize quality studies. However, qualitative research is grounded in a different philosophical perspective than quantitative research; therefore, the goal of critical appraisal for qualitative research is not to minimize bias. Applying criteria from a quantitative paradigm to appraise qualitative research is inappropriate, and one must use different criteria to judge the rigor of quantitative and qualitative designs.

Differences in the Quantitative and Qualitative Paradigms

The quantitative paradigm is grounded in the concept of logical positivism with the belief that the world is made up of observable, measurable facts. The focus is on measurement and analysis of causal relationships between variables, prediction, and generalization of findings (Golafshani, 2003) and, to this end, the approach is reductionistic—attempting to fragment and delimit phenomena into measurable or common categories. The focus is on defining concepts and operationalizing measures that represent the concepts. Thus, validity and reliability take on central importance in this paradigm (Devers, 1999).

Qualitative research uses a naturalistic approach, and the goal is to understand phenomena within the real context, without any attempt to manipulate the phenomenon of interest. The qualitative research paradigm is grounded in constructivism or interpretivism, which views knowledge and meaning as dynamic, contextual, and socially constructed from the interaction between human beings and their world (Devers, 1999). The goal of qualitative research is illumination, generating understanding of phenomenon within specific contexts and extrapolation to similar situations or contexts (Golafshani, 2003). In qualitative research, the researcher is the instrument, and the credibility of qualitative research depends on the ability and effort of the researcher.

Criteria for Qualitative Appraisal

Although there are numerous appraisal tools for qualitative research, there is no clear-cut definitive list of criteria. The aim of appraisal is to ensure that there is enough breadth and depth of the resorted data to suggest that the findings are trustworthy (Jones, 2004).

Cohen and Crabtree (2008) did a cross-publication content analysis of journal articles and texts that discussed criteria for rigorous qualitative research. They identified seven criteria for good qualitative research: (a) carrying out ethical research, (b) importance of the research, (c) clarity and coherence of the research report, (d) use of appropriate and rigorous methods, (e) importance of reflexivity or attending to researcher bias, (f) importance of establishing validity or credibility, and (g) importance of verification or reliability. They concluded that there was consensus on the first four criteria and divergent opinion on the remaining three, because qualitative researches have mixed views on whether it is appropriate for applying concepts such as bias, validity, and reliability (even though the criteria have been adapted to be appropriate to the qualitative paradigm) to qualitative work.

There have been many attempts to translate the concepts of validity, bias, and reliability to the qualitative paradigm. To this end, the concepts of rigor, trustworthiness, plausibility, and credibility have been the qualitative equivalent of validity, dependability, the corollary of reliability, and confirmability reflecting the process to decrease bias. The goal of qualitative work is not generalization, rather transferability—a term capturing the contextual similarity—is a more appropriate concept (Lincoln & Guba, 1985). Understanding these concepts is important to qualitative critical appraisal. Table 7.2 provides further explanation of these translated concepts and strategies that can be used to ensure them.

Validity in Qualitative Research

Hannes et al. (2010) focused their efforts not on translation but on clarifying what qualitative researchers do to establish validity and identification of the threats to validity. They define qualitative appraisal *criteria* as the standards to be upheld as ideals in qualitative research and define *techniques* as the methods used to minimize threats to validity. Using Maxwell's framework, which stresses that validity is based on the kinds of understanding we have of the phenomena under study, the authors described and compared appraisal tools on five types of validity: (a) descriptive, (b) interpretive, (c) theoretical, (d) generalizability, and (e) evaluative validity. They propose that descriptive, interpretive, and theoretical validity are central to qualitative research. It should be noted, however, that these categorizations are not discrete but overlapping concepts.

TABLE 7.2
Critical Appraisal From a Qualitative Paradigm

Concept	Definition/Explanation	Techniques to Facilitate Achieving the Concept
Credibility	■ The extent to which findings and conclusions are supported by data/study evidence. The findings/conclusion makes sense and has a coherent logic. ■ Includes credibility of researcher, method, and findings	
Credibility of researcher	■ Researcher must be credible, and any experiences that could influence interpretation of the phenomenon should be identified.	■ Are researchers' qualifications, experiences, perspectives, and assumptions identified? ■ Are there any personal connections between the researcher and the topic or participants?
Credibility of method	■ Strategies can be built into data collection to enhance credibility of findings such as prolonged engagement for observation or interview methods. ■ Triangulation (using multiple methods or data sources) to study the phenomenon of interest	■ Was there sufficient engagement for the researcher to gather trustworthy data? ■ Was more than one method used in data collection? ■ Were the data sources used sufficient to gather a full perspective of the phenomenon of interest?
Credibility of findings	■ Use of a second researcher to analyze and confirm data and to ask questions about methods, meanings, and interpretation of the data ■ Having participants from the study review the findings and give their views regarding the credibility of the interpretations and findings enhances credibility. ■ Triangulation uses multiple data sources, investigators, methods, or theories to provide corroborating evidence to substantiate the findings. ■ Search for disconfirming evidence ("deviant" or "negative" cases). Actively search for cases that do not fit the pattern and refine the theory and working hypotheses in light of this evidence.	■ Was a second researcher used for peer review? ■ Was peer debriefing used? ■ Was member checking used? ■ Was triangulation used? ■ Were approaches to seek disconfirming evidence identified?

(Continued)

TABLE 7.2

Critical Appraisal From a Qualitative Paradigm *(Continued)*

Concept	Definition/Explanation	Techniques to Facilitate Achieving the Concept
Transferability (also referred to as applicability and fittingness)	■ Transferability addresses the extent to which the findings can be applied to other contexts. ■ Thick description and purposive sampling are strategies to enhance transferability. ■ Providing a detailed description of the context facilitates decisions about transferability.	■ Was the sample and context clearly defined?
Dependability (reliability)	■ Achieved through the use of an audit trail or data archiving—allows an independent examiner to track the decisions made and the steps taken in the study ■ Use of a skeptical peer review where another individual skilled in the research approach asks questions about the methods, meanings, and interpretation of the data	■ Did the study describe methods to identify transparency in decision making during the analysis process? ■ Was the analysis confirmed by a second researcher? ■ Was a tape recorder or other mechanical device used to record the interviews?
Confirmability (objectivity, bias reduction)	■ Use of triangulation ■ Use of skeptical peer review or audits ■ Search for disconfirming evidence or negative cases ■ Reflective journal keeping by the researcher chronicling how his or her personal characteristics, feelings, and biases may be influencing the work, and what strategies have been used to manage them	■ Was triangulation used? ■ Did the study describe methods to identify transparency in decision making during the analysis process? ■ Was the analysis confirmed by a second researcher? ■ Did the researcher document a reflexive approach?

Adapted from Beck, 1993; Devers, 1999; Patton, 2002.

Descriptive validity is "the degree to which descriptive information such as events, subjects, setting, time, and places are accurately reported" (Hannes et al., 2010, p. 5). It captures criteria that ask the reviewer to determine the impact of the investigator and whether the context was adequately reported. The manuscript should provide an understanding of the context in which the research was carried out. This helps in understanding the phenomenon as well as in decision making about transferability of the findings. Components of context include the physical setting as well as the investigator's role in the setting. Because the researcher is the instrument, one must appreciate that the interaction of the researcher and setting influences the nature and types of data collected. Any events over time that could have changed the nature of the study or affected the results should be reported. To this end, appraisal criteria that address context could determine if there is a statement locating the researcher culturally or could ask the questions, "What role does the researcher adopt within the setting?" and "Are the findings interpreted within the context of other studies and theory?" Criteria focusing on the impact of the investigator could ask "whether the influence of the researcher on the research and vice versa has been made clear," "Has the relationship between researchers and participants been adequately considered?" "Are the researcher's own position, assumptions, and possible biases outlined?" and "Is there evidence of reflexivity—that the researcher has reflected on his or her potential personal influence in the collection and analysis of data?"

Interpretive validity is "the degree to which participant's viewpoints, thoughts, intentions, and experiences are accurately understood and reported by the qualitative researcher" (Hannes et al., 2010, p. 5). Using the words of the informants as building blocks, researchers construct interpretive accounts of the phenomenon. The primary question is the "believability" of this account. Appraisal criteria may ask "whether participants, and their voices, are heard," or "is there adequate evidence provided to support the analysis?" Techniques to enhance interpretive validity include member checking, participant feedback, close collaboration with participants, peer debriefing, methods and analytic triangulation, and self-reflection by the researcher on potential biases, preconceptions, assumptions, and reference frameworks (Hannes et al., 2010).

Theoretical validity is "the degree to which a theory or theoretical explanation informing or developed from a research study fits the data and is, therefore credible and defensible" (Hannes et al., 2010, p. 5). Criteria capturing theoretical validity include items on the theoretical framework (i.e., "Is there congruency between the stated philosophical perspective and the research methodology?" and "What theoretical framework guides or informs the study?") and on evaluation/outcome criteria (i.e., "Do conclusions drawn in the research report appear to flow from the analysis, or interpretation, of the data?" or "Is the conclusion justified given the conduct of the study?). Techniques to enhance theoretical validity include prolonged engagement such that there is "sufficient time to study the subjects and setting and to create a set of patterns and relationships that are stable and contribute to an understanding of why these occur" (Hannes et al., 2010, p. 6). Theory triangulation and searching for disconfirming or negative cases are also approaches to ensuring theoretical validity.

Generalizability (external validity) is "the degree to which findings can be extended to other persons, times, or settings than those directly studied" (Hannes et al., 2010, p. 5). In appraisal tools, the criterion addressing this concept falls under the criterion value and implications of research. Items identified assessing this criterion include the following: "How valuable is the research?" "To what setting and population are the study findings generalizable?" and "What are the implications for policy and practice?"

Evaluative validity is "the degree to which an evaluative framework or critique is applied to the object of the study" (Hannes et al., 2010, p. 5). It establishes the "degree to which a certain phenomenon under study is legitimate, justified, or raises questions, and involves the application of an evaluative framework to the phenomenon under study" (Hannes et al., 2010, p. 3). Critical appraisal criteria, which have an item on "outcome/evaluation," may capture a component of evaluative validity; however, qualitative researchers do not attempt to evaluate the phenomenon under study.

Evaluation of the Quality of Study Design

Consistent with all research, the research design should be appropriate for the question of interest. Sampling approaches, data collection methods, data types and sources, data analysis methods, and reporting of findings are criteria that can be used to facilitate an overall judgment of the quality of the research and whether the researchers who conducted the research are consistent with standards of qualitative research (Hannes et al., 2010). Qualitative analysis, unlike quantitative analysis, does not follow a strict formula and rules-oriented approach to analysis, rather, uses a more creative process, which depends on the insights and conceptual capabilities of the analyst (Patton, 1999). It requires the research to recognize patterns, which, in part, is an intuitive process. However, complementing the intuitive process is technical rigor, which is a systematic process. The qualitative researcher needs to report sufficient details related to data collection and the processes of analysis used in order for readers to judge the quality of the resulting product. In qualitative research, designs evolve during data collection and analysis. The paper should clearly indicate how and why the study design changed.

Strategies for Enhancing Rigor

There are several strategies that can be employed by qualitative researchers to enhance study rigor and methods for gathering high-quality data that are carefully analyzed and, consequently, have more confidence in the findings. Some of these strategies have been presented in Table 7.2 but will be expanded on in the text that follows.

Triangulation is an approach that corroborates that the research findings accurately reflect people's perceptions. There are different types of triangulation: researcher, method, source, and theoretical. Using multiple observers/researchers, recording and describing the participants' behavior and context allow for cross-checking of observations and enhances descriptive validity. Using multiple methods broadens the understanding of the phenomenon. Its usefulness arises from the logic that no single method ever adequately solves the problem of rival explanations. Because each method reveals different aspects of empirical reality, multiple methods of data collection and analysis provide cross-data validity checks enhancing confidence in the trustworthiness of the findings/explanations and, therefore, enhance interpretive validity. Examining the consistency of different data sources within the same method is triangulation of sources. Theoretical triangulation uses multiple perspectives or theories to interpret and explain the data. Patton reminds us, however, that the goal is not to find the same result but to test for consistency in the results. Different kinds of day may yield somewhat different results, because different modes of inquiry are sensitive to different real-world nuances, and better understanding of these inconsistencies is illuminative (Patton, 1999).

Analysis or documentation of evaluator's effects is considered important to establishing credibility or validity of qualitative research. There are four ways in which the researcher can influence the findings of a study: (a) the participants may react differently because of the researcher; (b) the researcher may change during the course of the data collection or analysis; (c) the researcher brings forward predispositions, selective perceptions, and/or biases; and (d) the researcher's level of training or preparation may influence the ability to collect and analyze the data (Patton, 1999, 2002). Not only must these areas of concern be addressed in the study, but also there are collection and analysis techniques that minimize this threat. Ensuring that there is sufficient or prolonged engagement allows for a period for researcher and participants to get used to each other. Keeping daily field notes and monitoring observer effects by either direct questioning or observation demonstrates the researcher's awareness of this threat. Similarly, daily field notes with attention to shifts in one's own attitudes and behaviors monitor researcher change. Addressing researcher predispositions or biases involves declaring any personal connections between the researcher and the topic or participants, stating up front prior interpretations or experiences with the phenomenon, as well as maintaining a posture of empathic neutrality in which the researcher is caring toward the people under study but neutral or impartial about the findings. Lastly, the issue or researcher competence is closely tied to perceived credibility of the findings. The study should document what verification or validation procedures were used to establish quality of the analysis. Use of an audit trail or data archiving allows for an independent examiner to track the decisions made and steps taken in the analysis of the data. Having a "skeptical peer review" where another researcher skilled in the research approach asks questions about the methods, meanings, and interpretation of the data, or having an independent researcher analyze samples of the data to compare interpretations are techniques to enhance the trustworthiness of the findings. The analysis process and findings in terms of patterns, linkages, and plausible explanations should be clearly described, and the report should provide information on approaches taken to test these findings by searching for disconfirming evidence or negative cases.

Transferability is the degree to which the findings from qualitative research can be transferred or generalized to other contexts or settings. Transferability can be enhanced by thoroughly describing the research context (study participants, demographics, contextual background information) and providing thick description on the sending and receiving context. In this way, readers can make informed decisions about "to whom the results might be generalized or to which groups the findings can be transferred" (Hannes et al., 2010, p. 6).

CRITICAL APPRAISAL OF SYSTEMATIC REVIEWS

The purpose of a systematic review is to provide reliable evidence summaries. The quality of the review and what tends to set systematic reviews apart from narrative reviews is in part based on the degree to which systematic methods were used to reduce the risk of error and bias. A systematic review becomes systematic through development and adherence to an explicit and auditable protocol for review (O'Mathúna, Fineout-Overholt, & Kent, 2008; Sandelowski, 2008). The protocol, as described in Chapter 3, sets forth the background for the review, the review question (generally, using the PICO or PICo formats), and the inclusion and exclusion criteria that will guide the study selection, the search strategy, the approach to appraisal of the studies, and the approach to analyze and synthesize the findings. Although a published manuscript may not provide the total protocol/proposal, it should at least be referred to in the published manuscript giving evidence of an a priori plan for the process.

Even when using an established protocol, the reality is that not all systematic reviews are of equal quality, and it is critical for the user of research to critically appraise the systematic review for its degree of rigor. As for single studies, there are many approaches to critical appraisal of systematic reviews. Used here is an adaptation of the Joanna Briggs Institute's (2000) guide for systematic review appraisal. The questions described in Table 7.3 follow the general review process ending with reporting of the findings, conclusions, and recommendations.

The *research's question* should be clearly and explicitly stated. If not clearly stated, the utility of the remainder of the study is questionable. A systematic review tends to have narrow or focused questions, but many systematic reviews have been broader using several subquestions. Using the PICO format in quantitative research, the question

TABLE 7.3
Critical Appraisal of a Systematic Review

Review question	Is the review question clearly and explicitly stated?
Search strategy	Were comprehensive search methods used to locate studies?
	Was a thorough search done of appropriate databases and were other potentially important sources explored?
Inclusion criteria	How were studies selected?
Critical appraisal	Was the validity of studies assessed appropriately?
Similarity of studies	Were the populations of the different studies similar?
	Was the same intervention/phenomenon of interest evaluated by the individual studies?
	Were the same outcomes used to determine the effectiveness of the intervention being evaluated?
	Were reasons for differences between studies explored?
Reporting of findings	Are review methods clearly documented?
	Is the review question clearly and explicitly stated?
	Was the search strategy reported?
	Was the inclusion criteria reported?
	Was the criteria for appraising studies reported?
	Were the methods used to combine studies reported?
Conclusions and recommendations	Is a summary of findings provided?
	Are specific directives for new research proposed?
	Were the recommendations supported by the reported data?

Source: Adapted from The Joanna Briggs Institute (2000). Appraising systematic reviews. *Changing Practice: Evidence Based Practice Information Sheets for Health Professionals.* (Suppl 1), 1–6.

encompasses the components of (a) population of interest and condition, (b) intervention, (c) comparison or control intervention, and (d) outcome of interest. Setting and time may also be part of the question. For qualitative reviews, the mnemonic PICo captures the components of (a) population, (b) phenomena of interest, and (c) context.

A clear, transparent, and comprehensive *search strategy* is a critical component of a systematic review (Manchikanti, 2008; O'Mathúna et al., 2008). The search strategy should be transparent so that it is reproducible, not only by other researchers, but also by the primary author so that the review can be updated. The aim of a comprehensiveness search is to locate as much of the completed research on the topic as possible (The Joanna Briggs Institute, 2000). This involves not only searching multiple databases and the grey literature, but also using additional search strategies such as footnote chasing and key author and organization identification to identify missed papers—both published and unpublished. Appraisal of the search strategy captures whether the appropriate bibliographic databases were used, whether there was follow-up from reference lists, whether personal contact with experts was made, whether unpublished studies were identified, and whether non-English language studies were searched.

Inclusion and exclusion criteria operationalizes the review question and reduces selection bias by specifying a priori the boundaries, rather than including/excluding studies based on their results. These criteria define the scope of the review and should specify which type of study designs will be included in the review as well as specifying the parameters for the population, intervention, and outcomes. Additionally, temporal and linguistic constraints should be identified (Manchikanti, 2008). By establishing these criteria a priori, it limits the risk of selection bias.

As clearly highlighted earlier in this chapter, in the systematic review process, *critical appraisal* is done of each potential study's research design to ensure the validity prior to the final determination to include or exclude the study. Because the goal is to pool data, the purpose of critical appraisal is to exclude lesser quality studies, thereby minimizing the risk of error and bias in the systematic review findings. Thus, when appraising a systematic review, it is necessary to determine whether the validity of studies was assessed appropriately. Appraisal should have been completed by two reviewers. Appraisal criteria vary by research design, but the review criteria used should be clearly documented. The review should provide a table of included and excluded studies. For included studies, an aggregated table of characteristics should be provided.

Reporting of findings or data synthesis provides the summary of results from the different studies in order to obtain an overall evaluation of the effectiveness of an intervention or a more in-depth representation of a phenomenon of interest. Quantitative results are reported in terms of treatment effects and precision. An overall evaluation of the effectiveness of an intervention or treatment can be determined with a meta-analysis. A meta-analysis takes similar measures from comparable studies, and when possible, the measures of the effect are combined. Methods for combining the studies should be reported. Studies are not pooled when there are differences in the population, intervention or how outcomes were measured, or when findings differ significantly. Thus, the reports should specify whether the populations of the different studies were similar; whether the same interventions were evaluated; whether the same outcomes were used to determine effectiveness; and whether the reasons for differences between studies were explored. The characteristics and results of each study should be clearly displayed in an included studies table. When pooling is not possible, a narrative table can be used presenting focused results. For qualitative systematic reviews, the process of data extraction should be clearly documented with a clear depiction of how findings were interpreted into a new coding structure and synthesis.

Conclusions, recommendations, and *implications* for research and clinical practice flow from the findings of the review. For effectiveness studies, the main result and the size and confidence of that result guide recommendations and implications. For all designs, the authors should provide a summary of the findings, suggest new directions for research, and make recommendations for practice that are supported by the reported data.

SUMMARY

Critical appraisal is one of the more important steps of a systematic review. The determination to include or exclude a paper from the review can mean the difference between a good review and a mediocre review. There are many tools available to assess the validity and relevance of a research article. By using one of these, the reviewer has a foundation on which to choose only the most relevant, high-quality studies available for inclusion in the review.

EXERCISES

Read the following systematic review. Write a letter to the editor of the journal regarding the adequacy of the critical appraisal process that was used to determine what articles to include in the review: Cummings, G., Lee, H., MacGregor, T., Davey, M., Wong, C., Paul, L., & Stafford, E. (2008). Factors contributing to nursing leadership: A systematic review. *Journal of Health Services Research & Policy, 13*(4), 240–248. doi:10.1258/jhsrp.2008.007154

REFERENCES

Beck, C. T. (1993). Qualitative research: The evaluation of its credibility, fittingness, and auditability. *Western Journal of Nursing Research, 15*(2), 263–266.

Boccia, S., La Torre, G., Persiani, R., D'Ugo, D., van Duijn, C. M., & Ricciardi, G. (2007). A critical appraisal of epidemiological studies comes from basic knowledge: A reader's guide to assess potential for biases. *World Journal of Emergency Surgery, 2*, 7.

Cohen, D. J., & Crabtree, B. F. (2008). Evaluative criteria for qualitative research in health care: Controversies and recommendations. *Annals of Family Medicine, 6*(4), 331–339.

Cummings, G., Lee, H., MacGregor, T., Davey, M., Wong, C., Paul, L., & Stafford, E. (2008). Factors contributing to nursing leadership: A systematic review. *Journal of Health Services Research & Policy, 13*(4), 240–248. doi:10.1258/jhsrp.2008.007154

Devers, K. J. (1999). How will we know "good" qualitative research when we see it? Beginning the dialogue in health services research. *Health Services Research, 34*(5 Pt 2), 1153–1188.

Evans, D. (2001). Systematic reviews of nursing research. *Intensive & Critical Care Nursing, 17*(1), 51–57.

Evans, D., & Pearson, A. (2001). Systematic reviews: Gatekeepers of nursing knowledge. *Journal of Clinical Nursing, 10*(5), 593–599.

Fineout-Overholt, E., O'Mathúna, D. P., & Kent, B. (2008). How systematic reviews can foster evidence-based clinical decisions. *Worldviews on Evidence-Based Nursing, 5*(1), 45–48.

Golafshani, N. (2003). Understanding reliability and validity in qualitative research. *The Qualitative Report, 8*(4), 597–607.

Greenhalgh, T. (2006). *How to read a paper: The basics of evidence-based medicine* (3rd ed.). Oxford, UK: Blackwell.

Hammick, M., Dornan, T., & Steinert, Y. (2010). Conducting a best evidence systematic review. Part1: From idea to data coding. BEME Guide No. 13. *Medical Teacher, 32*(1), 3–15.

Hannes, K., Lockwood, C., & Pearson, A. (2010). A comparative analysis of three online appraisal instruments' ability to assess validity in qualitative research. *Qualitative Health Research, 20*(12), 1736–1743. doi:10.1177/1049732310378656

Higgins, J. P. T., & Green, S. (2008). *Cochrane handbook for systematic reviews of interventions.* West Sussex, UK: John Wiley & Sons.

Hoffmann, T., Bennett, S., & Del Mar, C., Eds. (2010). *Evidence-based practice across the health professions.* New South Wales, Australia: Elsevier.

The Joanna Briggs Institute. (2000). Appraising systematic reviews. *Changing Practice: Evidence Based Practice Information Sheets for Health Professionals*, (Suppl 1), 1–6.

The Joanna Briggs Institute. (2008). *Joanna Briggs Institute reviewers' manual: 2008 edition.* Adelaide, Australia: Author.

Jones, M. L. (2004). Application of systematic review methods to qualitative research: Practical issues. *Journal of Advanced Nursing, 48*(3), 271–278.

Lincoln, Y. S., & Guba, E. G. (1985). *Naturalistic inquiry.* Newbury Park, CA: Sage.

Magarey, J. M. (2001). Elements of a systematic review. *International Journal of Nursing Practice, 7*(6), 376–382.

Manchikanti, L. (2008). Evidence-based medicine, systematic reviews, and guidelines in interventional pain management, part I: Introduction and general considerations. *Pain Physician, 11*(2), 161–186.

Margaliot, Z., & Chung, K. C. (2007). Systematic reviews: A primer for plastic surgery research. *Plastic and Reconstructive Surgery, 120*(7), 1834–1841.

O'Mathúna, D. P., Fineout-Overholt, E., & Kent, B. (2008). How systematic reviews can foster evidence-based clinical decisions: Part II. *Worldviews on Evidence-Based Nursing, 5*(2), 102–107.

Patton, M. Q. (1999). Enhancing the quality and credibility of qualitative analysis. *Health Services Research, 34*(5 Pt 2): 1189–1208.

Patton, M. Q. (2002). *Qualitative research and evaluation methods* (3rd ed.). Thousand Oaks, CA: Sage.

Rochon, P. A., Gurwitz, J. H., Sykora, K., Mamdani, M., Streiner, D. L., Garfinkel, S., . . . Anderson, G. M. (2005). Reader's guide to critical appraisal of cohort studies: 1. Role and design. *British Medical Journal, 330*(7496), 895–897.

Sandelowski, M. (2008). Reading, writing and systematic review. *Journal of Advanced Nursing, 64*(1), 104–110.

SUGGESTED READINGS

Mason, D. J. (2005). The evidence of things not seen: It takes good research and more to practice evidence-based nursing. *American Journal of Nursing, 105*(9), 11.

Mishra, L. D., & Agarwal, A. (2010). The art of critically reviewing a medical article. *The Indian Anaesthetists' Forum.* Retrieved from http://www.theiaforum.org/Article_Folder/Critical-Review-Medical-Article.pdf

PART IV

Methods for Systematic Reviews

CHAPTER EIGHT

Systematic Review of Experimental Evidence: Meta-Analysis

Cheryl Holly

OBJECTIVES

Upon completion of Chapter 8, you will be able to:

- Define meta-analysis
- State the purposes of a meta-analysis
- Assess and identify threats to the internal validity of a meta-analysis
- Identify sources of variation
- Interpret results of a meta-analysis

IMPORTANT POINTS

- A meta-analysis is the statistical analysis of findings from two or more primary studies for the purposes of amalgamating the results across the studies, with the same methodological rigor applied to primary research.
- The purpose of a meta-analysis is to pool the results of primary studies to determine effect size.
- Meta-analysis of experimental evidence involves the extraction of data from randomized controlled trials.
- Meta-analysis can play an important role in developing research studies, setting policy, and/or making decisions at the point of care.

INTRODUCTION

In 1952, Hans Eysenck concluded that psychotherapy did not work and using it as a treatment modality was a waste of time. This started a debate that lasted until 1978 when Gene Glass, working with his colleague, Mary Lee Smith, statistically aggregated the findings of 375 psychotherapy outcome studies and concluded that psychotherapy did indeed result in positive outcomes. Glass called his method *meta-analysis*. Today, meta-analysis is an accepted form of research that provides the foundation for determining best practice, and allows an individual health care practitioner to make up-to-date decisions at the point of care (Lipsey & Wilson, 2001). In fact, Chalmers (2006) claimed that almost any intervention will be tested repeatedly and that it is imperative to look at a body of evidence, rather than individual studies. Meta-analysis refers to the statistical method for reviewing, pooling, and summarizing available quantitative findings from several primary research studies to produce an overall understanding of empirical knowledge, rather than collecting data from individual subjects (Littell, Corcoran, & Pillai, 2008). Borenstein, Hedges, Higgins, and Rothstein (2009) contended that the pooling and summarizing of these studies can only be meaningful if done systematically (i.e., within the context of a systematic review). A systematic review of experimental evidence can contain multiple meta-analyses, including subgroup analysis of the main review focus or separate analysis of effects of different outcomes within the same review. In effect, a systematic review pools all of the available findings on a given topic from smaller studies with few subjects into one larger study with many subjects. A meta-analysis of interventions can be understood as a survey of a series of research reports, rather than a survey of a group of people, where each report is interviewed (extracted and appraised) and the resulting data are analyzed (Lipsey & Wilson, 2001). Meta-analysis changes the focus from statistical significance to the direction and magnitude of the effects across studies by combining individual sample sizes and results, referred to as a *combined effect*. As such, it provides a more powerful and precise understanding than separate estimates from individual, smaller studies alone (Lipsey & Wilson, 2001). Meta-analysis can be conducted if studies have the same population, use the same intervention, and measure the same outcomes. The focus of this chapter is on the pooling of experimental evidence extracted from randomized controlled trials (RCT), which will be referred to as meta-analysis (i.e., a meta-analysis of interventions), although a meta-analysis can also be conducted with nonexperimental evidence (see Chapter 9) or in a nonrandomized manner (see Table 8.1).

META-ANALYSIS

Meta-analysis is used to analyze the major trends and variations across all of the studies included in the analysis (Littell et al., 2008). Its main purposes are to explore the relationship between two variables and the effect one has on the other, to determine the degree of variability between the variables, and to explain any identified variance.

In meta-analysis, the results of similar, but individual, studies are combined to determine the overall effect of an experiment (usually called the intervention or the treatment) when compared to either standard of care or a control intervention (which may be a placebo or nothing). In meta-analysis, the effect size and weight of each study are calculated so that results from different studies, which use different measures of the same construct or report results in different ways, can be pooled (Littell et al., 2008). The effect size indicates whether the results favor the treatment or the control (referred to as the direction and magnitude), whereas the weight indicates the amount of influence each individual study has on the overall results when all of the studies in the analysis are pooled (Pearson, Field, & Jordan, 2007).

TABLE 8.1

Types of Controlled Trials

Type of Controlled Trial	Level of Evidence	Randomization	Experimental Group	Control Group	Comments
Uncontrolled	Weak				No concurrent comparison exists. Controls are implicit.
Nonrandom-ized	Reliable if confirmed by an RCT or meta-analysis		X	X	Allocation to groups are nonrandom.
Randomized	Strongest	X	X	X	Subjects are allocated by a random method to the standard treat-ment group and one or more treatment groups.

Note: RCT = randomized controlled trial.
Source: Adapted from Stanley, K. (2007). Design of randomized controlled trials. *Circulation, 115*, 1164–1169.

Meta-analysis is a three-stage process, each with a distinct series of steps as seen in Table 8.2. Following the formulation of a review question, performance of a literature search, and selection of potential studies for appraisal, the first stage in the meta-analysis is the appraisal and extraction of data from each of the selected RCT studies. Extracted data are used to determine a summary estimate of effect and chance variation, called a *confidence interval*. All statistics are converted into a common metric. A summary statistic provides an overall estimate of the strength of relationship between independent and dependent variables, whereas a confidence interval indicates the precision of the estimate. The second stage involves entering data into a data management program and calculating a weighted mean across studies. Greater weight is given to some studies than others based on how precise the results are. Those studies with greater precision carry more weight, regardless of sample size. One criticism of meta-analysis is that it is additive in terms of results and simply calculates a summary statistic as if it is one large study. In reality, a meta-analysis calculates a weighted average by taking into account the results within each individual study. Unlike a narrative review where the weight or importance of a study for inclusion in a review is determined by unknown criteria, the weights assigned to each study in a systematic review are determined by mathematical criteria (Borenstein et al., 2009). The third stage is the generation and interpretation of a forest plot. A forest plot is a graphical representation of the relative strength of treatment effects in a meta-analysis of RCTs.

TABLE 8.2

Stages of Meta-Analysis

Preliminary Stages
Formulate a clinical question that demonstrates a comparison
Develop a search strategy for randomized controlled trials
Select studies for possible inclusion in the review
Stage 1
Appraise the selected studies for actual inclusion in the review using a prespecified study appraisal method
Develop a coding manual and data extraction form
Stage 2
Extract and code data using a prespecified data extraction tool
Enter data into a prespecified data management program
Calculate a pooled average
Stage 3
Generate and interpret the forest plot
Draw conclusions about best practice

Advantages and Disadvantages of a Meta-Analysis of Experimental Evidence

The results of a systematic review of experimental evidence can assist in discriminating between therapies and interventions that work from those that do not or those that may produce risk; they substitute speculation with a more reliable approximate of how well things function (Pearson et al., 2007). An advantage of this type of review is that it takes into account both studies that had significant results and studies that failed to find statistical significance, which may not have been published because of a lack of statistical power or a small sample size. By using both types of studies, external validity is increased (Borenstein et al., 2009; Pearson et al., 2007). Many studies that are strong in internal validity (design characteristics) do not use a representative sample of subjects. This limits the generalizability of results. Including many studies of varying sample size and levels of significance increases the variation of the sample and strengthens external validity. On the other hand, meta-analysis requires a good deal of effort, loses the qualitative distinctions between studies, and can include flawed studies. Meta-analysis is conducted with empirical research studies that produced quantitative findings. Theoretical and policy papers and qualitative forms of research cannot be subjected to a meta-analysis (Lipsey & Wilson, 2001). The most frequent criticism of meta-analysis, however, is that it combines "apples and oranges," what Polit and Beck (2004) refer to as the "fruit problem" (p. 697), the possibility of combining studies that conceptually are not comparable. For example, a series of studies on the effect of oral care on the development of ventilator-associated pneumonia (VAP) could be analyzed for its effect in preventing pneumonia. It would not be appropriate to analyze the effect of oral care on development of pneumonia and the gender differences of those on a ventilator, because the focus is on the relationship between oral care and VAP. Synthesizing studies that might differ on both independent and dependent variables brings into question the utility of the findings. Furthermore, many studies may have similar independent and dependent variables but differ in the strength of the design, allowing for potential inclusion of flawed studies in the review. Finally, even though the statistics used in meta-analysis are quite sophisticated, the end product will never be better than the individual studies that make up the whole meta-analysis (Lipsey & Wilson, 2001). The individual or primary studies that make up a meta-analysis are RCTs, a research design in which there is a treatment group and a control or comparison group. A clinical trial is a prospective scientific experiment that uses human subjects. A treatment is introduced and evaluated. In an RCT, each human subject participant is assigned (allocated), through a chance method, to receive either the treatment to be evaluated or to be in the control group (Stanley, 2007). RCTs sit near the top of the evidence hierarchy, clearly acknowledging their importance to evidence-based practice. Systematic reviews are at the apex.

RANDOMIZED CONTROLLED TRIALS

A RCT is considered the gold standard for testing the effectiveness of treatments and/or interventions. The principle underlying these trials is one of control, which works to segregate the effect of the intervention, keeping all other extraneous effects in check (Salmond, 2008). Some RCTs are stronger or better designed than others. Those that use historical controls are weaker than those where the control is simultaneous with the intervention (Littell et al., 2008). The two more commonly used types of RCT are parallel and crossover studies. In a parallel study design, each subject is randomized to only one treatment, although there may be more than one treatment group. For example, Ersek, Turner, Cain, and Kemp (2004) randomized adults, aged 65 years and older, to assess the effectiveness of a training group intervention for pain self-management, as compared with an education-only control condition.

In a crossover trial, each subject receives more than one treatment in a predetermined sequence. Upon completion of a course of one treatment, subjects are then switched to another. It is a repeated-measures study with a within-subjects design. This means that each subject acts as his or her own control. The assumption of crossover trials is that patients usually have a stable condition that will not vary between the first and second treatments (Joanna Briggs Institute [JBI], 2009), and the comparison groups are equal because they are the same people (Polit & Beck, 2004). For example, in a study of the effects of butter and margarine on lipid profiles, Chisholm et al. (1996) randomized subjects to a 6-week butter diet followed by a 6-week margarine diet, or the reverse sequence. Treatment periods were separated by 5 weeks' washout in which patients returned to their usual diet. The impact on lipids was then measured by blood sample.

In the more common parallel randomized trial, the unit of randomization is usually the individual subject, although nursing units, hospitals, and classrooms can also be randomized. It is the ideal design for an experimental study of the effects of an intervention because it determines the effect of an intervention compared with another treatment option, whether it be placebo, another treatment, or the usual care

(Polit & Beck, 2004). RCTs can determine the existence of a cause–effect relationship between a treatment and an outcome and are used to evaluate how effective a new treatment/therapy/intervention is for patients with a certain condition (JBI, 2009). An RCT is characterized by manipulation, control, randomization, blinding, and sampling.

Manipulation refers to the process of doing something to the intervention or experimental group, usually called Group A. In an RCT, manipulation is referred to as the *treatment* or *intervention*. The process manipulated is thought to have an influence on the outcome and is the independent variable. For example, the independent variable can be the administration of a cancer drug (new vs. old), attempting a new method of teaching (e.g., podcasts vs. traditional lecture), or providing methods of chronic pain relief (e.g., herbal supplements vs. opioids).

Control refers to the process of isolating the intervention so that confounding (rival) influences do not sway the outcome when comparing the intervention (Group A) to something else, usually the standard of care. This group is generally known as Group B. The results of Group B on the outcome variable are used to determine how well the intervention worked (JBI, 2009). For example, if the effect of complementary methods of pain relief (massage) on laboring women was the focus of interest, Group A would receive massage, Group B would receive the usual care, and both groups would be evaluated for pain. In this example, the effect of massage on pain can be more clearly understood.

Randomization refers to assigning subjects to either the treatment or control group and is an essential element of an RCT. Randomization ensures that all groups are comparable at the beginning of the study. Confounding factors (variables), such as age, race, or comorbidities, which may impact the results, are spread evenly across groups to ensure that treatment arms (groups) are as equal as possible prior to receiving the intervention. Thus, properly designed and performed RCTs reduce the risk of bias, the influence of confounding factors, and the occurrence of results by chance. Randomization is founded on the logic that groups must be as alike as possible. For example, if a greater number of healthier patients were in one group and sicker patients in another, the observed effect could be biased in favor of the healthier group, rather than serving as an assessment of the treatments (Stanley, 2007). Randomization can be achieved simply by pulling names from a hat or rolling a die, or by using more complex processes such as computer-generated sequences. There is no guarantee that randomization will result in completely alike groups; it tends to produce groups that are "on the average" alike. Stratification can be used as an added method to achieve as much balance between treatment and control groups as possible. Stratification can be accomplished by forming risk groups (strata) based on prognostic factors, such as hypertension or obesity, or demographic factors, such as age, gender, race, or socioeconomic factors. A separate randomization is done for each stratum forcing a balance between groups (Stanley, 2007). Randomization can also assist in preventing an overestimation of effectiveness through attention to the intention to treat principle (ITT). ITT is a strategy for analysis in an RCT that evaluates patients in the groups to which they were originally randomly assigned, regardless of whether they completed the trial. Because RCTs are conducted on the premise that treatment groups are similar, apart from random variation, the randomization feature is lost if analysis is not performed on the groups produced by the randomization process. ITT is considered the standard for preserving the integrity of randomization and guarding against any risk of bias that may occur if subjects who were randomized are not included in the analysis of outcomes (Polit & Gillespie, 2009). For example, Hollis and Campbell (1999) explained that in a trial comparing medical and surgical treatment for stable angina pectoris, some patients allocated to the surgical intervention died before the surgical treatment (an operation) could be provided. If these deaths are not attributed to the surgical intervention group using an ITT analysis, the surgical intervention would have a falsely low mortality.

Blinding is a method used to eliminate bias. Blinding is relevant for individuals included in the trial as well as the investigators, data collectors, and assessors. Blinding ensures that those involved in the trial do not know which treatment has been assigned to what group or to what person. *Single-blind* and *double-blind* are terms used to describe the extent of the blinding. If blinding has occurred at both the subject and study participant levels, the study is said to be double-blind; if only one of these, for example, the subject, is blinded about the group assignment, the study is single-blind. Stanley (2007) believes that all RCTs should be double-blinded so that neither the patients' nor the caregivers' desire for favorable outcomes bias the results. However, it may not be possible to use blinding in some RCTs (e.g., those evaluating invasive interventions).

Sampling is the process of selecting individuals or groups from the target population and including them in the trial. The target population is the group of people to whom the results of the trial will be relevant or applicable. Inclusion/exclusion criteria are set a priori (before the study) to define a specific study group for the trial. The most important issue to consider when selecting a sample is that the sample is representative of the target population. There are different methods of sampling from the population that can be used. *Probabilistic (random) sampling* is the random sampling of individuals from the target population. This ensures that different individuals in the population all have an equal chance of being involved with the trial. *Cluster or multistage sampling* can be used when a large sample is required, for example, where a random sample of hospitals is drawn, and then a random sample of nursing units, and then random patients from each unit. *Consecutive sampling* is the successive sampling of every patient who meets the inclusion criteria from the population over a period. *Systematic sampling* occurs when samples are decided on a system, such as every third patient is to be enrolled in the trial. This may be hazardous if the investigator can affect the order in which patients are seen. *Convenience sampling* is sampling by handiness or ease. This sample technique will save time and money and is quite simple, but may not be representative of the target population (Polit & Beck, 2004). A group of students in a classroom testing a new teaching strategy is a convenience sample.

Assessing Study Quality

There are several available tools to assess (appraise) a study for inclusion in a systematic review of interventions, as presented in Table 8.3. In addition, four essential

TABLE 8.3

Examples of Critical Appraisal Tools for Randomized Controlled Trials

Name	Type	Number of Items	Suggestions for Scoring
CASP	Checklist	10	No
Joanna Briggs Institute	Checklist	10	No
QUORUM	Checklist	14	No
CEBM	Checklist	17	No
Jadad	Flow diagram	5	Yes

Note. CASP = Critical Appraisal Skills Program; CEBM = Centre for Evidence-Based Medicine; QUOROM = Quality of Reporting of Meta-Analyses.

questions to ask when appraising an RCT for a systematic review of experimental evidence are suggested by the JBI (2009):

1. Can results from populations differing in race, age, or gender be combined?
2. Can results of the same construct, measured in different ways, be combined?
3. Are the interventions provided to the experimental or treatment group similar enough to be combined for a meta-analysis?
4. Are the control groups in each of the studies receiving treatment similar enough to be combined for a meta-analysis?

These questions are often difficult to answer and can involve subjective decision making and the need for expert judgment. Experienced systematic reviewers should be consulted in situations where opinions are varied and a decision needs to be made (JBI, 2009).

In addition, Littell et al. (2008) suggest that attention is needed to determine the presence of any bias in the studies being considered for inclusion. *Bias* is the result of errors in the research process that leads to results deviating from the truth. An RCT attempts to eliminate sources of bias, where feasible, through randomization, control, blinding, and sampling methods as described previously; however, these processes may not always be as effective as hoped. There are four primary forms of bias that can affect the outcomes of an RCT: selection bias, performance bias, attrition bias, and detection bias.

Selection bias occurs when the groups in a research study are different. In other words, an error was made in choosing subjects for a study and the sample is not representative (i.e., all potential participants did not have an equal chance of being assigned to either the control or the intervention group). A selection bias can cause a real effect to appear nonexistent, or cause a nonexistent effect to appear real (Littell et al., 2008). For example, calling patients at home in the evening to determine their satisfaction with a hospital stay tends to underrepresent those who work nights or who have two jobs, and who are more likely to be in a lower socioeconomic group.

Performance bias refers to differences in care provided to patients if the caregiver is aware of whether a patient is in a control or treatment group. For example, in a study of the effect of music therapy on preprocedural anxiety, nursing staff in the waiting area were comforting the control group subjects by talking more softly, patting them on the back, and telling them that the procedure would go well—activities they did not normally perform. It was known who was in the intervention group because these patients were wearing headphones to listen to music, whereas the control group patients were not (Heck-Kanellidis, 2010). Littell et al., (2008) refer to this as *contamination of treatment*.

Attrition bias refers to the differences between control and treatment groups in terms of patients dropping out of a study, or not being followed up as thoroughly as others in the group. Attrition, also called mortality or loss of follow-up, occurs when the subjects are no longer available to the study. Attrition may be related to a refusal to continue to participate, a change in health status, a move out of the area, or practical barriers, such as lack of transportation or change in employment hours, or death (Littell et al., 2008).

Detection or assessor bias occurs if outcomes are measured differently for patients depending on whether they are in the control or treatment group. A detection bias generally occurs when the assessor (the one determining the outcome results) knows whether the subject is in the control or intervention group (Littell et al., 2008).

Data Extraction and Coding

A critical step in meta-analysis is extracting and coding data so that the variables of interest can be compared as in primary research (Lipsey & Wilson, 2001). *Data extraction* refers to the process of pulling out relevant results from the original (primary) research studies to be included in the systematic review, and preparing (coding) these data for inclusion in the meta-analysis (JBI, 2009). Extracted data provide a link between the primary studies and the review, with a focus on information to identify the studies, research process, description of interventions, outcomes, and any raw data needed to calculate an effect size (Littell et al., 2008). Data can be extracted onto forms or directly into a computer program. If data are extracted onto paper forms, they must be entered into a computer for analysis at some time, preferably by trained coders.

The JBI has developed standard data extraction tools suitable for meta-analysis, which can be viewed on their website (www.joannabriggs.edu.au). Other examples can be found in the appendices of the books by Lipsey and Wilson (2001) and Littell et al. (2008). In addition, spreadsheet software, such as Excel, and database programs, such as Access, can be formulated for data extraction for meta-analysis. Borenstein and colleagues have developed an easy-to-use meta-analysis program based on an Excel spreadsheet, which can be tested at www.statistics.com. However, even the best tool is not a panacea, as Gøtzsche, Hróbjartsson, Marić, and Tendal (2007) found a 37% data extraction error rate in 27 meta-analyses reviewed. Whichever method of data extraction is used, attention to detail is extremely important.

Most forms have several sections and begin with information that identifies the study (author, year) and the extractor (initials). It is helpful to give each study a review number (e.g., 001), and the date of the extraction should be recorded. Table 8.4 provides some of the essential elements to be extracted.

TABLE 8.4
Study Elements for Data Extraction and Coding

Study Description
   Study ID #
   Coders' initials
   Date of extraction/coding
   Author(s) of study being extracted
   Year of publication
   Type of publication (e.g., journal, dissertation)
   Source of the publication (e.g., name of journal, website address)

Background Information
   Country where study was conducted
   Study setting (e.g., hospital, community center)
   Sample characteristics (e.g., average age, gender, ethnicity, educational level, disease/
     conditions)

Study Information
   Identified sources of bias
   Sampling procedures
     Allocation concealment methods
   Method of assignment to groups (allocation)
   Group description and sample size
     Intervention A (experimental)
     Intervention B (control)
   Data collection methods for each outcome variable
   Attrition

Comments
   Authors' conclusions
   Coders' comments

Source: Adapted from Joanna Briggs Institute (2009). *Study guide for module 2*. Adelaide, Australia: Author; and Lipsey, M. W., & Wilson, D. W. (2001). *Practical meta-analysis*. Thousand Oaks, CA: Sage.

In some cases, all of the raw data required for a systematic review may not be available in the selected study. Data may have only been reported in the aggregate or two different populations may have been combined (e.g., adults and children with Type 2 diabetes) when only one population is needed in a review (e.g., children with Type 2 diabetes). In these instances, the standard approach is to make contact with the authors of the publication and seek their assistance in providing the raw data (JBI, 2009; Littell et al., 2008).

Coding refers to a method of ensuring that all extracted variables are defined and described using the same terms or abbreviations. Each item to be extracted and coded needs to be precisely defined so that coding is similar across coders. Coding structures should be developed before the review begins and then pilot tested with those who will be extracting the data. At this time, a coding manual should also be developed. The manual will serve as a resource or guide for coders. The goal of coding is to build a database for eventual statistical analysis, and a sufficiently detailed manual will eliminate any ambiguity that will interfere with the analysis of findings (Lispey & Wilson, 2001). Coders (those who are extracting and coding the data) must be able to reliably and consistently extract complex information. The use of a coding form that reflects the information in the coding manual can increase reliability and make the process more efficient and timely. Coding can also be done directly into the computer. It is useful to provide space for comments on either type of form to eliminate the necessity of returning to the original study. Software programs, such as FileMaker Pro, Microsoft Access, or FoxPro, allow for the development of screens for entering data. Data entered in this way can then be downloaded and imported into a statistical analysis program (Lipsey & Wilson, 2001; Littell et al., 2008; Haywood, Hargreaves, White, & Lamb, 2004).

Because the overall intent of a systematic review is to determine effect size (the statistical index used to represent study findings in a meta-analysis), Lipsey and Wilson (2001) provided a list of items to be extracted and coded that can support the determination of the effect size. These include the following:

- The variable of the principal interest to be reflected in the effect size
- The total sample size
- The effect size sample
- Standard deviation or variances
- Means or proportions

To increase the rigor of a systematic review and eliminate any ambiguity, two coders should extract data independently and then compare results. Any discrepancies can be discussed, and if necessary, resolved with a third coder or reviewer (JBI, 2009; Littell et al., 2008). Table 8.5 presents the steps for a good coding procedure.

TABLE 8.5
Steps in Coding

1. Decide which characteristics you want to code and the abbreviation for each characteristic. Define each variable.
2. Decide exactly how you will code each characteristic. If you decide to use a continuous scale, specify the units. If you decide to use categories, specify what groups you will use.
3. Write down the specifics of your coding scheme in a code book. The code book should contain explicit instructions on how to code each characteristic, including specific examples where necessary.
4. Pilot the coding scheme and train the coders.
5. Meet with the coders to correct ambiguities in the scheme.
6. Determine interrater reliability among the coders.
7. Check with the coder's frequently to resolve any issues.

Source: Adapted from Littell, J., Corcoran, J., & Pillai V. (2008). *Systematic reviews and meta-analysis.* New York, NY: Oxford University Press.

Data Analysis

In a meta-analysis, effect size metrics are calculated to analyze the results of pooled studies. In combination, these provide an understanding of the effectiveness of an intervention. The effect size is what makes a meta-analysis possible. It provides a common metric and standardizes the results across findings so that they can be compared. An effect size is a measure of strength (magnitude) and direction of a relationship between variables (Lipsey & Wilson, 2001). According to Lipsey and Wilson (2001), any standardized statistical index can be an effect size (e.g., standardized mean difference, correlation coefficient, odds ratio) as long as it meets the following criteria:

- It is comparable across studies.
- It represents the magnitude and direction of the relationship of interest.
- It is independent of sample size.

Different effect size measures are used for dichotomous and continuous data. Dichotomous variables are those that have only two categories (e.g., yes/no, absent/present, negative/positive, pass/fail). Continuous variables take on a range of values and are expressed on a scale (e.g., length of stay, test scores, temperature). More commonly, continuous variables are used as outcome measures in a meta-analysis (Littell et al., 2008). When data such as these are used to estimate population parameters, they are called point estimates (i.e., they provide an approximation of the principal variable of interest). Meta-analysis is based on the possibility that point estimates collected from multiple samples are scattered around the population parameter, so that the direction of the effect size can be determined. However, all estimates are approximate. A confidence interval is necessary to evaluate the level of certainty. When the confidence interval includes zero, the estimate is not significant (Borenstein et al., 2009; JBI, 2009; Littell et al., 2008).

Effect Size for Dichotomous Variables

The most commonly used effect size estimates for dichotomous variables is the odds ratio (OR). Odds is a chance that something will happen or will not happen and is based on probability theory. According to Littell et al. (2008), for example, in a control group, if four people experience a headache (the event) following administration of a placebo and 16 people do not experience a headache, the odds are 4/16 (0.25) that someone in the group of 20 will experience a headache. If a second group of 10 subjects is added and eight people experience a headache after being provided with medication, the odds are 8/12 (0.67). The OR can now be reported as a comparison between the intervention group and the control group by dividing the odds for the intervention group (Group A) by the odds for the control group (Group B): 8/12 divided by 4/16 is equal to 2.67. Essentially, the odds of experiencing a headache (the event) after being given a new medication (the exposure or treatment) is 2.67

TABLE 8.6

Effect Sizes for Dichotomous Variables (Example)

	Event	No Event	Total *N*	Odds	Risk
Treatment group	8	12	20	8/12 = 0.67	8/20 = 0.40
Control group	4	16	20	4/16 = 0.25	4/20 = 0.20
OR = (8/12)/(4/16) = 2.67					
RR = (8/20)/(4/20) = 2.0					
RD (ARR) = Risk A − Risk B = 0.20					
NNT = 1/RD = 1/.20 = 5					

Note. OR = odds ratio; RR = risk ratio; RD = risk difference; ARR = absolute risk reduction; NNT = number needed to treat.
Source: Adapted from Littell, J., Corcoran, J., & Pillai V. (2008). *Systematic reviews and meta-analysis.* New York, NY: Oxford University Press.

times more likely than if a placebo (the control) were given. This is known as the OR. If the OR were 1.0, there would be no difference between the groups (Littell et al., 2008; see Table 8.6).

Dichotomous Variables

The risk ratio (RR), or relative risk, can also be used. Similar to the OR, the RR compares the chance of an event in one group with that same event in another group. The risk is the number of people in a group who experience an event divided by the total number in the group. Therefore, those in Group A, which was mentioned previously, have a relative risk of experiencing a headache of 0.4 or 40%. This is accomplished by dividing 8 by 20 (8/20). The risk of the control group is 4/20 or 0.20 (20%). Note that the risk of experiencing a headache in the treatment group (Group A) is twice that of the control group (Group B; Littell et al., 2008). An RR of 1.0 indicates that there is no difference between the groups. Misinterpretation of the differences between an OR and an RR can result in an overestimation of effect size, suggesting that the treatment may be better or worse than it is (JBI, 2009).

A third way to evaluate the results of a meta-analysis with dichotomous data is to use the risk difference (RD), or absolute risk reduction (ARR). This measure is calculated by subtracting the risk of Group A (0.40) from the risk of Group B (0.20), meaning that there is a 20% less risk of experiencing a headache in Group B (Littell et al., 2008).

Finally, the RD can be transformed into a measure called the number needed to treat (NNT), which denotes the number of people who must be treated to obtain one more case with a positive outcome. The NNT is the reverse of the RD (1/RD). A decrease in the RD means an increase in the NNT. Using the aforementioned example, the NNT is 1/0.20 or five people (Littell et al., 2008). Therefore, at least five more people would have to be added to the study to have one more person experience the event.

When deciding what effect size measure to code and extract, it is important to remember that most clinicians can understand the concept of being at risk for something, so the RR is the preferred measure (JBI, 2009).

Effect Size for Continuous Variables

There are several types of effect size, based on either difference scores or correlations that can be used with continuous variables. These include mean differences and changes over time (e.g., pretest/posttest measures) and correlational coefficients (r). The mean difference is the difference between the average of the treatment group (Group A) and the control group (Group B) when the outcome measures are reported using the same scale—in other words, the arithmetic mean. For example, in a study of pain intensity, if the pain is reported using a 10-point categorical scale, the mean difference between groups can be compared. Alternatively, if two different measures of pain intensity were used, such as a visual analog scale and the 10-point categorical scale, a standardized mean difference (SMD) or Cohen's *d* is useful. This metric is used when scores are reportedly different for the same construct. The SMD is the mean difference divided by pooled standard deviation (SD) of the two groups. The pooled SD can be calculated by any statistical software program, such as the Statistical Program for the Social Sciences (SPSS) or Excel (Lipsey & Wilson, 2001; Littell et al., 2008), or with the free web calculator, Hyperstat Online. These effect sizes indicate the mean difference between two variables expressed in SD units. A well-known guide offered by Cohen (1988), as presented in Table 8.7, maintains that a result of 0.8 is a large effect, 0.5 is a moderate effect, and 0.2 is a small effect.

Correlations (r) can also be used as an effect size metric. Correlational and standardized mean effect sizes cannot be directly compared, but they can be converted for purposes of comparison to a Fisher's z score, which is not to be confused with the z score used for significance testing. A Fisher's z score makes variables comparable for analysis (see Lipsey and Wilson, 2001, for a more detailed description). The standard product moment correlation is calculated on two continuous variables, such as length of stay and socioeconomic status, or blood pressure and weight. Studies that do not use a control group report changes in one group between the pretest and the posttest. The mean score obtained pre- and post-test is known as the *unstandardized mean score gain*. This score is divided by the pooled SD of the pretest and posttest scores to obtain a standardized mean score gain (Littell et al., 2008). Gain scores should not be confused with SMD, since gain scores are derived from one group and SMD are derived from two groups (JBI, 2009).

TABLE 8.7
Cohen's Interpretation of Effect Sizes

ES Metric	Large Effect	Medium Effect	Small Effect
OR	4.3	2.5	1.5
SMD	0.8	0.5	0.2

Note: ES = effect size; OR = odds ratio; SMD = standardized mean difference.
Source: Based on Cohen, J. (1988). *Statistical power analysis for the behavioral sciences* (2nd ed.). New York, NY: Academic Press.

TABLE 8.8
Data Synthesis Choice

Dichotomous data	Odds ratio (OR)	Relative risk (RR)	Risk difference (RD)
Continuous data	Mean (M)	Mean difference (MD)	Standardized mean difference (SMD)

Combining Continuous and Dichotomous Data

Occasionally, review authors may include studies that have examined the same outcome using both continuous and dichotomous measures. For example, one study may measure the A1c levels directly (continuous), whereas another study only indicates whether the person met a predetermined level, which is then used to determine a high or normal level of A1c (dichotomous). In this case, if the raw data are available from the study authors, it could be possible to convert the continuous data into a dichotomous scale (whether patients had high levels of A1c) using the same predetermined high and normal scores (JBI, 2009; see Table 8.8).

Data Synthesis

Variation and Heterogeneity

Systematic reviews combine studies that pool the results of the same outcome from samples and settings that are different. Such diversity, or variation, can result in statistical heterogeneity. Heterogeneity can be related to patient conditions, setting, age, sex, diagnosis or disease severity, or dose or intensity of the intervention. Additionally, heterogeneity can also be related to the methods used, for example, differences on how the studies were conducted, the study quality, or data analysis (Higgins, Thompson, Deeks, & Altman, 2002).

When used in relation to meta-analysis, the term *heterogeneity* refers to the amount of variation in the results of included studies, which may impact results. It is important to determine the degree of statistical heterogeneity so that a single effect size can be appropriately reported. Statistical heterogeneity is assessed with a chi-square statistic that uses estimates of each individual study's weight and effect size, in combination with the overall effect size (JBI, 2009). A test for heterogeneity is actually a test to determine homogeneity, using the null hypothesis. If results demonstrate an insignificant p value (more than the level of .05), there is little variation (no heterogeneity) and a single effect size can be reported. A significant p value (equal or less than the level of .05) indicates limited homogeneity; rather, heterogeneity is present, and there is not a single treatment effect. Although some variation between the results of studies will always occur because of chance alone, heterogeneity is said to occur if there are significant differences between studies, and under these circumstances, the meta-analysis is not valid. A quick way to identify heterogeneity is to compare the chi-square statistic with its degrees of freedom. If the chi-square result is larger than its degrees of freedom, heterogeneity is present. This is a low-power test, however, that can fail to detect significant differences if only a few studies are in the meta-analysis. Consequently, the confidence level should be narrowed to 99% (a p value of $< .01$) when there are few studies included in the meta-analysis to protect against the possibility of falsely stating that there is no heterogeneity present (JBI, 2009; Lipsey & Wilson, 2001; Littell et al., 2008; Baujat, Mahe, Pignon, & Hill, 2002).

Deeks, Higgins, and Altman (2006) provide six alternatives to conducting meta-analysis when heterogeneity is indicated.

1. Double-check the data extracted and enter these data into the software program being used to be sure that everything is correct. Consider setting the program up with a double data entry feature.
2. Do not proceed with the meta-analysis. Consider alternatives such as summarizing the results of included studies in a narrative summary.
3. Explore the heterogeneity through subgroup analysis.
4. Perform a random-effects meta-analysis if this was not done first.
5. Check to be sure the correct effect measure was used and change the measure if necessary.
6. Exclude studies that may be causing the heterogeneity and rerun the analysis (see the succeeding topic, "Sensitivity Analysis").

Sensitivity Analysis

Sensitivity analysis is used to determine the accuracy of decisions made during the review. The purpose of a sensitivity analysis is to determine whether the results are consistent under different assumptions—in other words, to establish the consistency of results. For example, a study that was deficient in some way (e.g., poor study design, high attrition rates) can be dropped from the analysis, the effect size recalculated, and the results reanalyzed to examine the effect of this study on the overall results (JBI, 2009).

What Model to Use

Meta-analysis can be based on either of two statistical models: a fixed-effects model or a random-effects model. In a fixed-effects model, it is assumed that all of the study results come from the same population and produce estimates of one effect size (Littell et al., 2008). In fact, Borenstein et al. (2009) prefer to call it a fixed-effect model (singular) because there is only one true effect. Essentially, the difference between treatment and control is the same (or fixed) in each study (JBI, 2009). Observed differences would be due only to chance. Variation equally affects variables across studies and is caused by sampling error alone (Borenstein et al., 2009). The term *sampling error* is used to describe the situation in which, for example, not all sample sizes are equal in each study so some errors or variations occur, and because this influences all studies in the same manner, the effect is fixed. However, Borenstein et al. (2009) believe that this situation is highly unlikely and suggest that the random-effects model should be used in most situations. A random-effects model is based on the logic that the effect size can vary across studies. The effect size may be random because of variation in participants (some older, some younger), intensity of health condition (some severe, some moderate), or differences in study design (parallel vs. crossover trials), among others. There is limited consensus about whether a fixed or random model should be used in meta-analysis, although Borenstein et al. (2009) contend that a random-effects model should always be used because there is always variation across studies. In many cases when heterogeneity is absent, the two methods will give similar overall results. When heterogeneity is present, the random-effects estimate provides a better estimate of the effect size. However, the random-effects model does not eliminate heterogeneity and should not be considered as a substitute for an investigation into the reasons for the heterogeneity and the conduct of subgroup analysis if appropriate (JBI, 2009). The decision about what model to use, therefore, for the meta-analysis requires discussion and judgment on the part of the reviewers and is based on the type of data extracted and the objectives of the review. This decision should be made prior to the beginning of review. A fixed-effects model should be used if all of the studies in the review are identical and if the goal of the review is to generalize to the review population. Studies conducted by a wide range of researchers, however, are not likely to be identical. Accordingly, the random-effects model is more commonly used (Borenstein et al., 2009; JBI, 2009; Littell et al., 2008), and according to Borenstein et al. (2009), it should always be used.

The Forest Plot

A forest plot is a graphical display of the results of the meta-analysis. Presented in Figure 8.1 is a forest plot for a meta-analysis of the effects of chocolate on diastolic and systolic blood pressure (Ried, Sullivan, Fakler, Frank, & Stocks, 2010). At the top of the plot is usually the title of the review and a brief description of the treatment and comparison variables. The left-hand column lists the names of the studies. These will be either in chronological order from the top downward or alphabetical. The results of each study listed are divided by treatment and control group in the next six columns, including the total number of the review samples and the change in blood pressure following the treatment (chocolate). The totals for each column are at the bottom. The eighth column provides the weight or influence of each study to the meta-analysis. The weight is determined by the size of the sample. The next column provides the confidence interval and tells that a random-effects model was used for analysis. The far right-hand column is a plot of the measure of effect (e.g., an OR) for each of these studies (often represented by a square) incorporating confidence intervals represented by horizontal lines. The overall measure of effect is represented as a vertical line. This effect size is seen as a diamond, which represents the pooled treatment effect. In this case, the diamond is to the left of 0, indicating that chocolate decreases blood pressure. At the lower right-hand area of the forest plot is a determination of heterogeneity. Most often, an I^2 is used, a numerical value from 0% to 100%, which is an estimate of the heterogeneity present. If the I^2 is 85% or greater, the results of the meta-analysis are questionable and should not

A) SBP all studies

Study	Treatment N	ΔSBP	SD	Control N	ΔSBP	SD	Weight	Mean Difference Random, 95% CI
Taubert 03	13	-4.7	3.28	13	0.4	3.28	10.1%	-5.10 [-7.62, -2.58]
Murphy 03	13	2	10.04	15	3	6.86	5.1%	-1.00 [-7.47, 5.47]
Engler 04	11	-1	13.18	10	-2.8	6.5	3.4%	1.80 [-6.97, 10.57]
Fraga 05	14	-6	8.23	14	-2	8.23	5.5%	-4.00 [-10.10, 2.10]
Grassi 05a	15	-7	6.29	15	-0.5	6.21	7.3%	-6.50 [-10.97, -2.03]
Grassi 05b	20	-12	4.28	20	-0.7	4.07	10.0%	-11.30 [-13.89, -8.71]
Taubert 07	22	-2.9	1.6	22	-0.1	1.6	11.9%	-2.80 [-3.75, -1.85]
Crews 08	45	-3.6	10.81	45	-3.1	10.88	7.3%	-0.50 [-4.98, 3.98]
Grassi 08	19	-3.8	3.01	19	-0.1	2.76	11.0%	-3.70 [-5.54, -1.86]
Muniyappa 08	20	-2	9.84	20	-1	9.84	5.5%	-1.00 [-7.10, 5.10]
Davison 08a	12	-1.9	6.85	11	4.2	8.62	5.2%	-6.10 [-12.50, 0.30]
Davison 08b	13	1.1	5.31	13	-0.5	8.29	6.3%	1.60 [-3.75, 6.95]
Shina 09	20	4.6	10.16	19	4	11	5.0%	0.60 [-6.06, 7.25]
Ried 09a	11	-2	9.71	10	-4.9	13.42	2.8%	2.90 [-7.20, 13.00]
Monagas 09	42	0	19.14	42	-3	20.08	3.7%	3.00 [-5.39, 11.39]
Total (95% CI)	**290**			**288**			**100%**	**-3.16 [-5.08, -1.23]**

Heterogeneity: Tau² = 7.86; Chi² = 54.06, df = 14 (P < .00001); I² = 74%
Test for overall effect: Z = 3.22 (P = .001)

B) DBP all studies

Study	Treatment N	ΔDBP	SD	Control N	ΔDBP	SD	Weight	Mean Difference Random, 95% CI
Taubert 03	13	-1.6	3.68	13	0.3	3.4	8.7%	-1.90 [-4.62, 0.82]
Murphy 03	13	1	8.99	15	0	6.07	3.8%	1.00 [-4.77, 6.77]
Engler 04	11	0.9	6.16	10	-0.1	4.76	5.1%	1.00 [-3.69, 5.69]
Fraga 05	14	-5	5.99	14	-1	5.99	5.4%	-4.00 [-8.44, 0.44]
Grassi 05a	15	-4.2	4.23	15	-0.3	4.32	7.9%	-3.90 [-6.96, -0.84]
Grassi 05b	20	-7.8	4.11	20	-0.2	3.76	9.3%	-7.60 [-10.04, -5.16]
Taubert 07	22	-1.9	1	22	0	1.8	12.9%	-1.90 [-2.76, -1.04]
Crews 08	45	-0.5	6.31	45	-0.6	6.29	9.0%	0.10 [-2.50, 2.70]
Grassi 08	19	-3.9	3.54	19	-0.2	2.89	10.3%	-3.70 [-5.75, -1.65]
Muniyappa 08	20	-3	9.84	20	-4	9.84	3.5%	1.00 [-5.10, 7.10]
Davison 08a	12	-1.8	5.2	11	2.8	5.64	5.4%	-4.60 [-9.05, -0.15]
Davison 08b	13	-0.5	3.61	13	-0.2	5.41	6.9%	-0.30 [-3.84, 3.24]
Shina 09	20	6.6	9.04	19	5.2	10.36	3.5%	1.40 [-4.72, 7.52]
Ried 09a	11	0.9	8.93	10	-0.5	7.55	2.8%	1.40 [-5.65, 8.45]
Monagas 09	42	-2	10.4	42	-3	10.4	5.4%	1.00 [-3.45, 5.45]
Total (95% CI)	**290**			**288**			**100%**	**-2.02 [-3.35, -0.69]**

Heterogeneity: Tau² = 3.40; Chi² = 36.75, df = 14 (P = .0008); I² = 62%
Test for overall effect: Z = 2.97 (P = .003)
Note: N, number of participants; ΔSBP/ΔDBP, difference in mean SBP/DBP between start and end of intervention; SD, standard deviation; CI, confidence interval; DBP, diastolic blood pressure; SBP, systolic blood pressure.

FIGURE 8.1

A meta-analysis of the effects of chocolate on blood pressure.

Source: Ried, K., Sullivan, T., Fakler, P., Frank, O., & Stocks, N. (2010). Does chocolate reduce blood pressure? A meta-analysis. *BMC Medicine, 8*, 39. doi:10.1186/1741-7015-8-39. This is an open access article.

be used because the studies are too different to combine. If the I² is between 40% and 84%, there are moderate levels of heterogeneity present. I² results of less than 40% represent very low levels of heterogeneity. See Table 8.9 for suggestions on how to interpret this and other forest plots (Borenstein et al., 2009; JBI, 2009; Littell et al., 2008).

TABLE 8.9

Assessing a Forest Plot

Question to Ask	Hints to the Answer
1. How many studies were used in the review?	1. Count the number of studies in the right-hand column. These will be either in alphabetical or chronological order or based on the weight assigned to the study. Studies will be identified by author name or other identifying factor.
2. What is the range of years for the studies in the review?	2. Look at the year next to each author name in the first column to determine the range of years.
3. How large is the total sample of the review?	3. Add the sample sizes for both the treatment and control groups for each of the studies (n). The total will give you the review sample size (N).[a]
4. Which is the largest study?	4. Review the column that identifies the number of participants, or determine which of the studies has the largest black box.[a]
5. Which is the smallest study?	5. Review the column that identifies the number of participants, or determine which of the studies has the smallest black box.
6. Which study influenced the study the most?	6. Determine the study with the highest weight percentage.
7. Which study influenced the review the least?	7. Determine the study with the lowest weight percentage.
8. What is the confidence interval for the review as a whole?	8. The confidence interval is a determination of certainty associated with the parameter estimate. A narrow confidence interval is more precise. Look at the line going through each of the black boxes to determine the confidence intervals.
9. What are the confidence intervals for each of the individual studies?	9. Look at the middle of the forest plot at the lines extending from either side of the point estimate. Any confidence interval that crosses the mid-line (the line of no effect) is not statistically significant.
10. How would you interpret the confidence interval?	10. The vertical line through the middle of the forest plot is the line of "no effect," an odds ratio of 1. Any line that crosses the line of no effect is not statistically significant. Look at the diamond (pooled average) at the bottom of the graph. It is weighted using an inverse variance method. The inverse variance is a measure of precision, and is inversely related to the size of the confidence interval. A study with a smaller confidence interval (more precision) contributes more to the effect size than a study with a wide confidence interval (less precision).
11. How is the presence of heterogeneity determined?	11. Look at the I^2 result. If results are greater than 85%, there is too much difference between the studies to combine them. If results are between 40% and 84%, studies can be combined, but a random-effects model should be used for analysis.

(Continued)

TABLE 8.9

Assessing a Forest Plot *(Continued)*

Question to Ask	Hints to the Answer
12. What is the chi-square?	12. Chi-square is a test of heterogeneity, with a distribution of N-1 degrees of freedom (*df*). A significant *p* value associated with this index indicates significant levels of heterogeneity (more than would be expected from sampling error alone). This is a power test when there are only a few studies in the meta-analysis.
13. What does the z score tell you?	13. The *z* score is the test for overall effect. A *z* score greater than or less than 2.0 is significant.
14. What does the probability tell you?	14. The probability is another test for heterogeneity. An insignificant result tells you that the studies are homogeneous; a significant result indicates heterogeneity.
15. How would you know if it was safe to recommend the results of the review?	15. Look at the probability (it should be insignificant), the *z* score (it should be greater or less than 2.0), the confidence interval (it should not include 0), and the placement of the diamond (should be on the side that favors treatment); also look at the I^2 result to determine the percentage of heterogeneity and decide if any subgroup analysis is necessary.

[a]Any imbalance can be addressed with the use of a random-effects model so that one study does not unduly influence the results.
Source: Based on Borenstein, M., Hedges, L., Higgins, J., & Rothstein, H. (2009) and Lipsey, M. W., & Wilson, D. W. (2001).

Writing a Meta-Analysis Report

A meta-analysis should be reported in the same manner as a primary research report. There should be sections devoted to an abstract, background, methods, results, discussion and conclusion, and with implications for both practice and research. The report should describe the topic of the analysis and place that topic into a broader context. An explanation of why the meta-analysis was necessary is a critical ingredient. Relevant statistics should be used to support the importance of the topic. Anyone reading the report should be left with a precise understanding about why a systematic review on this topic was necessary, how it was conducted, and the effect of the intervention under study. In other words, transparency is crucial. See Table 8.10 for a suggested outline of a meta-analysis report.

SUMMARY

A meta-analysis is the statistical analysis of findings from two or more primary studies for the purpose of amalgamating the results across the studies with the same methodological rigor applied to primary research. Meta-analysis is considered the gold standard of integrative research because it allows the determination of best practice, allowing individual health care practitioners to make evidence-based and up-to-date decisions at the point of care.

TABLE 8.10
Outline for Writing a Meta-Analysis Report

Abstract: A 300-word abstract that includes the background, objectives, methods, search strategy, inclusion and exclusion criteria, data collection and analysis, key results, and conclusions.

Background:
  Describe the problem, supported by any relevant statistics.
  State why a meta-analysis on the topic is necessary and significant.
  Describe any supporting theoretical framework and salient previous research of the analysis.
  End the section with the purpose and objectives of the review.

Objectives: The goal of the review along with any subobjectives being considered.

Methods: The criteria for including studies in the review, including:
  Types of studies
  Types of participants
  Types of interventions
  Types of outcome measurements

Search strategy: Describe each of the following:
  Key words used
  Databases searched
  Grey literature searched
  Hand-searched journals
  Any attempt to contact authors

Data analysis and collection
  Selection of studies, how inclusion and exclusion criteria were applied, and how any disagreements were handled
  Data extraction strategies
  Assessment of methodological quality

Measures of treatment effect, choice of effect size metrics for dichotomous and/or continuous data
  Assessment of heterogeneity
  Assessment of any identified bias, including reporting bias
  Use of fixed- or random-effects model
  Plans for any subgroup analysis
  Sensitivity analysis

Results
  Results of the search with a flowchart of the search strategy
  Excluded studies and reasons for exclusion
  Description of included studies, including country of study origin
  Description of the aggregated sample for this review
  Description of overall quality of studies and quality assessment rating scales used, and allocation and blinding methods
  Key findings organized by overall objective and subobjectives

(Continued)

TABLE 8.10

Outline for Writing a Meta-Analysis Report *(Continued)*

Discussion

Summary of the primary results, with emphasis on benefits and harms

Discussion of quality and completeness of the evidence

Implications for practice

Suggestions for further research

EXERCISES

Review the forest plot in Figure 8.1, and answer the following questions:

1. Chi-square is 36.75, $df = 14$, $p = .0008$. How would you interpret this?
2. The z score 2.97 for overall effect, $p.003$. How would you interpret this?
3. Is there heterogeneity present? How do you know?
4. The diamond, which represents the overall effect size for the review, is to the left of the midline on the plot. What does that mean in terms of the review results?
5. Would you recommend consumption of chocolate/cocoa as a method to decrease blood pressure?

REFERENCES

Baujat, B., Mahe, C., Pignon, J.-P., & Hill, C. (2002). A graphical method for exploring heterogeneity in meta-analyses: Application to a meta-analysis of 65 trials. *Statistics in Medicine, 21*(18), 2641–2652.

Borenstein, M., Hedges, L., Higgins, J., & Rothstein, H. (2009). *Introduction to meta-analysis.* West Sussex, United Kingdom: Wiley & Sons.

Chalmers, I. (2006). *The scandalous failure of scientists to cumulate scientifically.* Abstract to paper presented at: Ninth World Congress on Health Information and Libraries, Salvador, Brazil. Abstract retrieved from http://www.icml9.org/program/activity .php?lang=en&id=36

Chisholm, A., Mann, J., Sutherland, W., Duncan, A., Skeaff, M., & Frampton, C. (1996). Effect on lipoprotein profile of replacing butter with margarine in a low fat diet: Randomised crossover study with hypercholesterolaemic subjects. *British Medical Journal, 312*(7036), 931–934.

Cohen, J. (1988). *Statistical power analysis for the behavioral sciences* (2nd ed.). New York, NY: Academic Press.

Deeks, J. J., Higgins, J. P. T., & Altman, D. G. (2006). Analysing and presenting results. In J. P. T. Higgins & S. Green (Eds.), *Cochrane handbook for systematic reviews of intervention.* Chichester, United Kingdom: Wiley & Sons.

Deeks, J. J., Higgins, J. P. T., & Altman, D. G. (2011). Analyzing and undertaking meta-analysis. Available at http://www.cochrane-handbook.org/

Ersek, M., Turner, J., Cain, K., & Kemp, C. (2004). Chronic pain self-management for older adults: A randomized controlled trial. *BMC Geriatric.* Online publication. doi:10.1186/1471-2318-4-7

Gøtzsche, P. C., Hróbjartsson, A., Marić, K., & Tendal, B. (2007). Data extraction errors in meta-analysis that use standardized mean differences. *Journal of the American Medical Association, 298*(4), 430–437.

Haywood, K. L., Hargreaves, J., White, R., & Lamb, S. E. (2004). Reviewing measures of outcome: Reliability of data extraction. *Journal of Evaluation in Clinical Practice, 10*(2), 329–337.

Heck-Kanellidis, J. (2010). Unpublished manuscript. Newark, NJ: University of Medicine and Dentistry of New Jersey, School of Nursing.

Higgins, J., Thompson, S., Deeks, J., & Altman, D. (2002). Statistical heterogeneity in systematic reviews of clinical trials: A critical appraisal of guidelines and practice. *Journal of Health Services & Research Policy, 7*(1), 51–61.

Hollis, S., & Campbell, F. (1999). What is meant by intention to treat analysis? Survey of published randomized controlled trials. *British Medical Journal, 319*(7211), 670–674.

Joanna Briggs Institute. (2009). *Study guide for module* 2. Adelaide, Australia: Author.

Lipsey, M. W., & Wilson, D. W. (2001). *Practical meta-analysis*. Thousand Oaks, CA: Sage.

Littell, J., Corcoran, J., & Pillai V. (2008). *Systematic reviews and meta-analysis*. New York, NY: Oxford University Press.

Pearson, A., Field, J., & Jordan, Z. (2007). *Evidence-based clinical practice in nursing and health care.* Oxford, England: Blackwell.

Polit, D. F., & Beck, C. T. (2004). *Nursing research: Principles and methods.* (7th ed.). Philadelphia, PA: Lippincott Williams & Wilkins.

Polit, D. F., & Gillespie, B. M. (2009). The use of the intention-to-treat principle in nursing clinical trials. *Nursing Research, 58*(6), 391–399.

Ried, K., Sullivan, T., Fakler, P., Frank, O., & Stocks, N. (2010). Does chocolate reduce blood pressure? A meta-analysis. *BMC Medicine, 8*, 39. doi:10.1186/1741-7015-8-39

Salmond, S. (2008). Randomized controlled trials: Methodological concepts and critique. *Orthopaedic Nursing, 27*(2), 116–122.

Stanley, K. (2007). Design of randomized controlled trials. *Circulation, 115*, 1164–1169.

SUGGESTED READINGS

Feuerbach, R. D., & Panniers, T. L. (2003). Building an expert system: A systematic approach to developing an instrument for data extraction from the literature. *Journal of Nursing Care Quality, 18*(2), 129–138.

Higgins, J. P. T., Thompson, S. G., Deeks, J. J., & Altman, D. G. (2003). Measuring inconsistency in meta-analyses. *British Medical Journal, 327*(7414), 557–560.

Lewis, S., & Clarke, M. (2001). Forest plots: Trying to see the wood and the trees. *British Medical Journal, 322*(7300), 1479–1480.

Shutta, K. M., & Burnett, C. B. (2000). Factors that influence a patient's decision to participate in a phase I cancer clinical trial. *Oncology Nursing Forum, 27*(9), 1435–1438.

Wilson, S. R., Yamada, E. G., Sudhaker, R. et al. (2001). A controlled trial of an environmental tobacco smoke reduction intervention in low-income children with asthma. *Chest, 120*(5), 1709–1722.

CHAPTER NINE

Systematic Review of Observational Evidence

Cheryl Holly

OBJECTIVES

Upon completion of Chapter 9, you will be able to:

- Describe the research designs used for observational systematic review
- Compare and contrast the benefits of observational and interventional meta-analysis
- Explain the various types of bias and confounding variables found in observational research studies

IMPORTANT POINTS

- The evidence available from randomized controlled trials will not answer all clinical questions.
- Because of the differing patient groups and settings used in observational studies, heterogeneity may present a challenge.
- The use of observational data is usually necessary to assess harm adequately and may provide the only data for assessing either benefit or harm in minority or vulnerable populations.
- Systematic reviews of observational data will always have confounding variables and bias, because the interventions studied were not deliberately chosen and randomized.

INTRODUCTION

Observation means to broadly make a judgment from what one has seen (Observation, 2010). According to Dahnke (2011), observation is a focused, intentional recognition—part of a formalized effort to acquire knowledge. A systematic review of observational data meet this characterization, with the ultimate goal of using acquired knowledge to determine best practice. A systematic review of observational data is conducted for essentially the same reason as a meta-analysis of interventions—to create estimates of performance based on all available and relevant evidence and to account for variation of findings between and among studies (Deeks, 2001). Although the randomized controlled trial (RCT) is considered the gold standard and principal research design for evaluation of interventions, procedures, and services, there are many aspects of care that cannot be tested or evaluated in a randomized fashion. In addition, RCTs are often time and labor intensive and expensive. Often, the RCT will confirm what has been found in the previous observational studies (Jepsen, Johnsen, Gillman, & Sorensen, 2004), but findings may also differ significantly, as in the inconsistent results found regarding cardiac risk in studies on the drug Avandia (Harris, 2010). Contradictory findings such as the one mentioned previously lend themselves to a systematic review, which pools all available evidence to determine best practice. Although it can be called a meta-analysis because of this pooling of data across studies, the results of an observational meta-analysis are less precise than a meta-analysis of interventions.

Much health care research is conducted using observational designs. Included among these are epidemiological study or risk factors, prognostic factors for the prediction of future events, or studies of diagnostic and screening accuracy. Observational studies are designed to understand the many different conditions and exposures experienced by people, which are not limited to treatment or intervention. In an observational study, the investigator takes a much less active role than in an RCT (The Joanna Briggs Institute [JBI], 2009). For example, questions about the consequences of choice such as "Does eating a diet high in unsaturated fat cause breast cancer?" cannot be tested in a randomized experiment (Egger, Smith, & Schneider, 2001).

For the purposes of this chapter, observational studies are defined as those in which the investigators did not assign an intervention. These studies include descriptive observational studies (prevalence surveys, case series, and case reports) and analytical observational studies (cohort, case-control, and cross-sectional studies) and studies of diagnostic and prognostic test accuracy. The investigators' role in these studies is to observe, record, and analyze results. See Table 9.1 for a depiction of these approaches.

SIGNIFICANCE IN OBSERVATIONAL STUDIES

Significance in research terms has nothing to do with importance. *Significance*, in statistical terms, refers to the probability that a relationship could be caused by chance; in other words, it is probably true or not true, but is not necessarily important. Significance in observational studies is determined through an evaluation of the p value, where p is understood to mean probability. In calculating a p value, it is assumed that there really is no difference. A p value of less than .05 is considered small; that is, there is a less than one in 20, or five in 100, chance of something happening. When p values are this small, the results of the study are interpreted to be significant (unlikely to have resulted through chance). Even smaller p values at the level of .01 are called *highly significant*. P values this small indicate that the results could occur less than once in 100 times (Davies & Crombie, 2009).

Confidence intervals (CI) can also be used to determine the significance of study results. A CI is the range of values that encompass a population parameter. Because it is impossible to measure a total population, the study sample is used to calculate

TABLE 9.1

Research Designs for Observational Studies

Study Design	Description	Data Collection	Advantages	Disadvantages
Prospective cohort study	A longitudinal study of a group of people who share a common characteristic, such as year of high school graduation or taking the same drug	Medical records Environmental or lifestyle questionnaires Physiologic measurement Interview data	Allows investigation of rare diseases or diseases with a long latency Can measure risk Large cohorts can minimize selection bias Aids in understanding causal associations Can test hypotheses	Subjects are not randomly assigned High attrition rates Expensive to conduct Long time to obtain useful data for analysis
Retrospective cohort studies	A historical study of a group of people who share a common characteristic, such as smoking and heart disease or working in a coal mine	Medical records	Less expensive and faster than a prospective cohort study Can test hypotheses	Lack of follow-up affects study validity
Case-control studies	A study of "cases" who have a condition or exposure in comparison with "control" cases who do not have the condition or exposure	Medical records Registry data Death certificates Population surveys	Allows understanding of risk factors Inexpensive Few personnel needed Useful for studying outcomes that take a long time to develop (e.g., cancer) Can test hypotheses	There is a better recall of information among exposed groups (recall bias) Odds ratios are used as a proxy measure for relative risk

(Continued)

TABLE 9.1

Research Designs for Observational Studies *(Continued)*

Study Design	Description	Data Collection	Advantages	Disadvantages
Case series/ case report	A tracking study of people given a similar treatment, such as the use of an automated external defibrillator for out-of-hospital cardiac arrest and survival	Medical records Detailed patient reports	Adverse events and side effects are identified Can be hypothesis generating	
Cross-sectional studies	A descriptive study of a group of people at one point in time; a "snapshot" Also called a prevalence study	Survey methods Secondary data	Provides a foundation for the stronger cohort or RCT designs Can be hypothesis generating	No control group Difficult to determine when the outcome of interest began because everything is measured at one time
Descriptive studies	Descriptive studies identify descriptive characteristics, which frequently constitutes an important first step in the search for determinants or risk factors that can be altered or eliminated to reduce or prevent disease		Hypothesis generating Can be useful in establishing trends or patterns	

Note. RCT = randomized controlled trial.

a range within which the population value will most likely fall. This is known as the 95% CI. The values at either end of the range are known as the confidence limits; the wider the CI, the less the accuracy; that is, there is less certainty that the strength of the association has been precisely estimated (Davies & Crombie, 2009).

The two definitions of statistical significance are compatible. If you have a *p* value of less than .05, it is the same as getting a 95% CI that does not overlap zero. In the reverse, a *p* value greater than .05 equates to a 95% CI that includes 1 (the null value), meaning that there is no effect (Davies & Crombie, 2009).

Significance of the study results or lack thereof, however, is less a concern in systematic review than in primary research. Systematic reviews are concerned with the combined or pooled results of individual primary studies. The process of systematic review involves searching for all available and relevant studies regardless of significance. Including studies that have significant or insignificant results changes the focus from statistical significance to the direction and magnitude of the result, which is important to the development of best practice recommendations. In an observational systematic review, more information may be gained from an in-depth review of any identified variance than from statistical computation (Egger et al., 2001).

DESCRIPTIVE AND ANALYTIC OBSERVATIONAL STUDIES

An *observational study* is a study in which the researcher does not intervene. Observational studies include descriptive studies and analytic studies. Studies of diagnostic accuracy and tests used for prognosis are also considered observational studies.

A *cohort study* is a longitudinal observational study whose focus is a clearly defined exposure or risk with a control group. The word *cohort* is used to mean a group of individuals followed forward over a period to examine an outcome of interest and map its long-term effects. Cohort studies follow two or more groups from exposure to outcome, and then compare the experience of the exposed group with that of the unexposed group. If the exposed group has a higher or lower rate on the outcome of study interest, an association between exposure and outcome is suggestive (Heffernan, 2010). For example, Chan et al. (2010) followed a group of adults who experienced in-hospital cardiac arrest to determine their survival rate to discharge following the use of an automated external defibrillator (AED). Results indicated that for cardiac arrests caused by shockable rhythms, AED use was not associated with survival (adjusted RR, 1.00; 95% CI, 0.88–1.13; $p = .99$).

Cohort studies can be prospective (future) or retrospective (past). *Prospective design* allows exposure to risk factors to be assessed directly over time. A *retrospective design* is effective for diseases with a long development time. Retrospective cohort studies should not be confused with case-control studies, which are also retrospective. Cohort studies track people forward in time from exposure to outcome, whereas case-control studies trace backward from outcome to exposure. Risk in cohort studies is measured by relative risk, absolute risk, and attributable risk (see Table 9.2; Davies & Crombie, 2009; Heffernan, 2010).

A *case-control study* is also an observational study with a control group. A particular disease or condition, such as food poisoning, is the starting point—the case—and the study looks backward to try to determine a cause and any associated

TABLE 9.2

Measures for Cohort Studies

Measure	Abbreviation	Description
Relative risk	RR	The likelihood or risk of those exposed to a condition will get the disease as opposed to the nonexposed group
Absolute risk	AR	The incidence rate of exposure
Attributable risk	ATR	The difference in incidence between the exposed and nonexposed groups

risk factors. The cases are known because they exhibit symptoms of the condition under study (e.g., the diarrhea that might be expected from a case of food poisoning). Controls must be similar to the cases, except that they do not have the outcome in question (i.e., no diarrhea). Results of a case-control study are reported using an *odds ratio* (OR): the ratio of exposed to nonexposed in the case group divided by the same ratio in the control group (Heffernan, 2010). For example, Suarez et al. (2010), using cases and controls from the large, multistate, population-based National Birth Defects Prevention Study, examined the relation between neural tube defects and maternal exposures to cigarette smoke, including passive smoke exposure. Results when adjusted for race/ethnicity and study center suggested that maternal exposure to passive smoking increased the incidence of neural tube defects in infants (OR, 1.7; 95% CI, 1.4–2.0).

A *case series* (also known as a clinical series) is an observational study that tracks patients with a known exposure who are given similar treatment or reviews their medical records for exposure and outcome. Thus, this study can be retrospective or prospective and usually involves a smaller number of patients than case-control studies (Heffernan, 2010). For example, Shellmer et al. (2011) reported on patients who completed cognitive and adaptive functioning testing preliver and 1- and 3-year postliver transplantation for maple syrup urine disease, which is associated with central nervous system damage, developmental delays, and neurocognitive deficits. Findings showed either no significant change ($N = 8$) or improvement ($N = 5$) in IQ scores preliver to postliver transplantation.

A *case report* is an anecdotal, yet, detailed report of the symptoms, signs, diagnosis, treatment, and follow-up of an individual patient (National Cancer Institute (NCI) Dictionary, 2010). Typically, case reports are constructed to describe an unexpected observation or association or an unexpected event, or to share findings on rare occurrences or adverse effects (NCI Dictionary, 2010). For example, Fraser, Estabrooks, Allen, and Strang (2010) provided a case example to illustrate how the case manager balances and weighs the factors that influence resource allocation decisions and discusses home care case manager resource allocation decisions.

The most commonly used observational study is the descriptive study. *Descriptive studies* are observational studies that describe patterns related to person, place, and time. Often, a descriptive study is the first step into research in a new area. Descriptive studies simply describe, explain, or explore a topic; they do not establish cause and effect. Descriptive studies are valuable, because they can highlight associations between variables or between or among variables. Descriptive studies do not have a comparison (control) group, which means that they do not allow for inferences to be drawn about associations (Heffernan, 2010). For example, Aznar et al. (2011) studied patterns of physical activity in Spanish children. Their findings indicated that few children achieved the exercise levels recommended for health; at particular risk were adolescent girls. They concluded that more effort needs to be devoted to promoting appropriate opportunities for Spanish girls during the day and to promoting physical activity during weekends for all children.

A *cross-sectional study* is a descriptive study that gathers information on both the condition and the exposure at the same time. Cross-sectional studies provide a "snapshot" of one point in time. This type of data can be used to assess the prevalence of acute or chronic conditions in a population. A cross-sectional study is sometimes called a prevalence study (Heffernan, 2010). For example, Chen, P. F. Liu, Liu, & Tsai (2010) examined the level of awareness of hypertension guidelines and associated factors among nurses in 10 hospitals in Taiwan using survey methods. Among the seven dimensions of the hypertension management questionnaire, the definition of hypertension, methods for blood pressure measurements, and impact of high blood pressure on cardiovascular disease had the lowest rates of correct answers. Multiple regression analysis revealed that the nurses' clinical experience, educational level, work setting, in-service education training on hypertension, and level of the hospital ($R = 35.4\%$, $F = 52.89$, $p < .001$) independently predicted the nurse's level of awareness. The authors concluded that a large proportion of the nurses in northern Taiwan had insufficient knowledge of the hypertension guidelines.

STUDIES OF DIAGNOSTIC ACCURACY

Studies of diagnostic accuracy are conducted to determine the exactness of tests used to diagnose conditions. The accuracy is plotted against a standard reference test. A diagnostic test is any test used in making a diagnosis based on presenting signs and symptoms or monitoring the progression of a disease or condition (Deeks, 2001). Diagnostic tests include blood tests, urine tests, psychological evaluations, or imaging studies, among others. However, diagnostic tests are not only used in health care. There are many educational tests used to diagnose learning disabilities, intellectual delays, and learning styles. The results of a diagnostic test are compared with the results of a reference standard in the same person or patient. The reference standard is the test or series of tests used to determine the presence or absence of the target condition in patients. Reviewers should define the reference standard that is going to be used in the review. Diagnostic test accuracy studies differ from prognostic studies in that prognostic accuracy studies test information used to identify patients who may experience a future event, such as disease recurrence or sudden death (Bossuyt & Leeflang, 2008). "What's the prognosis?" is a commonly asked question in health care.

A good diagnostic test is defined by its sensitivity and specificity. Sensitivity (positive results) and specificity (negative results) results are not static. They can vary based on the population or setting. According to the Joanna Briggs Institute:

> . . . due to the wide variation of human beings, (an ideal) test does not exist and what really happens is that a "normal" range of values is established for a particular test and the patient is compared to that range, with the outcome being a likelihood that the patient has/does not have the condition or disease. (p. 25)

A diagnostic test can have one of four outcomes: true positive, true negative, false positive, or false negative. Sensitivity and specificity can be calculated using the formula TP/(TP + FN). Specificity can be calculated using TN/(TN + FP) (see Table 9.3; JBI, 2009).

These measures, along with a likelihood ratio (LR) and receiver operating characteristic (ROC) curve, are used to determine the accuracy of a diagnostic test. Studies that test the accuracy of a diagnostic test using these measures are suitable for a systematic review. *Likelihood ratio* (LR) is a ratio of the probability that a particular result will occur in a patient with the disease, compared with the probability that someone without the disease would have the same result. It is calculated using the sensitivity and specificity results as follows (JBI, 2009):

Sensitivity/(1 − specificity) is a positive LR
(1 − sensitivity)/specificity is a negative LR

The *receiver operating curves* (ROC) are plots of the sensitivity and specificity data. These curves are used to determine the overall diagnostic accuracy of a test. An inaccurate test will have a line close to the rising diagonal. In a perfect test, the line will rise steeply and pass close to the top of the left-hand corner. Sensitivity is plotted on the vertical axis and 1 − specificity is plotted on the horizontal axis. Once a curve has been developed, the area between the curve and the x-axis can be determined and is called the *area under the curve* (AUC). This represents the accuracy of the diagnostic test. An AUC of 1 represents a perfect test and an AUC of 0.5 represents a useless test. A quick way to determine the utility of the AUC results is the traditional school grading system, where .9–1.0 is excellent (an A), .8–.9 is good (a B), and so on until .5–.6, which is failing (an F; JBI, 2009). For further information on the use of ROC and AUC in determining diagnostic accuracy see Zou, O'Malley, & Mauri (2007).

TABLE 9.3

Sensitivity and Specificity

	Disease Present	Disease Absent
Positive test result	True positive (TP)	False positive (FP)
Negative test result	False negative (FN)	True negative (TN)

STUDIES OF PROGNOSIS

The primary purpose of a study of prognosis is to predict outcomes with or without establishing causality (Glasziou, Irwig, Bain, & Colditz, 2001). For example, low slung ears may be predictive of Down's syndrome, but clearly, it is not a cause. According to Glasziou et al. (2001), there are two primary reasons to be interested in making predictions about the future status of patients. The first concerns the patient. Patients with a specific condition are interested in their future. They want to make plans and determine whether any adaptation to lifestyle and/or living arrangements might be necessary. The second concerns the physician. Physicians want to be able to classify patients as high or low risk for development of related symptoms and to appropriately determine therapy.

BIAS AND CONFOUNDING IN OBSERVATIONAL STUDIES

A meta-analysis of interventions is predicated on an unbiased effect of the intervention with random variation held in check by randomization and the intention to treat (ITT) principle. An observational study, on the other hand, can yield estimates that may prove misleading because of confounding factors, biases, or both. Egger, Smith, and Schneider (2001) report, for example, that any review assessing the effect of coffee on myocardial infarction must adjust for smoking because smoking and drinking large amounts of coffee have been found to be associated with heart disease, and smoking is a cause of coronary heart disease (CHD). However, even with adjustment for confounding factors such as these, the issue of bias always arises. Bias in an observational study is a deviation of a measurement from the truth, leading to either an underestimation or overestimation of significance (Glasziou et al., 2001) and can be related to the way in which the study was designed, conducted, or interpreted. Bias may result from poor diagnosis or poor diagnostic criteria, poor case choice, poor choice of controls, or variation in the way risk exposure data is collected or measured in case and controls. The internal validity of the study is affected by any bias present (Jepsen et al., 2004).

Two potential biases that may limit the suitability of an observational study are selection bias and information bias (Jepsen et al., 2004). Table 9.4 presents questions to ask to determine whether a bias is present in an observational study. *Selection bias* refers to differences between the sample studied and the larger population. In other words, the sample is not representative of the larger population. Selection bias is more common in case-control studies than in cohort studies. Examples of selection bias include self-selection, volunteerism, failure to follow the intention to treat principle, attrition, and lack of follow-up (Jepsen et al., 2004).

Information bias can occur in a cohort design. Information bias, also known as classification or measurement bias, refers to an error in measuring the exposure or outcome. Information bias can occur in various ways, including differences in the way information is gathered (in person vs. telephone), coded, entered, or interpreted. For example, an interviewer may ask unclear questions, fail to precisely follow the research protocol, or transcribe information inaccurately. In case control studies that

TABLE 9.4

Questions to Ask to Determine Bias in Observational Research

1. To determine if a selection bias is present, ask:

   In a cohort study, are participants in the exposed and unexposed groups alike in all key aspects except for the exposure?

   In a case-control study, are cases and controls alike in all key aspects except for the condition under study?

2. To determine if an information bias is present, ask:

   In a cohort study, is information about the obtained outcome asked in exactly the same way for both exposed and unexposed groups?

   In a case-control study, is information about collected exposure asked in the same way for cases and controls?

3. To determine if a confounding is present, ask:

   Could the results be accounted for by a factor that was not considered a priori (e.g., smoking, diet, activity level)?

Source: Adapted from Grimes, D. A., & Schulz, K. F. (2002). Bias and causal associations in observational research. *Lancet, 359*(9302), 248–252.

rely on memory of past experiences, information bias is referred to as recall bias, where those in the exposed group may have better recall or better information than the healthier controls (Grimes & Schulz, 2002; Jepsen et al., 2004).

A *confounding* is a clouding of results, such that the outcomes of a study cannot be clearly determined. Confounding variables are perplexing, because the design of the study did not take these variables into account, a priori, causing an incorrect interpretation of results. Whereas bias involves error in the measurement of a variable, confounding involves error in the interpretation of the measurement (JBI, 2009). According to Mann (2003), a confounding variable is independently associated with both the variable of interest and the outcome of interest. For example, lung cancer (outcome) is less common in people with asthma (variable). However, it is improbable that asthma provides protection against lung cancer. It is more likely that the occurrence of lung cancer is lower in people with asthma because fewer asthmatics smoke cigarettes (confounding variable; Mann, 2003). The only way to eliminate the possibility of a confounding variable is via a prospective randomized controlled study. In this type of study, each type of exposure is assigned by chance; therefore, confounding variables are equally present across all groups (Mann, 2003).

Observational Systematic Review

An observational systematic review is conducted when there are gaps in the RCT evidence and there is observational data available that can provide valid and useful information to answer the review question. Gaps in the RCT evidence can be identified at several points during the review: when scoping the review, when reviewing titles

TABLE 9.5

Dangers Inherent in Overreliance on the Randomized Controlled Trials

RCTs may be of short duration and may not be able to assess harm.
RCTs do not often include vulnerable or minority populations. Populations are homogenous such as women; elderly and minority groups are often excluded.
RCTs report efficacy (worth), not effectiveness.
RCT settings may not represent typical situations (e.g., research university hospital vs. community hospital).
Assessment of harm is a secondary consideration in an RCT.
Patients who are more susceptible to harm are often underrepresented.

Note. RCT = randomized controlled trial.

and abstracts, or when appraising the results of the RCT. In addition, trial data may be insufficient for several reasons as presented in Table 9.5. Other reasons for conducting a systematic review of observational data include developing a more precise understanding of etiology, particularly those with rate outcome; evaluating future outcome; and reviewing of public and community health services.

Systematic review of observational studies is useful to quantify sources of variability in results across studies. In addition, a systematic review of observational studies may also be the only available method for assessing the efficacy and effectiveness of some interventions (e.g., fluid resuscitation in the burn patient; Al-Shahi & Warlow, 2001).

Systematic review of diagnostic evidence is conducted to draw conclusions about the accuracy of tests used to make a diagnosis. The test that is being evaluated is known as the *index test*; several index tests can be evaluated within the same review. The index test is evaluated against a comparator (a reference standard) for a target condition (i.e., the condition of interest). The reference standard is usually the test representing the best available method of detecting the target condition (e.g., a chest X-ray is considered a clinical reference test for the diagnosis of tuberculosis). It is sometimes referred as the "gold standard" (Smidt, Deeks, & Moore, 2008).

Prognostic systematic review poses some challenges for the reviewers. According to Altman (2001), in most prognostic studies, the outcome of primary interest is the time to an event, often death, making meta-analysis difficult. Secondly, in many studies, more than one prognostic indicator is studied, and it is often difficult to isolate individual outcomes for each of the indicators. However, consideration must be given to the fact that the study of many variables simultaneously could result in development of a prognostic model for predicting the course of a disease or condition (JBI, 2009). Finally, Altman (2001) relates that many prognostic features are continuous variables, and researchers use a wide variety of methods of analysis, making pooling difficult. However, despite these shortcomings, there are several reasons to conduct a systematic review of prognostic evidence. Among these are to guide clinical decision making, improve understanding of the disease progress, to define risk based on prognosis, and to make accurate predictions about future events and outcomes (Altman, 2001).

Conducting the Review

The first step in conducting a systematic review of observational evidence is to develop a focused clinical question. For descriptive and analytic observational review, the question formulation should follow the typical PICO parts of patient (P), intervention or exposure (I), comparison (C), and outcome (O). For example, "What are the effects of economic and nutritional status on preterm births?"

Because a systematic review of diagnostic test accuracy is used to ascertain how well a test, or a series of tests, is able to correctly identify patients with the target condition (Bossuyt & Leeflang, 2008), the review question will vary slightly, as patient/condition of focus (P), index test (I), reference standard (C), and outcomes (O). For example, Doust, Glasziou, Pietrzak, and Dobson (2004) assessed the diagnostic accuracy of brain natriuretic peptide (BNP), including a comparison with atrial natriuretic peptide (ANP) in heart failure patients, finding that BNP is an accurate marker of heart failure.

Prognostic questions generally have only two parts: the population (P) and outcome (O). For example, Al-Shahi and Warlow (2001) were interested in the frequency and clinical course of arteriovenous malformations (AVM) in the brain of adults.

Search Strategy

The search strategy for a systematic review of observational evidence follows the same stages as presented in previous chapters with some minor variation. Reviewers may perform an initial search looking for both observational studies and RCTs, or searches can be performed sequentially, searching first for an RCT and then observational studies. In any review of quantitative evidence, RCTs are always included in the search; with observational evidence used as the default in the event there are no or limited numbers of RCTs found. The use of clinical filters is important for finding diagnostic and prognostic studies, and one way to accomplish this is to use PubMed's clinical inquiry fields.

The search for diagnostic studies should focus on cross-sectional studies, whereas a prognostic review should focus on retrieval of cohort studies. When conducting a review for either of these, a target condition should be specified. A target condition describes patients with a particular clinical history, examination, and test results (Bossuyt & Leeflang, 2008).

Appraising Studies

As discussed in the previous chapters, appraisal of retrieved studies and the decision to include a study in a systematic review is a crucial decision for reviewers. Any systematic review should include those available studies that are of the highest quality. Appraisal of each paper by two reviewers independently accomplishes this goal.

When appraising case control and cohort studies attention needs to be paid to the representativeness of the sample to the population under study, comparability of the sample's current health status, methods used to minimize selection bias, and strategies used to identify and deal with any confounding factors. It is necessary to determine if the outcomes of those who withdrew from the study were described (Intention to Treat Principle) and the appropriateness of all statistical methods used (JBI, 2008).

Appraisal of descriptive, case series and/or case reports should involve attention to inclusion criteria, methods of randomization, sufficient description of all groups used in any comparisons, and strategies used to identify and deal with any confounding factors. In addition, it is also necessary in these studies to determine if the outcomes of those who withdrew from the study were described (Intention to Treat Principle) and the reliability and appropriateness of all statistical methods used (JBI, 2008).

A more detailed description can be found in the JBI 2008 reviewers' manual at www.joannabriggs.edu.au

For a diagnostic systematic review, tools such as the STARD statement (Standards for Reporting of Diagnostic Accuracy; http://www.stard-statement.org) can be used. The STARD checklist comprised 25 items for evaluation related to the design of the study, study participants, test methods and results, statistical analysis, and an evaluation of the study discussion. The aim of the STARD initiative is to improve the accuracy and completeness of reporting of studies of diagnostic accuracy, to allow readers to assess the potential for bias in the study (internal validity), and to evaluate its generalizability (external validity). An easy-to-follow flow diagram that is useful in describing the study and the flow of patients is also available on the STARD website.

The Quality Assessment of Diagnostic Accuracy Studies (QUADAS) checklist can also be used for appraisal of diagnostic studies when doing a systematic review. The tool is organized into a checklist of 14 questions, which are answered *yes*, *no*, or *unclear* (see Table 9.6). Most items included in QUADAS relate to bias (items 3, 4, 5, 6, 7, 10, 11, 12, and 14), with only two items each relating to variability (items 1 and 2) and reporting (items 8, 9, and 13). A more detailed description of each item together with a guide on how to score each of the questions can be found at Whiting, Rutjes, Reitsma, Bossuyt, & Kleijnen (2003).

Notably, the following additional questions should be asked when appraising diagnostic studies to be sure that only the highest quality studies are included in the review (JBI, 2009):

What is the clinical spectrum of the patients in the study?
Was there blinded interpretation of the test and reference standard results?
If a prospective design, was there consecutive patient sampling?
Is there adequate description of the index test, the reference standard, and the study population and setting?

The appraisal of studies of prognosis is a bit different. Establishing an accurate prognosis is one of the most common tasks for the health care provider. Prognosis is also important in making inferences about quality of care, when comparing

TABLE 9.6

The Quality Assessment of Diagnostic Accuracy Studies (QUADAS) Tool

Was the spectrum of patients representative of the patients who will receive the test in practice?
Were selection criteria clearly described?
Is the reference standard likely to correctly classify the target condition?
Is the period between reference standard and index test short enough to be reasonably sure that the target condition did not change between the two tests?
Did the whole sample or a random selection of the sample receive verification using a reference standard of diagnosis?
Did patients receive the same reference standard regardless of the index test result?
Was the reference standard independent of the index test (i.e., The index test did not form a part of the reference standard.)?
Was the execution of the index test described in sufficient detail to permit replication of the test?
Was the execution of the reference standard described in sufficient detail to permit its replication?
Were the index test results interpreted without knowledge of the results of the reference standard?
Were the reference standard results interpreted without knowledge of the results of the index test?
Were the same clinical data available when test results were interpreted as would be available when the test is used in practice?
Were uninterpretable/intermediate test results reported?
Were withdrawals from the study explained?

Source: From Whiting, P., Rutjes, A. W., Reitsma, J. B., Bossuyt, P. M., & Kleijnen, J. (2003). The development of QUADAS: A tool for the quality assessment of studies of diagnostic accuracy included in systematic reviews. *BioMed Central Medical Research Methodology, 3*, 25. doi:10.1186/1471-2288-3-25 (Open access.)

outcomes in populations from different contexts and institutions (Carneiro, 2002). According to Carneiro (2002), there are three components of an appraisal: (a) a qualitative element (What are the possible outcomes?), (b) a quantitative element (What is the probability of these outcomes occurring?), and (c) a temporal element (Over what period might they occur?). Cardarelli and Oberdorfer (2007) refine this approach by suggesting nine questions to be asked:

1. Are the study subjects truly representative of the population?
2. Were the study subjects chosen at a common point in the disease course?
3. Was the follow-up period sufficiently long and complete?
4. Were the study subjects and investigators blinded to the measures of interest?
5. Were adjustments made for important prognostic factors?
6. How likely are the projected outcomes over time?
7. What is the precision of the relationship between the end point and the outcome?
8. Are the study subjects substantially different from your patient?
9. How important is the evidence for your specific patient?

Data Extraction

It is important in a systematic review of observational evidence to extract and code data according to a prespecified plan. (See Chapter 8 for a detailed description of coding and extracting data.) Specific data to be extracted for an observational review is presented in Table 9.7.

Data Synthesis

Although there is no consensus regarding how to synthesize data for an observational systematic review, the usual procedure is to use the same methods used in a systematic review of interventions (see Chapter 8), keeping in mind that there may be greater degrees of confounding, bias, and heterogeneity in a review of observational evidence. Caution needs to be taken in interpreting the results of an observational review in order not to fall victim to plausible but spurious results. The statistical combination of data should not, therefore, be a prominent feature of an observational review. More may be gained from a careful review of heterogeneity (Eggers, Smith, & Schneider, 2001).

Writing the Report

Standards for reporting the results of an observational systematic review must be maintained to allow proper evaluation of the quality and completeness of the meta-analysis (Stroup et al., 2000). The Meta-analysis of Observational Studies in

TABLE 9.7
Data to Be Extracted for a Systematic Review of Observational Data

Descriptive studies
Mean
Standard deviation
Confidence interval
Odds ratio
Relative risk
Correlations
Diagnostic studies
Results from both the index test and comparator
Sensitivity results
Specificity results
Likelihood ratio
Receiver operator characteristic
Prognostic studies
A numerical summary of prognostic strength such as a hazard ratio, survival curve, or odds ratio

Epidemiology (MOOSE) group, convened by the Centers for Disease Control and Prevention (CDC), developed the MOOSE reporting guidelines to address this issue. The guidelines were developed to address the problem of increasing diversity and variability that exist in reporting meta-analyses of observational studies in an easy-to-follow checklist format (see Table 9.8).

The Preferred Reporting Items for Systematic Reviews and Meta-Analyses (PRISMA; formerly called Quality of Reporting of Meta-analyses [QUOROM]) Statement can also be used. The PRISMA Statement provides an evidence-based set of 27 items in a checklist format. Table 9.9 presents an outline of the essential elements of the PRISMA Statement. Although it focuses on randomized trials, the PRISMA Statement can also be used as a basis for reporting any systematic reviews.

TABLE 9.8
Writing a Report of Meta-analysis of Observational Studies
Summary of MOOSE Guidelines

1. Background

The background should include a description of the problem and study outcomes and detail about the population to be studied and types of studies that were included.

2. Search Strategy

The search strategy should be as transparent as possible and include information on who conducted the search (e.g., librarians or investigators), the timeframe, key words and phrases used. A list of excluded studies and the reason for exclusion is necessary. All databases and registries that were searched, including grey literature, should be listed. A description of other search strategies used must be included, for example, author contact or hand searching of journals.

3. Methods

The rationale and method of coding data and how the data were coded is necessary to report. This includes the use and training of multiple raters, how blinding was realized, and any interrater reliability study. Methods used to select studies for inclusion including the methodological assessment and a description of any confounding variables are necessary.

4. Data Analysis

Methods to assess heterogeneity and any sensitivity analysis conducted must be described. A description of all statistical methods used and justification for chosen model of analysis (fixed effect vs. random effect) should be sufficient enough in detail to allow replication. Any subgroup analysis conducted must also be included. The discussion should detail quantitative assessment of bias (e.g., publication bias) and grading of the level of evidence of included studies.

5. Conclusions

Concluding remarks should include attention to any alternative explanations for observed findings and generalization of results. Recommendation for further research and the implications for practice should also be addressed.

Source: From Stroup, D. F., Berlin, J. A., Morton, S. C., Olkin, I., Williamson, G. D., Rennie, D., . . . Thacker, S. B. (2000). Meta-analysis of observational studies in epidemiology: A proposal for reporting. Meta-analysis of observational studies in epidemiology (MOOSE) group. *Journal of the American Medical Association, 283*(15), 2008–2012.

The entire MOOSE guideline can be accessed at http://www.editorialmanager.com/jognn/account/MOOSE.pdf

TABLE 9.9

**Outline of Preferred Reporting Items for Systematic Reviews and
Meta-Analyses (PRISMA) Statement**

Title
Identify the review as a systematic review
Abstract
Introduction
Rationale for the review
Objectives of the review
Methods
Protocol and registration
Eligibility criteria
Information sources
Eligibility criteria
Search
Study selection
Data collection process
Data items
Risk of bias in individual studies
Summary measures
Synthesis of results
Selection/Topic
Risk of bias across studies
Additional analysis
Results
Summary of evidence
Studies included
Study characteristics
Risk of bias within studies
Results of individual studies
Additional analysis
Discussion
Limitations
Conclusions
Funding

Source: Liberati, A., Altman, D. G., Tetzlafff, J., Mulrows, C., Gotzsche, P., Ioannidis, J. A., . . . Moher, D. (2009). The PRISMA statement for reporting systematic reviews and meta-analyses of studies that evaluate healthcare interventions: explanation and elaboration. *British Medical Journal, 339*, b2700. doi:10.1136/bmj.b2700

SUMMARY

Most health care research, and especially nursing research, is carried out using observational designs. This type of study is used to understand the many different conditions and exposures experienced by people, which are not limited to treatment or intervention or which may not be amenable to intervention. Although the researcher takes a much less active role than in an interventional study, the results of an observational study are not less important, because a systematic review of observational studies may also be the only available method for assessing the efficacy and effectiveness of some interventions.

EXERCISES

Read the observational systematic review listed in the following and answer the subsequent questions:

Bargarli, A., Davoli, M., Minozzi, S., Vecchi, S., & Percucci, C. (2007). *A systematic review of observational evidence on treatment of opioid dependence.* Can be found at: http://www.who.int/substance_abuse/activities/observational_studies_treatment.pdf

1. What are the advantages and disadvantages of using observational research compared with other research methods with this particular review?
2. What sources of bias are apparent and how do they impact the review findings?
3. What are the strengths and weaknesses in the validity of review findings using observational studies?

REFERENCES

Al-Shahi, R., & Warlow, C. (2001). A systematic review of the frequency and prognosis of arteriovenous malformation of the brain in adults. *Brain, 124*(Pt 10), 1900–1926.

Altman, D. G. (2001). Systematic reviews of evaluations of prognostic variables. *British Medical Journal, 323*(7306), 224–228. doi:10.1136/bmj.323.7306.224

Aznar, S., Naylor, P. J., Silva, P., Pérez, M., Angulo, T., Laguna, M., . . . López-Chicharro, J. (2011). Patterns of physical activity in Spanish children: A descriptive pilot study. *Child: Care, Health and Development, 37*(3), 322–328. doi:10.1111/j.1365-2214.2010.01175.x

Bargarli, A., Davoli, M., Minozzi, S., Vecchi, S., & Percucci, C. (2007). *A systematic review of observational evidence on treatment of opioid dependence.* Can be found at: http://www.who.int/substance_abuse/activities/observational_studies_treatment.pdf

Bossuyt, P. M., & Leeflang, M. M. (2008). Developing criteria for including studies. In, *Cochrane handbook for systematic reviews of diagnostic test accuracy* (Version 0.4). Oxford, UK: The Cochrane Collaboration.

Cardarelli, R., & Oberdorfer, J. R. (2007). Evidence-based medicine, Part 5. An introduction to critical appraisal of articles on prognosis. *Journal of the American Osteopathic Association, 107*(8), 315–319.

Carneiro, A. V. (2002). Critical appraisal of prognostic evidence: Practical rules. *Revista Portuguesa de Cardiologia, 21*(7–8), 891–900.

Chan, P. S., Krumholz, H. M., Spertus, J. A., Jones, P. G., Cram, P., Berg, R. A., . . . Nallamothu, B. K. (2010). Automated external defibrillators and survival after in-hospital cardiac arrest. *The Journal of the American Medical Association, 304*(19), 2129–2136.

Chen, H. L., Liu, P. F., Liu, P. W., & Tsai, P. S. (2011). Awareness of hypertension guidelines in Taiwanese nurses: A questionnaire survey. *Journal of Cardiovascular Nursing, 26*(2), 129–136.

Dahnke, M. D. (2011). Observation: The scientific gaze. In M. D. Dahnke & H. M. Dreher (Eds.), *Philosophy of science for nursing practice: Concepts and application* (pp. 153–172). New York, NY: Springer.

Davies, H. T., Crombie, I. K. (2009). *What are confidence intervals and p values?* 2nd Edition. Available at: www.whatisseries.co.uk

Deeks, J. J. (2001). Systematic reviews of evaluations of diagnostic and screening tests. In M. Egger, G. D. Smith, & D. G. Altman (Eds.), *Systematic reviews in health care: Meta-analysis in context* (2nd ed., pp. 248–280). London, UK: BMJ.

Doust, J. A., Glasziou, P. P., Pietrzak, E., & Dobson, A. J. (2004). A systematic review of the diagnostic accuracy of natriuretic peptides for heart failure. *Archives of Internal Medicine, 164*(18), 1978–1984.

Egger, M., Smith, G. D., Schneider, M. (2001). Systematic review of observational data. In M. Egger, G. D. Smith, & D. G. Altman. (Eds.), *Systematic reviews in health care: Meta-analysis in context* (2nd ed., pp. 211–227). London, UK: BMJ.

Fraser, K. D., Estabrooks, C., Allen, M., & Strang, V. (2010). The relational nature of case manager resource allocation decision making: An illustrated case. *Care Management Journals, 11*(3), 151–156.

Glasziou, P., Irwig, L., Bain, C., & Colditz, G. (2001). *Systematic reviews in health care: A practical guide.* New York, NY: Cambridge University Press.

Grimes, D. A., & Schulz, K. F. (2002). Bias and causal associations in observational research. *Lancet, 359*(9302), 248–252.

Harris, G. (2010, July 13). Diabetes drug maker hid test data, files indicate. *The New York Times.* Retrieved from http://www.nytimes.com/2010/07/13/health/policy/13avandia.html

Heffernan, C. (2010). Ask Dr. Cath. Retrieved from http://www.drcath.net/index.html

Jepsen, P., Johnsen, S. P., Gillman, M. W., & Sørensen, H. T. (2004). Interpretation of observational studies. *Heart, 90*(8), 956–960.

Joanna Briggs Institute (2008). *Joanna Briggs Institute reviewers' manual.* Adelaide, Australia: Author.

Joanna Briggs Institute (2009). *Study guide for Module 2.* Adelaide, Australia: Author.

Liberati, A., Altman, D. G., Tetzlafff, J., Mulrows, C., Gotzsche, P., Ioannidis, J. A., . . . Moher, D. (2009). The PRISMA statement for reporting systematic reviews and meta-analyses of studies that evaluate healthcare interventions: explanation and elaboration. *British Medical Journal, 339*, b2700. doi:10.1136/bmj.b2700

Mann, C. J. (2003). Observational research methods. Research design II: Cohort, cross sectional, and case-control studies. *Emergency Medicine Journal, 20*(1), 54–60.

MOOSE Guidelines for Meta-Analyses and Systematic Reviews of Observational Studies. (2000). Retrieved from http://www.editorialmanager.com/jognn/account/MOOSE.pdf

National Cancer Institute Dictionary. (2010). Retrieved from http://www.cancer.gov/dictionary

Observation. (2010). In Encyclopaedia Britannica. Retrieved from http://www.britannica.com/EBchecked/topic/424010/observation

Shellmer, D. A., DeVito Dabbs, A., Dew, M. A., Noll, R. B., Feldman, H., Strauss, K. A., Morton, D. H., . . . Mazariegos, G. V. (2011). Cognitive and adaptive functioning after liver transplantation for maple syrup urine disease: A case series. *Pediatric Transplantation, 15*(1), 58–64. doi:10.1111/j.1399-3046.2010.01411.x

Smidt, M., Deeks, J., & Moore, T. (2008). Chapter 5: Guide to a Cochrane review and protocol for diagnostic accuracy. In *Handbook for systematic reviews of diagnostic test accuracy* [Version 0.4]. The Cochrane Collaboration.

Stroup, D. F., Berlin, J. A., Morton, S. C., Olkin, I., Williamson, G. D., Rennie, D., . . . Thacker, S. B. (2000). Meta-analysis of observational studies in epidemiology: A proposal for reporting. Meta-analysis of observational studies in epidemiology (MOOSE) group. *Journal of the American Medical Association, 283*(15), 2008–2012.

Suarez, L., Ramadhani, T., Felkner, M., Canfield, M. A., Brender, J. D., Romitti, P. A., & Sun, L. (2011). Maternal smoking, passive tobacco smoke, and neural tube defects. *Birth Defects Research. Part A, Clinical and Molecular Teratology, 91*(1), 29–33. doi:10.1002/bdra.20743

Whiting, P., Rutjes, A. W., Reitsma, J. B., Bossuyt, P. M., & Kleijnen, J. (2003). The development of QUADAS: A tool for the quality assessment of studies of diagnostic accuracy included in systematic reviews. *BioMed Central Medical Research Methodology, 3*, 25. doi:10.1186/1471-2288-3-25

Zou, K. H., O'Malley, A. J., & Mauri, L. (2007). Receiver-operating characteristic analysis for evaluating diagnostic tests and predictive models. *Circulation, 115*(5), 654–657.

SUGGESTED READINGS

Benson, K., & Hartz, A. J. (2000). A comparison of observational studies and randomized, controlled trials. *The New England Journal of Medicine, 342*(25), 1878–1886.

Bossuyt, P. M., & Leeflang, M. M. (2008). Chapter 6: Developing criteria for including studies. In, *Cochrane handbook for systematic reviews of diagnostic test accuracy* (Version 0.4). Oxford, UK: The Cochrane Collaboration.

Clarke, M. (2000). The QUORUM statement. *Lancet, 355*(9205), 756–757.

Grimes, D. A., & Schulz, K. F. (2002). Cohort studies: Marching towards outcomes. *Lancet, 359*(9303), 341–345.

Grimes, D. A., & Schulz, K. F. (2002). Descriptive studies: What they can and cannot do. *Lancet, 359*(9301), 145–149.

Schulz, K. F., & Grimes, D. A. (2002). Case-control studies: Research in reverse. *Lancet, 359*(9304), 431–434.

Shamliyan, T., Kane, R. L., & Dickinson, S. (2010). A systematic review of tools used to assess the quality of observational studies that examine incidence or prevalence and risk factors for diseases. *Journal of Clinical Epidemiology, 63*(10), 1061–1070.

Zou, K. H., O'Malley, A. J., & Mauri, L. (2007). Receiver-operating characteristic analysis for evaluating diagnostic tests and predictive models. *Circulation, 115*(5), 654–657.

CHAPTER TEN

Qualitative Metasynthesis

Susan W. Salmond

OBJECTIVES

Upon completion of Chapter 10, you will be able to:

- Define metasynthesis
- State the purposes of a metasynthesis
- Discuss viewpoints on appropriateness of pooling qualitative findings
- Critically appraise qualitative research papers
- Extract data in the form of findings
- Compare and contrast approaches to synthesizing findings

IMPORTANT POINTS

- A qualitative metasynthesis integrates individual qualitative studies by bringing together and breaking down the findings of individual studies, elucidating the key features, and combining these findings into a transformed whole.
- Approaches to synthesis vary based on their degree of interpretation.
- Qualitative findings are appropriate to pool if one conceptualizes generalization as cross-case generalizations, made from, and about, individual cases.
- Generalization or transferability refers to the extent to which the results of qualitative research "fit" with or can be applied to other contexts or settings.
- In meta-aggregation, existing meanings are determined. Through a process of coding and categorization, findings are integrated across studies. The final synthesis statements are an interpretation of the findings and categories.
- In metaethnography, an interpretive synthesis is used where new meanings are generated and a model or explanatory theory developed.

INTRODUCTION

Qualitative research is an umbrella term for research approaches that seek to gain an in-depth understanding of some aspect of the social world (Dew, 2007). The focus of qualitative research is the "quality or nature of human experiences and what these phenomena mean to individuals" (Draper, 2004, p. 642). A naturalistic approach is used to observe subjects in their natural environment in an attempt to understand phenomena within the real context, the context within which they occur, without any attempt to manipulate the phenomenon of interest. It can uncover links among concepts and behaviors and is useful in generating and refining theory (Bradley, Curry, & Devers, 2007). This chapter presents the most commonly assessed qualitative research designs in a systematic review.

AIM OF QUALITATIVE RESEARCH

The aim of qualitative research is illumination, generating understanding of phenomenon within specific contexts and extrapolation to similar situations or contexts (Golafshani, 2003). Qualitative research questions are "what," "how," and "why" type questions. The answers to these questions are obtained through research methods that consist mainly of different types of interviews and observations, both of which yield textual or image data (Draper, 2004). The researcher is the instrument through which these data are obtained, and credibility of qualitative research depends on the ability and effort of the researcher.

Grounded in constructivism or interpretivism, an underlying assumption of the qualitative paradigm is that knowledge and meaning are dynamic, contextual, and socially constructed from the interaction between human beings and their world (Devers, 1999). Thus, understandings can change over time and differ across varying social contexts (Dew, 2007). Although this is the overall paradigm of qualitative research, there are several qualitative methodologies or research approaches that have their own specific theoretical orientation. These theoretical orientations are the distinct principles underlying the particular research approach and reflect views on the nature and categories of being (ontology), as well as how we come to know and understand the world (epistemology). Figure 10.1 illustrates the different qualitative methodologies and their orientation. Table 10.1 provides further description of four commonly used qualitative research approaches.

Similar to all forms of research, there is an a priori plan or proposal setting forth the elements of the research design. However, in qualitative research, this process is flexible or iterative. Naturalistic inquiry designs cannot usually be completely specified in an a priori manner. There will be an initial specification of plans for observations and initial guiding interview questions; however, this may change or shift emphasis and even direction as the process unfolds (Barbour & Barbour, 2003; Patterson, Thorne, Canam, & Jillings, 2001). Table 10.2 provides general information on research methods and qualitative research design. Readers should refer to qualitative textbooks for a full understanding of qualitative research design.

TO SYNTHESIZE OR NOT TO SYNTHESIZE

The aim of metasynthesis is to identify the key findings from qualitative studies that explore the same phenomenon of interest, then compare, contrast, and collate identifiable common themes and subthemes to synthesize a more in-depth description of the phenomenon (Annells, 2005). The appropriateness of combining qualitative find-

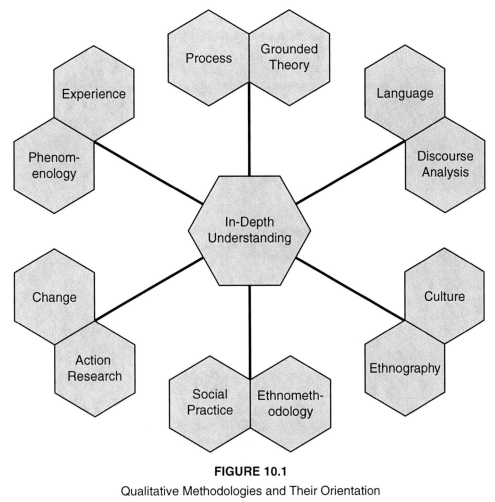

FIGURE 10.1

Qualitative Methodologies and Their Orientation

Source: Dew, K. (2007). A health researcher's guide to qualitative methodologies.
Australian and New Zealand Journal of Public Health, 31(5), 433–437.

ings in a metasynthesis has been a topic of debate for years. The argument against synthesis has been that qualitative research, with a focus on idiographic knowledge or knowledge of particulars, cannot be pooled because the "truth" from one study is only representative of that particular person or group, space, time, or context. Consequently, it was believed that the results could not be transferred to other individuals, groups, or contexts, and that summarizing qualitative findings destroyed the integrity of the individual projects (Sandelowski, Docherty, & Emden, 1997).

With the growing volume of qualitative research and the increased emphasis on evidence-based practice, how then can qualitative research inform practice? The value of qualitative research with a focus on an "N = 1 experience" is limited. Evidence from a single study is likely not to be sufficient to inform or change practice. Qualitative research conducted in isolation without making pragmatic links with prior research will rarely surface for use in contributing to nursing knowledge and practice (Estabrooks, Field, & Morse, 1994).

TABLE 10.1

Qualitative Research Methodologies

Methodology	Research Aim and Theoretical Orientation
Ethnography	■ Asks, "What is the culture of this group?" ■ Aims to explore in-depth how individuals in a specific culture or subculture make sense of their lived reality ■ Originating discipline: anthropology Assumptions ■ The social world should be studied in its naturalistic state. ■ Human actions are infused by social or cultural meanings. ■ People interpret stimuli within the context of their culture. ■ Members of a cultural group often do not have conscious awareness of the fundamental presuppositions or values that shape their view of the world or behavior. ■ To understand people's behavior, one must gain access to meanings. Methods Used ■ Participant observation, fieldwork: Situates the researcher in the setting through use of multiple methods of data collection, including observation, conversations, interviews, and archive/artifact analysis; the emic perspective of the peoples' beliefs and practices is documented. ■ Requires that the research be able to differentiate the "emic" (insider) and "etic" (outsider) perspective
Phenomenology	■ Asks, "What is the lived experience?" . . . the meaning, structure, and essence of this phenomenon for this person or group ■ Aims to understand and illuminate the "meaning, structure, and essence of the lived experience of a phenomenon for a person or group of people" (Patton, 2002, p. 482) ■ Aims to achieve in-depth understanding of the nature or meaning of our everyday experiences ■ Studies everyday experience from the subject's point of view ■ Originating discipline: philosophy Assumptions ■ There are two kinds of reality: (a) nomea—being in reality itself and (b) noesis—the phenomenon or appearance of reality in consciousness. ■ Consciousness of an object is not the real object but the individual's perception of the object; consciousness is the only access human beings have to the world. ■ Phenomenological reflection is retrospective or recollective of experience that has already passed or been lived through. ■ What is perceived varies based on experience, with one's orientation of wishing, willing, or judging. Methods Used ■ In-depth interviews with people who have direct experience (lived experience) with the phenomenon of interest.

(Continued)

TABLE 10.1

Qualitative Research Methodologies *(Continued)*

Methodology	Research Aim and Theoretical Orientation
	■ Researcher provides a window into other's experience (Dew, 2007).
	■ Researchers examine their own views toward the phenomenon and brackets or sets aside their own ideas and judgments and explores the phenomenon anew.
Grounded theory	■ Asks, "What theory emerges from systematic comparative analysis and is grounded in fieldwork so as to explain what has been and is observed?" (Patton, 2002, p. 125)
	■ Is a systematic approach to explore social processes in human interaction and generate theoretical constructs and/or concepts that illuminate human behavior and the social world.
	■ Aims to develop mid-range theory that is grounded or explained by the data collected
	■ Originating discipline: sociology
	Assumptions
	■ Theory is developed without being influenced by a priori assumptions.
	■ Draws from symbolic interactionism, which views behavior as developed through human interactions and an ongoing process of negotiation and renegotiation.
	Methods Used
	■ Begins with an inductive approach asking a broad question. As theoretical understanding develops, it guides further data collection and links induction and deduction through the constant comparative method.
	■ Theoretical comparison is a tool for looking at something and preserving some degree of objectivity.
	■ Theoretical sampling
	■ The researcher avoids using prior theoretical understandings.
Action research	■ Aims at solving specific issues or problems with the intent of improving the situation
	■ Explicitly becomes part of the change process as people from the organization or community are engaged in solving their problem
	■ Success comes not only from the degree of change but also from what has been learned from the experience.
	Assumptions
	■ The role of the researcher is to work with and for the people rather than undertake to study them.
	■ Participants are viewed as equals in the process.
	Methods Used
	■ Action–reflection spirals in which data are collected using a combination of methods, both qualitative and quantitative, and this data are analyzed and reflected on and fed back into the action cycle.

TABLE 10.2
Research Methods and Qualitative Research Design

Sample	*Goal:* Select informants who are able to provide rich description and insight into the phenomena of interest.
	Sample size: one that adequately answers the question. Often, size is determined by data saturation.
	Data saturation: The point in the research process when new themes, categories, or explanations no longer emerge from the data.
	Convenience sample: least rigorous approach where participants are chosen based on accessibility, ease, speed, and low cost.
	Purposive sample: purposively select specific information-rich cases, which will allow greater understanding or in-depth understanding of phenomena and will illuminate the questions under study. There are many approaches to purposive sampling and can include typical cases, deviant cases, or negative/disconfirming cases among others.
	Theoretical sample: When a theory is being built from the emerging data, the researcher selects a new sample to examine and elaborate on the theory.
Interviews	*Goal:* to facilitate description of one's personal perspective of a situation/experience/event to understand the participant's point of view and uncover the meaning of the experience.
	Question design: Open-ended interviewing with varying degrees of structure of the interview based on the underlying methodology and research question.
	Structured interview: provides set, detailed questions that are asked to all participants.
	General topic guide: provides broad questions and some additional probes that can be used.
	Introductory question: A very open-ended interview has only a broad opening question.
Focus groups	Small group of individuals chosen based on having some key common characteristics.
	Is a structured and informal approach that uses a small number of "focus questions" to stimulate recollection and dialog among group members.
Direct observation	Provides direct experience with how individuals interact with each other. The researcher does not become part of the context but tries to remain detached and unobtrusive.
Participant observation	The researcher has prolonged exposure with the participants in the natural setting. The researcher is part of the setting or process being examined. Uses unstructured observation, conversations, interviews, and artifact analysis.
Forms of data	Qualitative data describe and tell a story. Field notes, audio and videotapes, transcripts, documents, and artifacts (things subjects make or use) are sources of qualitative data.
Document review	Pull facts, situations, or series of events from formal documents

(Continued)

TABLE 10.2
Research Methods and Qualitative Research Design *(Continued)*

Data analysis	Data analysis may be an ongoing process and shapes the ongoing data collection with refining of questions, selecting new samples, or exploring new areas that emerge.
	Generally, verbal data are transcribed to text. Text is analyzed using some form of content analysis in which data are "indexed" or coded to reveal categories or themes. Data from each category/theme are identified and examined using constant comparison whereby each item is compared with the rest of the data to validate the categories.

Movement toward qualitative synthesis requires one to move away from the notion that qualitative research cannot be generalized. Sandelowski et al. (1997) stress that generalization should "not be narrowly conceived in terms of sampling and statistical significance" but to consider generalization in terms of "naturalistic or idiographic generalizations made about particulars" (p. 367). The generalizations are not grounded in the experimental paradigm that equates external validity with replication. It is not about generalizations that are predictive. Rather, the generalizations are cross-case generalizations made from, and about, individual cases, and generalization or transferability refers to the extent to which the results of qualitative research "fit" with or can be applied to other contexts or settings. In this sense, a naturalistic generalization can inform practice and support practice recommendations.

A qualitative metasynthesis integrates individual qualitative studies by bringing together and breaking down the findings (themes, metaphors, or categorizations) of individual studies, elucidating the key features, and combining these findings into a transformed whole—a single description of the findings that authentically represents all of the cases (The Joanna Briggs Institute [JBI], 2008; Schreiber, Crooks, & Stern, 1997; Zimmer, 2006). By producing a new and integrative interpretation of the findings, there is a more substantive understanding of the phenomenon than what was produced in individual studies. This contributes to "theory development, higher level abstraction, and generalizability to make qualitative findings more accessible for application in practice" (Zimmer, 2006, p. 313).

QUALITATIVE SYSTEMATIC REVIEW/METASYNTHESIS

As presented in earlier chapters, a systematic review is a descriptive research method where the subjects of the research are individual studies that are related to each other by the same phenomenon of interest. A *research question* and the specific inclusion criteria guide the process of study selection. Questions for a qualitative systematic review and accompanying *inclusion criteria* must be carefully considered because too broad of a question will result in an unmanageable amount of papers. Too narrow of a question, on the other hand, could result in a meaningless exercise because the phenomenon may not be captured. Generally, it is recommended that one begins with a tighter focus and make changes as needed as one begins to identify whether there are appropriate and sufficient papers.

The aim of the search is to retrieve all of the relevant studies in a field. To this end, multiple *approaches to searching* databases, grey literature, and additional strategies such as hand searching, footnote chasing, and author contact are conducted. These approaches are especially useful with qualitative research because most databases have only just begun to code qualitative methodology and because, oftentimes, titles of qualitative research are metaphorical in nature, Thus, a paper entitled *"On the Other Side of the Bed"* is actually a qualitative descriptive study of nurses who are family members of loved ones being cared for in critical care environments. The approaches to searching are described in depth in Chapters 5 and 6.

Study selection begins with an initial screen of study titles and abstracts, done independently by two reviewers, using the inclusion criteria to screen papers. Those determined to meet the inclusion criteria are retrieved for a second, more intense screening—the critical appraisal process.

The *critical appraisal* process, performed independently by two reviewers, examines each paper for validity and methodological congruency and rigor. Although there is debate whether qualitative research should be subject to critical appraisal, the approach supported in this text is that critical appraisal is a necessary component of a systematic review such that the ultimate pooling of findings is drawn from studies that are considered trustworthy. Qualitative work cannot, however, be appraised from a quantitative paradigm because the philosophical orientations are not congruent. Understanding the components of validity in qualitative work is critical to assuring that the qualitative methods used enhance the trustworthiness of the findings and, therefore, their utility to inform practice. Chapter 7 provides more discussion of qualitative critical appraisal.

Appraisers need a good understanding of qualitative research design to effectively appraise a study. One example of a qualitative critical appraisal tool is the JBI QARI Critical Appraisal Checklist for Interpretive and Critical Research. The tool is available at the JBI Connect website (http://www.jbiconnect.org/connect/downloads/QARI_crit_apprais.pdf). The JBI has adopted an inclusive, pluralistic approach to "what counts as evidence" and has developed methodologies for systematic reviews of qualitative evidence and metasynthesis. The JBI Critical Appraisal Checklist is part of the qualitative software package, the Qualitative Appraisal and Review Instrument (QARI). The 10 items examine different components of validity, methodological appropriateness, and ethical conduct of the study. Table 10.3 provides the criterion and rating schema used, as well as an explanation of how to interpret the criterion and perform the critique.

Based on the appraisal, the researchers make the decision whether to include or exclude the study from the synthesis. There is no set rule for an overall inclusion score. Rather, the researchers set a score or prioritize particular criterion that is critical for inclusion. The final report should provide information on this process, from retrieval through appraisal, showing what was included and excluded. Figure 10.2 provides a schematic illustration of this process from a comprehensive systematic review on transition out of intensive care unit (ICU). A table of excluded studies is developed for the final paper providing the rationale for excluding the paper. This transparency provides the necessary audit trail substantiating decision making.

There has been some debate whether studies that use different methodological approaches should be retrieved. Walsh and Downe (2005) argue that in the qualitative paradigm, which "sees truths as multiple, and knowledge as constructed, it is legitimate to include a variety of methodological approaches in a

TABLE 10.3

Joanna Briggs Institute's Critical Appraisal Checklist for Interpretive and Critical Research With Instructions on Interpretation

Criteria	Yes	No	Unclear	Interpretive Guide
1. Is there congruity between the stated philosophical perspective and the research methodology?				■ Methodology refers to the principles underlying particular research approaches ■ This information contributes to theoretical validity. ■ The underlying theoretical perspectives inform methodology, methods, and interpretation. ■ A simple statement that it is qualitative research is not sufficient. ■ Examples of theoretical perspectives may include positivist, interpretive, subtle realist, critical, and analytical, and each of these perspectives has associated with methodologies, which are congruent with the theoretical perspectives (for further information see the qualitative research project website project at the Robert Wood Johnson Foundation http://www.qualres.org/index.html) (Cohen & Crabtree, 2006). ■ The report should indicate the methodological approach used (e.g., phenomenology, ethnography, action research, grounded theory, etc.) ■ There should be congruence with the theoretical perspective and the methodology. For example, action research is congruent with the critical perspective. Phenomenology is congruent with the interpretive perspective.
2. There is congruity between the research methodology and the research question or objectives.				■ This criterion is examining the appropriateness or quality of the research design. ■ Identify the research question or objectives. The focus of most qualitative research is to explore the quality or nature of human experiences. Qualitative research questions generally use verbs such as explore, describe, and understand and attempt to explain the how and why of a phenomenon. ■ Identify the methodology or methodologies used. ■ Is the question congruent with the methodology? A question looking at cause and effect is not congruent with qualitative methodologies. A question that seeks to illuminate or understand experiences is congruent with interpretive methodologies. Questions that explore concepts of oppression, discrimination, and empowerment within identified populations are congruent with action research and feminist research.

(Continued)

TABLE 10.3

Joanna Briggs Institute's Critical Appraisal Checklist for Interpretive and Critical Research With Instructions on Interpretation *(Continued)*

Criteria	Yes	No	Unclear	Interpretive Guide
3. There is congruity between the research methodology and the methods used to collect data.				■ This criterion is examining the appropriateness or quality of the research design. ■ Methods encompass the techniques used to answer the question and include the sampling approach and data collection methods (i.e., survey, individual interview, focus group, etc.) and should reflect appropriate rigor ■ Has the paper *explicitly identified* the methods used for sampling? Are the participants appropriate for answering the research question? ■ Are the data collection approaches used appropriate for answering the questions and consistent with quality standards for the particular methodology? Is more than one data collection approach used? ■ Example: Combining survey techniques with interview/focus groups as well as document analysis is appropriate for action research but not for interpretive methodologies. ■ Example: Using purposive or theoretical sampling is appropriate for interpretive methodologies.
4. There is congruity between the research methodology and the representation of the analysis of data.				■ This criterion is examining the appropriateness or quality of the research design. ■ The paper should provide sufficient detail on the analysis approach used to be deemed credible. ■ Is the approach to thematic content analysis consistent with the methodology used; that is, for grounded theory methodology, one would expect description of codification and analysis in the constant comparative framework; for ethnography, one would expect it detailed how notes were taken during fieldwork. ■ Was data analyzed by more than one researcher? ■ Was data validated by participants? ■ Was there a search for negative or disconfirming evidence?

5. There is congruity between the research methodology and the interpretation of results.	■ This criterion is examining the appropriateness or quality of the research design. ■ Most qualitative work is inductive in nature and should clearly describe the main results so that the reader understands the themes, categories, or concepts. ■ Was there an audit trail substantiating the interpretation? ■ If a theoretical framework was used to guide the methods, has it been used in the data interpretations?
6. There is a statement locating the researcher culturally or theoretically.	■ This criterion supports descriptive validity. ■ Are the researcher's perspectives concerning the phenomenon and approach described? Are the researcher's own position, assumptions, and possible biases outlined? With the role of researcher as an instrument, these relationships and perspectives can influence all phases of the research process. ■ Are the findings interpreted within the context of other studies and theory?
7. The influence of the researcher on the research, and vice versa, is addressed.	■ This criterion supports descriptive validity. ■ The effect of the investigator on those researched and the effect of the research process on the investigator should be described. Has the relationship between researcher and study participants been adequately considered? Is there evidence of reflexivity—that the researcher has reflected on their potential personal influence during data collection? Is it reported how the researcher responded to events that arose during the study? ■ Is the relationship between the researcher and the study context of the study clearly and adequately described? ■ Has a reflective journal been kept?
8. Participants and their voices are adequately represented.	■ This criterion supports interpretive validity/believability. ■ Papers should provide illustrations to show the basis of their conclusions and to ensure that participants and their voices are represented in the report. Were there a reasonable number of quotations illustrating the theme? ■ Were techniques such as prolonged engagement and member checking used to confirm the believability of the voices?

(Continued)

TABLE 10.3

Joanna Briggs Institute's Critical Appraisal Checklist for Interpretive and Critical Research With Instructions on Interpretation *(Continued)*

Criteria	Yes	No	Unclear	Interpretive Guide
9. The research is ethical according to current criteria or, for recent studies, there is evidence of ethical approval by an appropriate body.				■ Was informed consent obtained? ■ Were measures taken to ensure confidentiality or anonymity? Or the ability to withdraw? ■ Was there appropriate support and referral available? ■ Was there an ethical board?
10. Conclusions drawn in the research report do appear to flow from the analysis or interpretation of the data.				■ This criterion contributes to theoretical and evaluative validity. ■ Were the conclusions appropriate and consistent with the data?

Source: Côté, L., & Turgeon, J. (2005). Appraising qualitative research articles in medicine and medical education. *Medical Teacher, 27*(1), 71–75. Hannes, K., Lockwood, C., & Pearson, A. (2010). A comparative analysis of three online appraisal instruments' ability to assess validity in qualitative research. *Qualitative Health Research, 20*(12), 1736–1743. doi: 10.1177/1049732310378656. The Joanna Briggs Institute. (2008). *Joanna Briggs Institute reviewer's manual: 2008 edition.* Adelaide, Australia: Author.

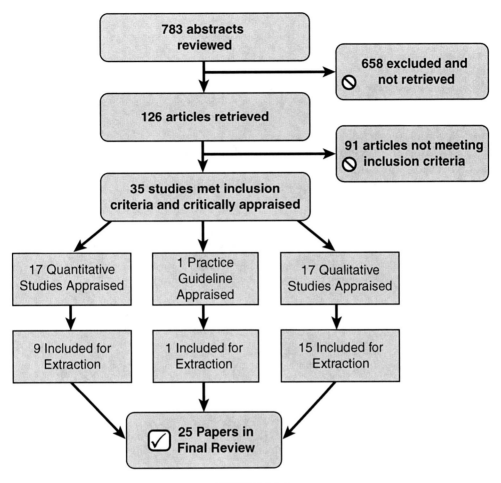

FIGURE 10.2

Algorithm of Study Selection Relocation Stress Following In-House Transfer out of ICU

metasynthesis" (p. 207). Sandelowski et al. (1997) also support multiple methodologies but suggests that the researcher may first want to group findings together from similar methodologies for initial examination before attempting any sort of synthesis between methods. The JBI approach stresses the fact that in the approach of meta-aggregation, the synthesis is of findings—not of primary data—and, therefore, multiple methodologies are appropriate for synthesis. The approach in this text is to support inclusion of various methodological approaches.

The included studies are then reviewed and the process of *data extraction* or identifying and recording relevant results begins. Data extraction is done independently by two people before conferring on the consistency of what was extracted. The intent of extraction is to reduce the findings of multiple studies into a single document. An agreed-upon data extraction instrument should be used so there is a standard approach used across all studies. This minimizes error, provides a historical record of decisions made about the data, and, ultimately, will become the data set for categorization and synthesis (JBI, 2008). Table 10.4 presents the JBI QARI Data Extraction Form for Interpretive and Critical Research with explanatory instructions. The form has been piloted and refined and is incorporated into the QARI software. As can be seen, the data extraction form first requires information on the methodological framework, research methods, contextual factors, and participants. The author's conclusions are abstracted, and the reviewer has an opportunity to record any issues about the paper they may have.

The final step in data extraction is to read and reread the paper and extract particular findings from the study along with illustrations from the text supporting the origin of the finding. These findings serve as the data for the synthesis. Findings appear as themes, metaphors, key concepts, or succinct summaries of findings. Sometimes, the finding is easy to identify and, in other cases, requires differentiation of what consti-

TABLE 10.4

Joanna Briggs Institute Qualitative Appraisal and Review Instrument Data Extraction Form for Interpretive and Critical Research

Page 1:

Methodology	Identify the research methodology used in the study.
	Example:
	Interpretive methodologies: phenomenology, ethnography, grounded theory
	Critical methodologies: action research, feminist research
Method	The way in which data is collected.
	Be specific (i.e., face to face, open-ended interviews, observation, etc). If multiple methods are used, list all methods.
Setting and context	Provide the specific location of the research in terms of local environment (i.e., acute care, long-term care, community dwelling). Be as descriptive as possible because this is a component in assessing transferability.
Geographical context	Location of the research: country, urban/rural/suburban
Cultural context	Cultural features in the study setting such as period, ethnic groupings, age-specific groupings, socioeconomic characteristics, employment, lifestyle, and so forth, which are associated with distinct values and beliefs.
Participants	Information related to inclusion and exclusion criteria
	Should provide the sample size and a description of the sample to include but not be limited to description of age, gender, sample size, participation rate, and ethnicity.
Data analysis	The specific method used for data analysis.
	Include software programs, type of analysis (i.e., contextual analysis, thematic analysis, discourse analysis, content analysis).
Author's conclusions	
Reviewer's comments	

(Continued)

TABLE 10.4

Joanna Briggs Institute Qualitative Appraisal and Review Instrument Data Extraction Form for Interpretive and Critical Research *(Continued)*

Page 2:

Findings	Illustrative Description	Pg #	Quality of Evidence Rating		
			Unequivocal	Credible	Not Supported
Findings are conclusions reached by the researcher after data analysis, often presented in the form of themes or metaphors but also can be as summary statements.	The informant's words or the author's observation or summary of the findings for that specific finding/theme. May have multiple illustrations describing different components of the theme.				

Source: The Joanna Briggs Institute. (2008). *Joanna Briggs Institute reviewer's manual: 2008 edition.* Adelaide, Australia: Author.

tutes a finding and what is data. Within each theme, there may be several different illustrations of different components of the finding. Each should be recorded separately. The illustrative text may be in the form of a direct quote, an observation, or a statement made by the author. Thus, after reviewing six papers, it may be that there are 36 findings.

In the JBI framework, the level of congruency between the finding and supporting data is graded for credibility. The three levels of credibility include: unequivocal, credible, and not supported. Unequivocal is not open to challenge and refers to evidence beyond reasonable doubt, and typically includes any directly reported quotation or observation. Credible equates with plausible and refers to evidence that can be logically inferred from the data but are interpretive in nature and, therefore, can be challenged. Not supported is designated when the finding/illustration is not supported by the data (JBI, 2008). Table 10.5 provides a small sample of findings/illustrations and credibility ratings for a comprehensive systematic review on transition out of ICU.

The final step in the systematic review process is the actual *synthesis*. This is an interpretive process that encompasses "comparison, translation, and analysis of original findings from which new interpretations are generated, encompassing and distilling the meanings" in the included studies (Zimmer, 2006, p. 312) into stronger and more generalizable knowledge claims (Thorne, 2009).

APPROACHES TO SYNTHESIS

For the purposes of this chapter, metasynthesis will be used as an umbrella term that captures a collection of approaches to synthesis. The aim of metasynthesis

TABLE 10.5

Findings/Illustrations and Credibility Ratings

Finding	Illustration	Credibility Rating
Sudden abandonment from abrupt transfer	"From a patient . . . You sort of feel like you've been kicked out. I was there such a long time. I think that when you get discharged, to a certain extent, it's you are finished, get out."	Unequivocal
Vulnerability	" . . . Everything was done for me [in ICU] . . . I found that when I went to the ward, they didn't seem to know anything about me."	Unequivocal
Vulnerability	" . . . For families, the sense of vulnerability was particularly associated with the significant responsibility they had to accept now the patients were in the ward."	Credible
Vulnerability	" . . . There were a lot of things I couldn't do. I couldn't even get out of bed."	Unequivocal
Unimportance	" . . . He couldn't do anything himself. It was just terrible. Nine weeks with one-on-one care and then he was put in a ward with six people."	Unequivocal

Source: Salmond, S., & Evans, B. (2010). *A systematic review of relocation stress following in-house transfer out of critical/intensive care units*. Adelaide, Australia: The Joanna Briggs Institute Library of Systematic Reviews.

is to assemble findings; categorize these findings into groups based on similarity in meaning; and to aggregate or interpret these findings to generate a set of statements that adequately represent the combined studies. These statements are referred to as *synthesized findings* and they can be used as a basis for evidence-based practice.

Metasynthesis involves the qualitative aggregation and/or interpretation of findings that have been extracted from topically related study reports. These findings are drawn from studies with varying qualitative methods and theoretical frameworks. The findings, in the form of themes, metaphors, and key concepts, are aggregated together and translated from one study to another using an idiomatic rather than a word-for-word translation (Reis, Hermoni, Van-Raalte, Dahan, & Borkan, 2007) creating a broader and deeper understanding of the phenomenon. The term *translation* refers to a process of "taking concepts from one study and recognizing the same concepts in another study, though they may not be expressed using identical words" (Thomas & Harden, 2008, p. 3).

As illustrated in Table 10.6, there are various approaches to metasynthesis. They vary in the degree of interpretation involved with approaches such as metastudy, metaethnography, and grounded theory being more highly interpretive, and metasummary and meta-aggregation being less interpretive and more integrative (Finfgeld-Connett, 2010). To illustrate the similarities and differences, the meta-aggregation and metaethnographic approaches will be

TABLE 10.6
Metasynthesis Approaches/Terminology

Term	Description
Grounded formal theory	Inductive research approach that uses findings from substantive grounded theory studies and systematically building conceptual links to synthesize a new grounded formal theory (Kearney, 1998; Thorne, Jensen, Kearney, Noblit, & Sandelowski, 2004)
Meta-analysis	Term frequently used to describe the statistical combining and analysis of results from multiple quantitative research studies (Egger, Smith & Phillips, 1997). Because of the term's common association with quantitative methods and data aggregation versus interpretation, its use in relationship to qualitative metasynthesis is discouraged. (Finfgeld, 2003)
Metastudy	Inductive research approach involving the analysis and interpretation of theory, methods, and research findings across qualitative studies, and the synthesis of this work to formulate new interpretations and theory (Finfgeld, 2003). Requires that the context and related assumptions behind the findings of each contributing report be taken into consideration and made visible in the final report (Thorne et al., 2004). Involves three distinct type of analyses from which a new theoretical interpretation is created.
Metadata analysis	Analysis and interpretation of findings across multiple qualitative research reports (Finfgeld, 2003)
Metamethod	Analysis and interpretation of methodological applications across multiple qualitative research reports (Finfgeld, 2003)
Metatheory	Analysis and interpretation of theoretical, philosophical, and cognitive perspectives, sources and assumptions, and contexts across multiple qualitative studies (Patterson et al., 2001)
Metaethnography	An interpretive synthesis (interpretation of interpretations) that arises from comparative translation. The synthesis can take many forms: reciprocal, refutation, and line of argument (Thorne et al., 2004). It is not limited to ethnographic studies.
Meta-aggregation	The aggregation or synthesis of findings to generate a set of statements that represent that aggregation, through assembling the findings rated according to their quality, and categorizing these findings on the basis of similarity in meaning. These categories are then subjected to a metasynthesis to produce a single comprehensive set of synthesized findings that can be used as a basis for evidence-based practice (JBI, 2008, p. 34).
Metasummary (descriptive metasynthesis)	An approach to synthesis of reports of primary qualitative studies containing findings in the form of topical or thematic summaries or surveys of the data the researcher had collected (Thorne et al., 2004). Is a quantitatively oriented aggregation of qualitative findings. They use low levels of interpretation and stay close to the findings of the original research and can be considered to be equal to the sum of the parts.

(Continued)

TABLE 10.6

Metasynthesis Approaches/Terminology *(Continued)*

Term	Description
Qualitative metasynthesis	An interpretative integration of qualitative findings from primary research that is interpretive in nature (Thorne et al., 2004). Goes beyond sum of the parts to providing new interpretations of findings.
Metasynthesis	Umbrella term referring to a complete study to produce new and integrative interpretations of findings that are more substantive than those resulting from individual studies (Finfgeld, 2003). The synthesis of findings across multiple qualitative reports to create a new interpretation.

described. As these processes are read, it must be remembered that the steps described are not mechanistic tasks and there is a creative and intuitive portion to the process.

Meta-Aggregation

In integrative approaches or meta-aggregations, the researcher deduces existing meanings. The reviewers do not reinterpret the primary research findings from each included paper but work with the interpretations primary researchers made in the first instance. It uses an integrative approach to summarizing the data, and the concepts that are extracted and synthesized are assumed to be largely secure and well specified.

Similar to all approaches, the researchers begin an iterative process by immersing themselves in the data. Reviewing all of the extracted findings and supporting illustrations prior to coding helps identify similar meanings and emergent themes/categories. Each finding/illustration is coded. *Codes* are tags or labels that help catalog or categorize the findings according to similarity in meaning and content. Some findings may have single codes and others may have multiple codes. Next, findings with common codes are grouped together or categorized based on similar meaning. By combining the codes, there is a translation of concepts from one study to another (Thomas & Harden, 2008). Table 10.7 provides a glimpse of the coding and categorization process in a systematic review on transition out of ICU. Sample findings and codings for two categories are presented. As can be seen, the original findings from different studies (each finding is numbered) were coded in the analysis process. Findings with different codes were analyzed to have similar meanings and were grouped together into categories.

The categories are then thematically grouped according to similar meaning, and these form the synthesized findings. This process is not simply aggregative, linear, and mechanistic but involves interpretation, albeit a more limited form of interpretation than approaches such as metaethnography. The aim is for the interpretation to be transparent and to maintain representativeness with the primary literature. The audit trail of decisions made throughout the review process enables this representativeness to occur.

TABLE 10.7

Findings/Illustrations, Codes, and Categories

Pooled Data Into New Category: Leaving the Protective Cocoon Engenders Vulnerability		
Findings	**Illustrations**	**Code**
12. Vulnerability	"Everything was done for me [in ICU] . . . I found that when I went to the ward, they didn't seem to know anything about me."	One among many
35. Adjustment	"You'd gone from this hugely protective critical care to this sort of hit and miss uncoordinated service."	ICU as a protective cocoon
42. Concerns about the ward environment	"So it was quite difficult and my relatives saw this and they knew that I'd gone from being in intensive care with my own nurse to suddenly being alone, really."	One among many
43. Concerns about the ward environment	"And even if you did buzz the nurses, they were obviously busy. They couldn't come as quickly as they could on the intensive care unit, you'd have to wait, which wasn't anybody's fault. But it would have been better if I could have done a bit more for myself."	One among many
94. Ambivalence	Although there was expression of fears about leaving the "safety" of critical care, the value of transfer to the ward was understood. " . . . going back on the ward it wasn't good at all, but, after a while, that didn't matter so much. But after having that wonderful care, and then to have to go back, which . . . is the sort of thing you should be trying to do, fend for yourself as soon as you can."	Reemergence of vulnerability

Pooled Data into New Category: Physical Debilitation Within Conflicting Expectations of Independence		
Findings	**Illustrations**	**Code**
29. Basic care: attention, rest, and personal care	When people felt they were unable to sleep and rest, and when they found themselves struggling to cope with mobility and personal care, particularly help with toileting, some became upset.	Physical debilitation
41. Concerns about the ward environment	"But I couldn't even walk; I couldn't get up and sit in a chair by myself. I could feed myself by that point, but I couldn't go to the toilet. I couldn't stand up; I couldn't get to the sink. If my glass was on a trolley at the bottom of the bed, I wouldn't have been able to reach that."	Physical debilitation
59. Physical problems	Tiredness, weakness, sleep difficulties, poor concentration or memory prevent functioning as before and cause stress.	Physical debilitation

(Continued)

TABLE 10.7

Findings/Illustrations, Codes, and Categories *(Continued)*

Pooled Data into New Category: Physical Debilitation Within Conflicting Expectations of Independence		
Findings	**Illustrations**	**Code**
26. Different levels of care	"But in a way, you need that because you need to start to do more for yourself, simple things were hard to do; for example, going to the toilet or having a wash. You realize you've got to get up and do it yourself, and I'd even have to wait for painkillers. But that's nobody's fault, that's just how it is."	Independence catalyst
30. Basic care: attention, rest, and personal care	"When I first got into the ward, I could hardly stand; in fact, almost couldn't stand without assistance. And I had an instance where I needed to go to the loo. And they brought a commode for me, which was fine, that was no issue. But because, if you can imagine I couldn't write properly and I couldn't use my arms properly, you can imagine what else I couldn't do. And subsequently, they didn't assist me with cleaning up properly, which left me in a less than clean or desirable position.	Unresponsive to functional dependence

Note. ICU = intensive care unit.

Source: Salmond, S., & Evans, B. (2010). *A systematic review of relocation stress following in-house transfer out of critical/intensive care units*. Adelaide, Australia: The Joanna Briggs Institute Library of Systematic Reviews.

Figure 10.3 captures this process of synthesis where findings are collapsed into categories and categories into synthesis statements.

As can be seen, there were a total of 18 findings that shared a common meaning and were categorized as "leaving the protective cocoon engenders vulnerability." Another category, "physical debilitation within conflicting expectations of inde-

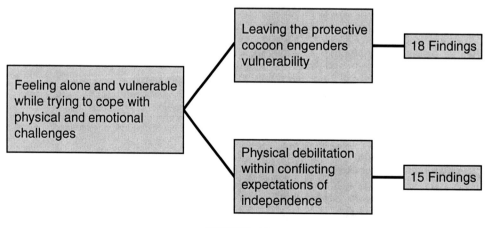

FIGURE 10.3

Findings are Collapsed Into Categories and Categories are Combined Into Synthesis Statements

pendence," captured the meaning of additional 15 findings. These categories were grouped into a synthesis statement "feeling alone and vulnerable while trying to cope with physical and emotional challenges." A subsequent table in the final report provides the numbered findings for each category, providing a clear audit trail that makes decision making transparent. The short synthesis statement can be further described to provide guidelines for practice. In this case, the broader synthesis statement was "change in the level of observation and care and lack of preparation for the physical debilitation and sleep disruptions stimulates a reemergence of vulnerability which is intensified when care routines are not responsive to individual deficits and needs" (Salmond, Evans, Hamdi, & Saimbert, 2011).

Metaethnography

In contrast to meta-aggregation, metaethnography is a form of interpretive synthesis in which the researcher tries to generate new meanings rather than deduce existing meanings. Findings are not aggregated but are analyzed and reinterpreted to generate new meanings in the form of explanatory, midlevel, or substantive theory. Proponents claim that this creates new knowledge. The goal is not explicitly to inform or provide recommendations for practice; rather, it aims to develop conceptual models of understanding. Figure 10.4 illustrates the steps of meta-aggregation and metasynthesis within the systematic review process.

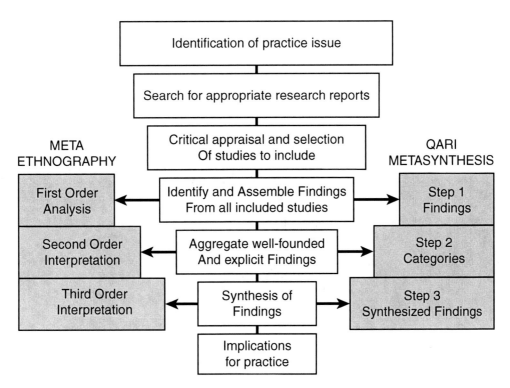

FIGURE 10.4
Metasynthesis of Qualitative Research Studies

There are different approaches to locating relevant studies within metaethnography. The first is similar to systematic review using meta-aggregation where the goal is to identify every possible relevant study. A second option is to use theoretical sampling until data saturation is reached (Atkins et al., 2008).

The steps common to metaethnography are described in Table 10.8 and comparable processes in meta-aggregation are presented to allow for comparison. The first two steps involve defining the topic and scope of the metaethnography. The third step begins the analysis process with data extraction of research design components, contexts, and main concepts. These three steps are very similar to the meta-aggregation process; however, subsequent steps in metaethnography are more interpretive than with meta-aggregation.

Then the next step is to determine how the studies are related or dissonant. Using a compare and contrast approach, the main concepts are juxtaposed against each other to determine how they are related—are they complementary, conflicting, or not at all related (and, therefore, not to be synthesized). Once the relationship has been determined, a second-order interpretation is developed by using a reciprocal translation where the main concepts from one paper are translated into the next through an iterative process, continuing until all papers are reviewed. The outcome of this step is the main explanation or theory arising from each paper (Britten et al., 2002). Table 10.9 provides a grid illustrating these steps. The grid describes the research design, context, main concepts illustrated in each paper, and the explanatory interpretation from each paper.

The last step in analysis is synthesizing translations, another level of higher order interpretation. In this creative, interpretive process, the second-order translations are filtered into more refined meanings and exploratory theories, and a line of argument synthesis is completed. In this process, an approach similar to grounded theory is used and a new interpretation is conceptualized (Flemming, 2007). This

TABLE 10.8

Steps in Metaethnography and Comparative Process in Meta-Aggregation

Step in Metaethnography	Description of Tasks Involved in Metaethnography Step	Comparative Process in Meta-Aggregation
1 Getting started	Topic identification Specifying the research question	Developing research question
2 Deciding what is relevant to the initial interest	In this step, the scope of the synthesis is defined and the studies that will be included are determined. This includes: ■ defining the focus of the synthesis ■ defining strategy ■ making decisions on inclusion ■ making decisions on quality assessment	Establishing inclusion criteria Developing search strategy Initial study selection followed by critical appraisal and final study selection

(Continued)

TABLE 10.8

Steps in Metaethnography and Comparative Process in Meta-Aggregation *(Continued)*

Step in Metaethnography	Description of Tasks Involved in Metaethnography Step	Comparative Process in Meta-Aggregation
3 Reading the studies	Reviewers read, reread, and become familiar with the studies. Data extraction of research methods and context Identification of main themes or concepts	Two-part data extraction 1. Research design and context 2. Findings and supporting illustrations
4 Determine how studies are related or dissonant	Using a compare and contrast approach, create a list of main concept or themes, then juxtapose them and determine how they are related. The aim is not to "force fit" themes but to determine if they are reciprocal, complementary, or conflicting.	Coding of findings
5 Translating studies into one another	Studies can be "added" together when there are similarities between them. Reciprocal translation begins by comparing concepts from two papers. This two paper synthesis is then compared to the next paper and this process is continued until all papers are translated. Themes are merged and categories collapsed in this process, keeping an open mind for emerging themes not identified in step 4. Deviant data should be considered in this process because it provides another perspective for understanding.	Collapsing of similar coded findings into categories of shared meaning
6 Synthesizing translations	Move to a higher order interpretation. Filter the translations into more than the parts along, but elucidate more refined meanings, exploratory theories, and new concepts and develop a line of argument synthesis.	The categories are thematically grouped according to similar meaning and these are interpreted to form the synthesized findings.
7 Expressing the synthesis	Different approaches to presenting the synthesis including the use of diagrams for illustrating the final hypotheses and models. Goal is to determine where the synthesis must be published to assure dissemination.	Preparation of report including best practice recommendations.

Source: Based on Atkins, S., Lewin, S., Smith, H., Engel, M. Fretheim, A., & Volmink, J. (2008). Conducting a meta-ethnography of qualitative literature: Lessons learnt. *BMC Medical Research Methodology, 8*, 21. doi: 10.1186/1471-2288-8-21. Britten, N., Campbell, R., Pope, C., Donovan, J., Morgan, M., & Pill, R. (2002). Using meta ethnography to synthesise qualitative research: A worked example. *Journal of Health Services & Research Policy, 7*(4), 209–215. Walsh, D., & Downe, S. (2005). Meta-synthesis method for qualitative research: A literature review. *Journal of Advanced Nursing, 50*(2), 204–211.

TABLE 10.9

Illustration of a Metaethnographic Grid

Methods and Concepts	Donovan and Blake	Morgan	Britten	Rogers et al.
Sample	Fifty-four patients with a suspected inflammatory arthropathy	Sixty White and Afro-Caribbean patients treated for hypertension for at least one year	Thirty patients, attenders, and non-attenders	Thirty-four patients with a diagnosis of schizophrenia or schizoaffective disorder
Data collection	Home interviews pre- and post-consultation; observation of consultations	Home interviews	Home interviews	Interviews
Setting	Three rheumatology units	Fifteen general practices	Two general practices	Different points in the mental health system
Types of medicine	NSAIDs and second-line drugs	Antihypertensive drugs	Unselected	Neuroleptic medication
Adherence/ Compliance	(Patients do not perceive compliance to be an issue)	Stable adherence and problematic adherence	Correct behavior and routine medicine-taking	Patients mentioned benefits of taking medicines
Self-regulation	Levels of noncompliance	Leaving off drugs	Preference for not taking drugs	Adjustment of medication, self-regulation
Aversion	Dislike of taking drugs, fear of side effects, weakness, dependence	Fear of side effects, addiction, harmful effects of drugs	Aversion to medicines, medicines as harmful	Wide range of side effects
Alternative coping strategies	Range of alternative remedies	Traditional (herbal) remedies	Use of alternative medicine	Alternative coping strategies
Sanctions	—	Patients warned by doctors and told severely about the need to take the tablets regularly	—	Coercion from significant others, fear of coercion from mental health professionals

(Continued)

TABLE 10.9

Illustration of a Metaethnographic Grid *(Continued)*

Methods and Concepts	Donovan and Blake	Morgan	Britten	Rogers et al.
Selective disclosure	Patients did not tell doctors of altered doses	—	—	Management of information to psychiatrists
Explanatory/ theory (second-order interpretation)	"Patients carry out a 'cost-benefit' analysis of each treatment, weighing up the costs/risks of each treatment against the benefits as they perceive them."	Medicine taking is influenced by cultural meanings and cultural resources.	Patients may not articulate views that they do not perceive to be medically legitimated.	"The self-regulation of medication appears to have been circumscribed or inhibited by the impact of the threat of social and professional sanctions."

Note. NSAIDs = non-steroidal anti-inflammatory drugs. *Source*: Britten, N., Campbell, R., Pope, C., Donovan, J., Morgan, M., & Pill, R. (2002). Using meta-ethnography to synthesise qualitative research: A worked example. *Journal of Health Services & Research Policy, 7*(4), 212.

final expression of the synthesis poses a hypothesis or presents models or explanatory, midlevel, or substantive theory (Walsh & Downe, 2005). Table 10.10 presents a synthesis table from a paper published by Britten et al. (2002) that uses four papers to illustrate a worked example of metaethnography. Main concepts are provided, along with second-order interpretations from each paper and the final synthesis or third-order interpretation.

From the analysis, it was determined that there are two types of medicine-taking practices: adherent medicine-taking and self-regulation. Self-regulation reflects aversion to taking medications, and the use of alternative coping strategies is one manifestation of this aversion.

> Sanctions from health professionals, such as warnings, coercion, or the threat of coercion, serve to inhibit self-regulation which can only flourish if sanctions are not severe. There is selective disclosure in the way in which patients manage the information they give to health professionals. Patients may not articulate views or information that they do not perceive to be medically legitimated, such as the use of alternative coping strategies. Fear of sanctions and guilt can produce selective disclosure. (Britten et al., 2002, p. 213)

This worked example has produced middle-range theories in the form of hypotheses that could be tested by other researchers.

TABLE 10.10

Synthesis, Including the Concepts and Second-Order and Third-Order Interpretations

Concepts	Second-Order Interpretations	Third-Order Interpretations
Adherence/compliance: stable adherence; correct behavior and routine medicine-taking	a. "Patients carry out a 'cost-benefit' analysis of each treatment, weighing up the costs/risks of each treatment against the benefits as they perceive them."	a. Self-regulation includes the use of alternative coping strategies.
Self-regulation: problematic adherence; levels of noncompliances; leaving off drugs; preference for not taking drugs; self-regulation	b. Medicine taking is influenced by cultural meanings and cultural resources.	—
Aversion: dislike of taking drugs; fear of side effects; aversion to medicines; harmful effects of drugs	c. Self-regulation is . . . inhibited by . . . the threat of social and professional sanctions	b. Self-regulation flourishes if sanctions are not severe.
Alternate coping strategies: range of alternative remedies; traditional remedies	d. Patients may not articulate views that they do not perceive to be medically legitimated.	c. Alternative coping strategies are not seen by patients as medically legitimate.
Sanctions: patients are warned by their doctors and told severely about the need to take the tablets regularly; coercion from significant others; fear of coercion from mental health professionals		d. Fear of sanctions and guilt produce selective disclosure.
Selective disclosure: patients do not tell doctors of altered doses; management of information to psychiatrists		

Source: Britten, N., Campbell, R., Pope, C., Donovan, J., Morgan, M., & Pill, R. (2002). Using meta-ethnography to synthesise qualitative research: A worked example. *Journal of Health Services & Research Policy, 7*(4), 213.

SUMMARY

This chapter has emphasized the importance of qualitative metasynthesis in using qualitative data findings in practice. The underlying debates on the appropriateness of pooling and appraisal in qualitative studies have been presented. The approach to qualitative systematic review using either meta-aggregation or metaethnography are presented and compared.

EXERCISES

Read the following qualitative research study and answers the questions: Kooienga, S., Stewart, V. T. (2011). Putting a face on medical errors: A patient's perspective. *Journal of Healthcare Quality, 33*(4), 37–41.

1. What is being investigated?
2. What is the role of the researcher? Is any researcher bias present?
3. What is the purpose of the study? What are the research questions?
4. What philosophical perspective is evident, if any?
5. Who are the participants?
6. What is the context or setting of the study?
7. What data were collected? Were they appropriate and related to the research question?
8. Are the conclusions of the study credible? Why or why not?

REFERENCES

Annells, M. (2005). A qualitative quandary: Alternative representations and meta-synthesis. *Journal of Clinical Nursing, 14*(5), 535–536.

Atkins, S., Lewin, S., Smith, H., Engel, M., Fretheim, A., & Volmink, J. (2008). Conducting a meta-ethnography of qualitative literature: Lessons learnt. *BMC Medical Research Methodology, 8,* 21. doi: 10.1186/1471-2288-8-21

Barbour, R. S., & Barbour, M. (2003). Evaluating and synthesizing qualitative research: The need to develop a distinctive approach. *Journal of Education in Clinical Practice, 9*(2), 179–186.

Bradley, E. H., Curry, L. A., & Devers, K. J. (2007). Qualitative data analysis for health services research: Developing taxonomy, themes, and theory. *Health Services Research, 42*(4), 1758–1772.

Britten, N., Campbell, R., Pope, C., Donovan, J., Morgan, M., & Pill, R. (2002). Using meta-ethnography to synthesise qualitative research: A worked example. *Journal of Health Services & Research Policy, 7*(4), 209–215.

Cohen, D., & Crabtree, B. (2006). Qualitative research guidelines project. Retrieved from http://www.qualres.org/index.html

Côté, L., & Turgeon, J. (2005). Appraising qualitative research articles in medicine and medical education. *Medical Teacher, 27*(1), 71–75.

Devers, K. J. (1999). How will we know "good" qualitative research when we see it? Beginning the dialogue in health services research. *Health Services Research, 34*(5 Pt. 2), 1153–1188.

Dew, K. (2007). A health researcher's guide to qualitative methodologies. *Australian and New Zealand Journal of Public Health, 31*(5), 433–437.

Draper, A. K. (2004). The principles and application of qualitative research. *Proceedings of the Nutrition Society, 63*(4), 641–646.

Egger, M., Smith, G. D., & Phillips, A. N. (1997). Meta-analysis: Principles and procedures. *British Medical Journal, 315*(7121), 1533–1537.

Estabrooks, C. A., Field, P. A., & Morse, J. M. (1994). Aggregating qualitative findings: An approach to theory development. *Qualitative Health Research, 4*(4), 503–511.

Finfgeld, D. L. (2003). Metasynthesis: The state of the art—so far. *Qualitative Health Research, 13*(7), 893–904.

Finfgeld-Connett, D. (2010). Generalizability and transferability of meta-synthesis research findings. *Journal of Advanced Nursing, 66*(2), 246–254.

Flemming, K. (2007). Synthesis of qualitative research and evidence-based nursing. *British Journal of Nursing, 16*(10), 616–620.

Golafshani, N. (2003). Understanding reliability and validity in qualitative research. *The Qualitative Report, 8*(4), 597–607.

Hannes, K., Lockwood, C., & Pearson, A. (2010). A comparative analysis of three online appraisal instruments' ability to assess validity in qualitative research. *Qualitative Health Research, 20*(12), 1736–1743. doi: 10.1177/1049732310378656

The Joanna Briggs Institute. (2008). *Joanna Briggs Institute reviewer's manual: 2008 edition.* Adelaide, Australia: Author.

Kearney, M. H. (1998). Ready-to-wear: Discovering grounded formal theory. *Research in Nursing & Health, 21*, 179–186.

Kooienga, S., Stewart, V. T. (2011). Putting a face on medical errors: A patient's perspective. *Journal of Healthcare Quality, 33*(4), 37–41

Patterson, B. L., Thorne, S. E., Canam, C., & Jillings, C. (2001). *Meta-study of qualitative health research: A practical guide to meta-analysis and meta-synthesis.* Thousand Oaks, CA: Sage.

Patton, M. Q. (2002). *Qualitative research and evaluation methods.* Thousand Oaks, CA: Sage.

Reis, S., Hermoni, D., Van-Raalte, D., Dahan, R., & Borkan, J. M. (2007). Aggregation of qualitative studies—from theory to practice: Patient priorities and family medicine/general practice evaluations. *Patient Education and Counseling, 65*(2), 214–222.

Salmond, S., & Evans, B. (2010). *A systematic review of relocation stress following in-house transfer out of critical/intensive care units.* Adelaide, Australia: The Joanna Briggs Institute Library of Systematic Reviews.

Salmond, S., Evans, B., Hamdi, H., & Saimbert, M. (2011). A Systematic review of relocation stress following in-house transfer out of critical/intensive care units. *JBI Library of Systematic Reviews, 9*(10).

Sandelowski, M., Docherty, S., & Emden, C. (1997). Focus on qualitative methods. Qualitative metasynthesis: Issues and techniques. *Research in Nursing & Health, 20*(4), 365–371.

Schreiber, R., Crooks, D., & Stern, P. N. (1997). Qualitative meta-analysis. In J. M. Morse (Ed.), *Completing a qualitative project: Details and dialogue* (pp. 311–326). Thousand Oaks, CA: Sage.

Thomas, J., & Harden, A. (2008). Methods for the thematic synthesis of qualitative research in systematic reviews. *BMC Medical Research Methodology, 8*, 45. doi: 10.1186/1471-2288-8-45. Retrieved from http://www.biomedcentral.com/1471-2288/8/45

Thorne, S. (2009). The role of qualitative research within an evidence-based context: Can metasynthesis be the answer? *International Journal of Nursing Studies, 46*(4), 569–575.

Thorne, S., Jensen, L., Kearney, M. H., Noblit, G., & Sandelowski, M. (2004). Qualitative metasynthesis: Reflections on methodological orientation and ideological agenda. *Qualitative Health Research, 14*(10), 1342–1365.

Walsh, D., & Downe, S. (2005). Meta-synthesis method for qualitative research: A literature review. *Journal of Advanced Nursing, 50*(2), 204–211.

Zimmer, L. (2006). Qualitative meta-synthesis: A question of dialoguing with texts. *Methodological Issues in Nursing Research, 53*(3), 311–318.

SUGGESTED READINGS

Beck, C. T. (2003). Initiation into qualitative data analysis. *Journal of Nursing Education, 42*(5), 231–234.

Orb, A., Eisenhauer, L., & Wynaden, D. (2000). Ethics in qualitative research. *Journal of Nursing Scholarship, 33*(1), 93–96.

Schofield, J. W. (1990). Increasing the generalizability of qualitative research. In E. W. Eisner & A. Peshkin (Eds.), *Qualitative inquiry in education: The continuing debate* (pp. 201–232). New York, NY: Teachers College Press.

Sofaer, S. (1999). Qualitative methods: What are they and why use them? *Health Services Research, 34*(5 Pt. 2), 1101–1118.

CHAPTER ELEVEN

Systematic Review of Economic Evidence

Cheryl Holly

Upon completion of Chapter 11, you will be able to:

- Differentiate among models of economic analysis
- Define health care economics
- Identify areas for systematic review of economic evaluation

IMPORTANT POINTS

- The term economics comes from the Greek word *oikonomia* meaning rules of the household. Economics is about choice and the decisions that must be made on how to best use available resources.
- The aim of economics is to be sure that chosen activities have benefits that are reasonable given the available resources.
- Economic evaluations have a common composition that involves measurement of input (cost) and outcome (benefit).
- Health economics applies the principles of economics to health care situations. It is concerned with the choice, the scarcity of health resources, and the cost of health-related interventions, treatments, and procedures, and the relationships among these.
- A systematic review of economic evidence seeks to describe the overall cost (including consequences) and benefits arising from alternative interventions, services, or treatments.

INTRODUCTION

All decisions have consequences. To make the best decisions, health care decision makers must be knowledgeable about related costs, clinical effectiveness, and the lost opportunities associated with provided or potential services. Economics provides a framework to assist in weighing alternative courses of action when making decisions given the available resources (Mugford, 2007). Economics is the study of how people

TABLE 11.1
Definitions of Economics

Economics is the study of people in the ordinary business of life. . . . Thus, it is on one [side] the study of wealth, and on the other, more important side, the study of man (Marshall, 1890, para. 1).

Economics is the science which studies human behavior as a relationship between given ends and scarce means which have alternative uses (Robbins, 1932, p. 35).

Economics is the study of how societies use scarce resources to produce valuable commodities and distribute them among different people (Samuelson, 1970, para. 2).

Economics is founded on the principle of scarcity, where more is wanted of goods and services than is available to individuals or the population (Culyer, 2005, p. 106).

Economics is all about humanity's struggle to achieve happiness in a world full of constraints . . . how to get the most out of limited resources (Flynn, 2006, p. 10).

Economics provides a framework to assist in weighting alternative courses of action when making decisions given the available resources (Mugford, 2007, p. 419).

choose their resources (American Economic Association, 2010). According to Culyer (2005), economics is concerned with the influence of human behavior on the consumption of resources, which may or may not be scarce, and which may have more than one use. These resources are the inputs of production: land, labor, and capital. As seen in the various definitions of economics presented in Table 11.1, economists seek to understand how decisions are made by various units, such as individuals, families, firms, and households (microeconomics), and also to aggregate outcomes related to money supply, income, unemployment, and the associations among them (macroeconomics). In principle, economics can be applied to most organizations. However, most of the economic theory centers on how goods are bought and traded (The History of Economic Thought [HET], 2010). The "invisible hand" of supply and demand, a phrase coined by Adam Smith in the 18th century, dominates these transactions. Smith, revered as the father of modern economics, posited that the self-regulatory nature of the marketplace (the "invisible hand") creates a fusion of forces of self-interest, competition, and supply and demand, which allows how resources should be allocated and the competition that underlies this determination (Kennedy, 2009).

DEFINITIONS OF ECONOMICS

In the late 20th century, the paradigm in economic thinking shifted from a price-based model to attention to incurred risk (HET, 2010). The study of risk has been influential in understanding that a focus on output alone may not generate sufficient revenue to cover operating costs and to repay debt obligations (Investor Words, 2010). Assessment of risk involves variations in price over time as more important than the actual price. This particularly applies to health care economics where risk-return trade-offs are among crucial decisions made when caring for patients or deciding what services to close or expand (HET, 2010).

The study of economics is important in developing an understanding about decisions that arise when people have unlimited wants, but limited resources; in other words, when resources are scarce. Scarcity, within an economic context, refers to limited resources, not a lack of riches. For example, because our resources are limited in comparison to our wants and needs, decisions need to be made on what goods and services are important, feasible, and affordable. Economics is a part of everyday life when decisions are made about which house to buy: the larger one in the average school district or the smaller one in a better school district. The decision is based not only on a comparison of the cost of housing in the two different school districts, but also on the benefits that can be provided by the individual schools and the quality of life in each of the neighborhoods, as well as other costs such as work commute or the nature and extent of local shopping. This distinction between financial cost (the cost of the house in monetary terms) and the economic cost (everything else) is important because much of the discourse of economics is dominated by notions of cost. Although the idea of financial cost is familiar, the economic cost has more far reaching effect, and may not be as familiar. Hayward (2009) explains that within the health care system, the time spent by patients and their families in a hospital waiting room represents a cost to them—despite the fact that no financial cost arises. Families in waiting rooms are unavailable for anything else—except waiting—and the benefit that may have accrued from other activity is lost. In economics, these lost outcomes are referred to as opportunity costs. In other words, the true cost of any endeavor, such as buying a house or waiting in a hospital, can only be understood by valuing all of the consumed resources.

Health care economic studies use a wide range of cost variables as presented in Table 11.2. It is necessary to understand which costs were included in an economic study because this provides information on the perspective of the study. Cost increases as the perspective widens. The ideal perspective is societal because it analyzes costs from the viewpoint of society. Cost from a societal perspective would involve indirect costs, such as time lost to illness or time spent to caring for an ill relative, and intangible costs, such as anxiety, pain, or suffering associated with an illness or treatment as well as the opportunity cost of lost productivity. Other perspectives include health insurance industry perspective, social services perspective, primary care perspective, hospital perspective, or patient perspective (Joanna Briggs

TABLE 11.2
Range of Costs Used in Economic Studies

Direct Costs are directly associated with the intervention.
Examples include mediations, medical devices, equipment and supplies
Screening costs, immunizations, radiology, and laboratory testing
Indirect Costs are those that are increased by decreased productivity.
Examples include caregiver time, transportation, treatments for adverse reactions, lost work days, hospice care
Fixed Costs are those that do not vary.
Examples include overhead, capital building costs
Intangible Costs are those that differ for each person.
Examples include pain, fatigue, suffering, anxiety
Opportunity Costs are benefits lost and not available for other uses.
Examples include waiting time

Institute [JBI], 2009). For example, from the viewpoint of the hospital, it would be useful to establish the cost perspective on staffing a new emergency department fast track with nurse practitioners or physicians with both cost and outcomes measured for each; and from the perspective of the health insurance industry, the monetary effect of such changes in staffing would be important should the nurse practitioner have similar outcomes at a lower cost. Understanding the perspective of the study will allow a more focused and useful interpretation of the data, as well as an identification of any inherent bias in the study.

ECONOMIC EVALUATION FOR HEALTH CARE

Economic evaluation is the study of the costs and consequences of interventions, services, or programs (Drummond, Sculpher, Torrance, O'Brien, & Stoddard, 2005). There are two types of economic evaluation: partial and full. A partial evaluation is a study of a single intervention or service. This type of evaluation makes no comparisons. It simply describes the costs associated with the one intervention or service under study, such as administration of a drug. A cost-minimization study is an example of a partial evaluation study. Cost-minimization evaluation is designed to determine the least costly intervention among multiple interventions with similar outcomes. There is no attempt to measure risks or other outcomes except cost. All outcomes are considered to be equivalent across intervention groups and only the monetary cost of the intervention is important. In the case of drug administration, the least costly drug would be preferred. For example, if two drugs were believed to be equivalent in terms of actions and outcomes, only the differences in cost would be compared in an effort to choose the one that provides the best value. Gray et al. (2001), in a study of atenolol versus captopril in patients with type 2 diabetes, found that the treatment of hypertensive patients with type 2 diabetes using atenolol or captopril was equally effective. However, total costs were significantly lower in the atenolol group.

A full economic evaluation is the comparison of at least two different courses of action in relation to both costs and consequences (Drummond et al., 2005). There are several schema of full economic evaluation: cost effectiveness, cost utility, and cost benefit. Table 11.3 provides details on these three types of full economic evaluation as well as the partial evaluation, cost-minimization analysis (CMA). Cost benefit and cost utility methods are concerned with outcomes and, therefore, provide information on the worth of treatments; cost-effectiveness methods assume that the intervention is valuable, and the focus is predominately the total cost of the intervention (Cunningham, 2001). These evaluations differ in the way in which consequences are measured. Cost-utility studies seek to establish benefit measured by quantity and quality of life (quality-adjusted life years [QALYs]). Cost-benefit studies seek to identify a specific ratio, such as cost benefit or gain loss. Outcomes typically focus on medical costs that were avoided. Cost-effectiveness studies are concerned with interventions that achieve similar outcome, but have different resource requirements. Clinical endpoints and their associated costs are the focal point for these analyses. The outcomes are determined in monetary units per clinical improvement, thus, allowing expenditure decisions to be made. See Table 11.3 for further examples of each of these types of economic evaluation.

TABLE 11.3

Methods of Economic Evaluation

Type of Evaluation	Aims of the Evaluation	Advantages	Important Points to Consider	Questions to Ask
Cost-minimization analysis (CMA)	To determine the least costly method with the best benefit	A comparison of the outcomes of two interventions with the same efficacy to determine which has a lesser cost.	The cheapest alternative found is generally preferred. All cost expenditures must be measured.	Is the cheapest alternative the best method in the long term?
Cost-effectiveness analysis (CEA)	To determine the best way of implementing an intervention* that has proved effective	Assumes that an intervention is effective. Outcomes are expressed in cost per unit of effect (e.g., how many life years gained; how many premature births averted; how much is pain reduced).	It is not possible to compare the outcomes of interventions with differing clinical effectiveness. The effect measure must be common to all alternatives, but may differ in degrees of effectiveness. Costs are measured in natural units (e.g., mortality rates, cholesterol levels).	How much does it cost to achieve clinical effectiveness? What is the extra cost to get improved effectiveness rates?
Cost-utility analysis (CUA)	To determine the level of well-being in terms of quality-adjusted life years (QALY)	Should be the method of choice when quality of life is an outcome of interest. The ideal method when the intervention is thought to effect morbidity or mortality.	Costs are measured in monetary units. Effects are measured in healthy years given the value placed on health. Allows for a consideration of differences in interventions, which involve quality and quantity of life. Outcomes are reported as improvements in health status.	What is the quality of life in terms of, for example, mobility, depression, pain, incontinence, self-care, and so forth.

(Continued)

241

TABLE 11.3

Methods of Economic Evaluation (Continued)

Type of Evaluation	Aims of the Evaluation	Advantages	Important Points to Consider	Questions to Ask
Cost-benefit analysis (CBA)	To determine the efficiency of the intervention relative to the standard or status quo	Most comprehensive of the evaluation methods. Allows analysis of one program or a comparison of several program outcomes. Seeks to determine a monetary ratio in terms of profit and loss. Is the only economic evaluation method that seeks to determine if the benefits of the intervention exceed the cost. Outcomes are measured as resource savings.	Financial cost, benefit and consequences are all valued in monetary units. If only one intervention can be funded, the activity with the highest excess financial benefit over costs is chosen based on this analysis. Effects measured are not necessarily common to all alternatives. The outcomes of a CBA are dependent on accurate costs and benefits of the intervention. Complex and expensive to conduct.	How much is the public willing to pay for benefits or willingness to pay to avoid consequences.

*Intervention is used here to refer broadly to any treatment, procedure, or service under study.

HEALTH ECONOMICS AND SYSTEMATIC REVIEW

The study of health economics reflects a widespread need to obtain maximum value for money by ensuring not just clinical effectiveness, but also cost effectiveness (Hayward, 2009). Health economics is a branch of economics that was first discussed by Arrow (1963) who was concerned with the uncertainty of medical care. In broad terms, health care economists consider issues related to scarcity in the allocation of health and health care, the cost of health behaviors, and conditions such as smoking, drug addiction, or hospital-acquired infections and the effectiveness of their treatments. The evaluation associated with these conditions is microeconomic in nature because they look at the effectiveness of individual treatments. A systematic review of economic evidence on the cost and effectiveness of these conditions involve the aggregation of both effectiveness of outcomes and cost. A systematic review of economic evidence can be conducted primarily to inform population-based decision making when a new intervention, service, or program is being implemented or evaluated or when decisions need to be made on the best and most cost effective alternative to choose. Theoretically, the costs and benefits from an economic evaluation could be pooled in a meta-analysis; however, there are no currently agreed-upon means to do this (JBI, 2009), although there are some examples in the literature (see, for example, Bower et al., 2003).

Health economics is studied primarily through the use of cost-effectiveness and cost-utility studies, with cost-effectiveness study dominating (Talmor, Shapiro, Greenberg, Stone, & Neumann, 2006). Because the ability of the health care system to provide care with an array of technologically sophisticated and expensive procedures exceeds the ability of the systems to pay for these services, choices need to be made (Hayward, 2009). In general, the concept of cost effectiveness is concerned with how to achieve a predetermined objective at the least cost or to maximize benefit with limited resources (Hayward, 2009). Cost-effectiveness analysis (CEA) is a method for comparing the expected benefits of an intervention with its total, or net, cost. This relationship is expressed in terms of a ratio calculated by dividing the incremental cost of the treatment by its incremental benefit, usually measured in lives saved. The disadvantage of this method, according to Talmor et al., (2006), is that not all saved life years are of equal value. For example, if a patient's life is saved by an intervention that leaves that patient unable to walk, the proposed intervention is not the same as another intervention that does not inhibit mobility. Additionally, cost-effectiveness outcome can be measured by blood pressure in millimeters of mercury, cholesterol levels, symptom-free days, infection rates, or mortality among others. A cost-effectiveness outcome can be derived from any natural unit that can be reported numerically.

Cost-utility analysis (CUA) is a type of CEA that examines the costs and effectiveness of interventions using the QALY as its measurement for effectiveness. Its purpose is to assist decision makers and policy planners to compare the value of different interventions with different benefits. CUA specifies a value for health states. The primary outcome of a CUA is a cost per QALY, or incremental cost-effectiveness ratio. A QALY places a weight on time in different health states. For example, a year of perfect health is worth one QALY and a year of less than perfect health is worth less than one QALY. Death is considered to be equivalent to zero (0; Phillips, 2009).

When combined with the costs of providing the interventions, QALYs indicate the additional cost necessary to have a year of perfect health. These ratios indicate the additional costs required to generate a year of perfect health (one QALY). Priorities can be developed based on the cost per QALY. In doing so, the process of resource allocation based on one QALY (one year of perfect health) can be established in a transparent fashion (Wailoo, Tsuchiya, & McCabe, 2009; Phillips, 2009).

CUA examines the effects of interventions on both quantity and quality of life, allowing comparison across various interventions for the same condition, as well as across different conditions (Talmor et al., 2006). As a general rule, CEA and CUA require only health care costs to be collected. Cost-benefit analysis (CBA) requires collection of data related to all costs and benefits (Shemilt et al., 2008). See Table 11.4 for examples of economic evaluation for further study.

A systematic review of economic evidence in health care is most advantageous if the answers to the following questions are already known (Drummond et al., 2005):

1. Can the procedure or treatment work? (Its efficacy in ideal situations)
2. Does the procedure or treatment work? (Its effectiveness in actual practice)
3. Is the intervention getting to those who need it? (Its availability or access in the real world)
4. Should the treatment or procedure be used given other priorities? (Its policy implications)

TABLE 11.4

Examples of Economic Evaluation

Type of Evaluation	Example
Cost-effectiveness analysis	Taylor, R. S., Taylor, R. J., Van Buyten, J. P., Buchser, E., North, R., & Bayliss, S. (2004). The cost effectiveness of spinal cord stimulation in the treatment of pain: A systematic review of the literature. *Journal of Pain Symptom Management, 27*(4), 370–378.
Cost-utility analysis	Stein, K., Dalziel, K., Walker, A., Jenkins, B., Round, A., & Royle, P. (2003). Screening for hepatitis C in genitourinary medical clinics: A cost utility analysis. *Journal of Hepatology, 39*(5), 814–825.
Cost-minimization analysis	Daucourt, V., Sicotte, C., Pelletier-Fleury, N., Petitjean, M. E., Chateil, J. F., & Michel, P. (2006). Cost-minimization analysis of a wide-area teleradiology network in a French region. *International Journal of Quality in Health Care, 18*(4), 287–293.
Cost-benefit analysis	Hillestad, R., Bigelow, J., Bower, A., Girosi, F., Meili, R., Scoville, R., & Taylor, R. (2005). Can electronic medical record systems transform health care? Potential health benefits, savings, and costs. *Health Affairs, 24*(5), 1103–1117

The purpose of doing a systematic review, then, would be to develop a decision-making model based on cost and effectiveness, including risk-benefit trade-offs. Potential areas for systematic review of health care economic evidence include the following:

An analysis of market share and competition for health services
The cost and consequences of health insurance
The demand for health services
The cost and effectiveness of services provided

WRITING THE SYSTEMATIC REVIEW PROTOCOL

A protocol that details the methods to be used in the systematic review is the first step in conducting a systematic review of economic evidence. As described in previous chapters, the protocol provides enough detail to understand exactly how the systematic review will be conducted. The protocol should follow the basic outline provided in Chapter 3, adding the essential elements for an economic evidence review as presented in Table 11.5.

TABLE 11.5
Essential Elements for Systematic Review of Economic Evidence Protocol

1. The title should indicate the type of review (e.g., cost-effectiveness, cost-utility, etc.), the intervention or outcome studied, and the setting.
For example: A systematic review of the cost effectiveness of two different wound dressing change protocols for diabetic patients at home.
2. The background needs to clearly describe why the review is necessary and the variables to be included in the review. The background should avoid making statements about cost because this is what the review will determine. In addition, the background should describe the perspective of the analysis to be conducted.
3. The review question should be stated using the PICO mnemonic.
For example: What are the cost advantages and disadvantages to using tegaderm versus wet dressing for diabetic patients at home with leg ulcers?
4. Inclusion criteria
Types of study to be included should be identified as cost-effectiveness, cost-minimization, cost-utility, or cost-benefit analysis, or some combination.
Types of interventions should be described in detail including who is doing the intervention and where it is done.
Types of outcomes should be described in relation to the type of review, for example, cost effectiveness.
5. Types of studies
The specific economic studies that will be included in the review. These need to be clearly indicated as CMA, CUS, CBA, CEA.

Note. CBA = cost-benefit analysis; CEA = cost-effectiveness analysis; CMA = cost-minimization analysis; CUS = cost-utility analysis; PICO = patient/problem, intervention, comparison, outcome.

A systematic review of economic evidence is constructed to answer one of two questions: (a) Is this procedure worth doing when compared with other procedures using the same resources; that is, how should we spend our money?, or (b) Are we satisfied that health care resources should be spent in this way and not some other way; that is, is our money being spent well (Cunningham, 2001)?

Whereas the search strategy should follow the same basic processes provided in previous chapters, there are databases specific to economic evidence that should also be searched. The comprehensiveness of the search strategy for economic evidence will lend credibility to the findings of the review. Economic databases that can be searched include the following:

Health Economics Evaluation Databases (HEED)
Health Technology Assessment
Database of Abstracts of Review and Effect (DARE)
Federal Reserve Economic Data (FRED)

As described in preceding chapters, the main purpose of an appraisal is to determine a study's quality and to decide if the study is worthy of inclusion in the systematic review. The basics of economic evaluation involve identifying, measuring, valuing, and comparing the costs and benefits of at least two different interventions for their clinical effectiveness. The measurement of cost is similar regardless of the type of analysis used. Costs can be considered direct, such as staff salaries or price of necessary equipment; indirect, such as loss of productivity because of illness; or capital, such as a need to construct a new laboratory or operating room (JBI, 2009). Benefits, on the other hand, have to do with improvements in health and can be tangible, such as lives saved, illnesses prevented, return to productivity; or intangible, such as reduction in pain and suffering.

However, the real cost of any health care intervention is the opportunity cost. Questions need to be asked about what will be lost from other programs or services by putting resources into a new intervention. For example, will staff be reassigned rather than new positions allocated? Will families have a waiting area close to the unit where their loved ones are? Opportunity costs in health care are based on the economic principles of choice and scarcity. Choices have to be made about what interventions will be undertaken, and which should not be undertaken or allowed to wither. For example, allocation of space would be a major determinant in how close a waiting room was to an inpatient in a hospital. The aim of an economic evaluation of health care interventions is to ensure that the benefits of a program are greater than the opportunity costs (JBI, 2009).

The scheme for reviewing economic evaluations should be transparent and involve (a) using unambiguous criteria to determine what studies are to be included in the review; (b) use of an abstraction form to extract data and adjust study results for analysis; and (c) provision of a summary of the economic information for each of the interventions assessed (Carande-Kulis et al., 2000). See Table 11.6 for the standard inclusion criteria for an economic evaluation.

To meet this need for transparency, several authors have devised sets of appraisal questions that can be used when deciding which study to include in an evaluation (see Table 11.7). Whichever appraisal tool is used, the purpose of the

TABLE 11.6

Standard Inclusion Criteria for an Economic Systematic Review

1. Primary studies that provide evidence of clinical effectiveness

2. Type of analytic method used

   Cost-effectiveness analysis

   Cost-benefit analysis

   Cost-minimization analysis

   Cost-utility analysis

3. Provision of sufficient detail for secondary analysis related to the identification, cost, measurement, valuing, and comparison of the costs and benefits of at least two interventions

appraisal is to establish the validity of the economic measurements and determine whether or not to include the study in a systematic review of economic evidence. For the review of all studies for inclusion in any type of systematic review, there needs to be a well-defined clinical question. In an economic review, there also needs to be a comprehensive description of the alternatives with all relevant costs associated with the alternatives identified.

TABLE 11.7

Two Guides to Critical Appraisal of Health Economic Studies: Questions to Ask

Joanna Briggs Institute (2009)	Greenhalgh (2006)
Is there a well-defined question?	Are the analyses based on a study which answers a clearly defined clinical question about an economically important issue?
Is there a comprehensive description of alternatives?	
Has clinical effectiveness been established?	Whose viewpoint are costs and benefits being considered from?
Are all important and relevant costs and outcomes for each alternative identified?	Have the interventions being compared been shown to be clinically effective?
Are costs and outcomes measured accurately?	Are the interventions sensible and workable in the settings where they are likely to be applied?
Are costs and outcomes valued credibly?	Which method of economic analysis was used and was this method appropriate?
Are costs and outcomes adjusted for differential timing?	How were costs and benefits measured?
Is there an incremental analysis of costs and consequences?	Were incremental, rather than absolute, benefits compared?
Were sensitivity analyses conducted to investigate uncertainty in estimates or costs or consequences?	Was health status in the "here and now" given precedence over health status in the distant future?
Do study results include all issues of concern to users?	Was a sensitivity analysis performed?
Are the results generalizable to the setting of interest in the review?	Were "bottom line" aggregate scores used?

Importantly, because cost-effectiveness studies are the more common type of economic analysis in health care, the effectiveness of the intervention must have been determined before the costs were studied, and this should be evident in each study selected for inclusion in the systematic review.

If there is any uncertainty regarding the outcomes reported—that is, if estimates of cost were used rather than actual costs—a sensitivity analysis should be reported. A sensitivity analysis involves examining estimates of key variables on study results. If effectiveness is based on clinical trial data, for example, then the usual measures of effect size can be used in a sensitivity analysis (JBI, 2009). A sensitivity analysis tests the conclusions of an economic analysis under varying assumptions and can be a one-way, two-way analysis, or a scenario analysis. In other words, the cost effectiveness of an intervention is recalculated with different values (Mugford, 2007). In a one-way sensitivity analysis test, only one variable is changed at a time, all other variables are kept at their baseline value. This provides an assessment of the effect of the change for each variable. A multivariant or a two-way analysis is used when there might be more than one uncertain parameter in the analysis, and involves varying two or more input values at the same time. This method can be used to assess patient risk thresholds (Mugford, 2007). A scenario analysis varies parameters by prestudy judgment relating to the alternative scenario being considered, which might include the best and worst cases. For example, a one-way sensitivity analysis on the usual costs, and then adding the cost of caregiver benefits was associated with cost effectiveness estimates ranging from 31,000 to 43,000 per QALY gained (Andronis, Barton, & Bryan, 2009).

EXTRACTING DATA FOR ECONOMIC EVALUATION

Data extraction for economic evaluation follows the same general principles as discussed in preceding chapters. This includes information related to the citation or study being reviewed (e.g., author, date, journal), and recording the method used. In the case of an economic systematic review, the method of evaluation needs to be identified as CBA, CUA, CMA, or CEA. A general description of the setting (e.g., hospital or nursing home), population (e.g., age, gender, race, and cultural background), and geographical location (e.g. city, state, country) is also necessary. Following this, data extraction is related to the question being asked in the review. Of importance, data that are concerned with clinical effectiveness results and economic results must be extracted. A summary of the author's conclusions is also necessary.

When extracting data related to clinical effectiveness, a description of the intervention and any comparators, or control groups, used in the study need to be fully explained. Important data to extract for each of these are the sample size, type of analysis and design used in the original study, and the results of the clinical outcome (e.g., cholesterol levels, blood pressure results, level of pain reduction) both before and after the intervention (JBI, 2009).

Extracting economic results requires details on the measurements (or benefits) used in each of the selected studies. Data should be extracted concerning the dollar value of costs or the health outcomes achieved (or both). Direct and indirect costs of the intervention or program are also necessary elements of extraction. Any sensitivity or alternative scenario analysis conducted should be described. Estimated benefits to the intervention or comparison, as well as a summary of cost findings and a synthesis of costs and results, are also necessary (JBI, 2009).

DATA SYNTHESIS

The synthesis of economic data does not follow the same pattern as other systematic reviews. Economic results can be reported in a narrative summary, sorted into tables by comparisons or outcomes, or tabulated in a matrix (JBI, 2009). The choice of synthesis depends on the quality and quantity of evidence found. The JBI has developed a permutation matrix called Analysis of Cost, Technology, and Utilization Assessment and Review Instrument (ACTUARI). The matrix uses a dominance rating, where each intervention is placed in a position on a grid depending on whether it is preferred over its comparator. The matrix has three possible outcomes, which are determined by the reviewer's rating of the economic evidence and presented visually. These ratings can be for either the intervention or the comparison.

1. The process is less expensive or more clinically effective (strong dominance).
2. Interventions are comparable or equal for cost or clinical effectiveness. There is weak dominance that supports either clinical effectiveness or cost effectiveness, but not both.
3. The intervention is less expensive. Nondominance exists where the intervention of interest is less effective or more costly.

REPORTING THE ECONOMIC SYSTEMATIC REVIEW

When reporting the results of a systematic review of economic evidence, clarity is of utmost importance. Whereas there is no generally agreed standard for economic systematic reports, three sections are essential to understanding the results. The first section should detail the background and significance of the review and provide the purpose of the review. Three criteria that need to be addressed in this section are (a) the economic importance of conducting the review in terms of resource implications; (b) consideration of both cost and consequences; and (c) the perspective of the review. It is advantageous to take a broad societal perspective whenever possible. This is because the data can be disaggregated at any point and analyzed from differing viewpoints. Therefore, key decision makers who would find the review useful should be identified early in the report (Drummond & Jefferson, 1996). The rationale for choice of the alternative or comparison intervention(s) should be given. The alternative intervention should be described in sufficient detail to assess the relevance to other settings (Drummond & Jefferson, 1996).

The second section should describe the methods of the review. Included in this section should be the aims of the review, the search strategy and its results, and the inclusion and exclusion criteria. The selection of the economic evaluation method should be described here and a justification as to why this was the method under study. The primary outcome measure should be clearly stated (e.g., life years, mortality rates, QALY, willingness to pay).

The third section addresses the analysis and interpretation of results. The alternatives being compared should be described in enough detail to anyone to relate the information on costs and outcomes to the alternative courses of action. The use of decision trees and flow diagrams can help to clarify the alternative paths being followed and provide a framework for incorporating cost and outcome data. Clear definition of alternative treatment paths and their probabilities, cost, and outcomes allow decision makers to use those parts of the review that are relevant to their perspective (Drummond & Jefferson, 1996). A discussion of costing and discounting is an important part of this section. Costing involves estimating the resources used, for example, days in intensive care—and their prices (unit costs; Drummond & Jefferson, 1996). Discounting is the estimate of the present value of costs and benefits against other periods (e.g., what is the cost of the intervention in 10 years).

SUMMARY

A systematic review of economic evidence seeks to describe the overall cost (including consequences) and benefits arising from alternative health care interventions, services, or treatments. To make the best evidence-based decisions, those who make decisions regarding the allocation of resources must be knowledgeable about related costs, clinical effectiveness, and the lost opportunities associated with provided or potential services. Economic systematic review provides a foundation to assist in weighing alternative courses of action.

EXERCISES

Watch an episode of a health care-based television program (e.g., *House, Nurse Jackie*) or watch the very old movie *Hospital*, and think about the following:

1. What are the lost opportunities portrayed?
2. Do a cost-benefit analysis on a patient care decision that was made in the program.
3. What outcomes were used to determine courses of action related to patient care or organizational issues?

REFERENCES

American Economic Association. (2010). Retrieved from http://www.aeaweb.org/AboutAEA/gen_info.php

Andronis, L., Barton, P., & Bryan, S. (2009). Sensitivity analysis in economic evaluation: An audit of NICE current practice and a review of its use and value in decision-making. *Health Technology Assessment, 13*(29), iii, ix–xi, 1–61.

Arrow, K. J. (1963). Uncertainty and the welfare economics of medical care. *The American Economic Review, 53*(5), 941–973.

Bower, P., Byford, S., Barber, J., Beecham, J., Simpson, S., Friedli, K., . . . Harvey, I. (2003). Meta-analysis of data on costs from trials of counseling in primary care: Using individual patient data to overcome sample size limitations in economic analysis. *British Medical Journal, 326*(7401), 1247–1252.

Carande-Kulis, V. G., Maciosek, M. V., Briss, P. A., Teutsch, S. M., Zaza, S., Truman, B. I., . . . Fielding, J. (2000). Methods for systematic reviews of economic evaluations for the guide to community preventive services. Task force on community preventive services. *American Journal of Preventive Medicine, 18*(1 Suppl.), 75–91.

Culyer, A. (2005). Health economics dictionary of health economics-Edward Elgar. Retrieved from http://www.4shared.com/document/mabuWoeM/Health_Economics-_Anthony_Culy.htm?aff=7637829

Cunningham, S. J. (2001). An introduction to economic evaluation of health care. *Journal of Orthodontics, 28*(3), 246–250.

Drummond, M. F., & Jefferson, T. O. (1996). Guidelines for authors and peer reviewers of economic submissions to the BMJ. The BMJ Economic Working Party. *British Medical Journal, 313*(7052), 275–283.

Drummond, M. F., Sculpher, M. J., Torrance, G. W., O'Brien, B. J., & Stoddard, G. I. (2005). *Methods for the economic evaluation of health care programmes* (3rd ed.). Oxford, United Kingdom: Oxford University Press.

Flynn, S. M. (2006). *Economics for dummies.* Hoboken, NJ: Wiley Publishing.

Gray, A., Clarke, P., Raikou, M., Adler, A., Stevens, R., Neil, A., & UKPDS Group. (2001). An economic evaluation of atenolol vs. captopril in patients with type 2 diabetes (UKPDS 54). *Diabetic Medicine, 18*(6), 438–444.

Greenhalgh, T. (2006). *How to read a paper: The basics of evidence based medicine* (3rd ed.). Oxford, United Kingdom: Blackwell Publishing.

Hayward, A. (2009). *What is health economics?* (2nd ed.). London, England: Hayward Group Ltd.

The History of Economic Thought. (2010). Retrieved from http://www.homgepage.newschool.edu/het

Investor Words. (2010). Retrieved from http://www.investorwords.com/1646/ecnomic_risk.html#ixzz0yfQT9mGo

Joanna Briggs Institute. (2009). *Manual for module 5. Economic evaluation.* Adelaide, Australia: Author.

Kennedy, G. (2009). Adam Smith and the invisible hand: From metaphor to myth. *Economic Journal Watch, 6*(2), 239–263.

Marshall, A. (1890). *Principles of economics: An introductory volume.* London, England: MacMillian. Retrieved from http://www.marxists.org/reference/subject/economics/marshall/index.htm

Mugford, M. (2007). Using economic evaluation for systematic reviews. In M. Egger, G. D. Smith, & D. Altman (Eds.), *Systematic reviews in health care* (2nd ed., pp. 419–428). London, England: BMJ Publishing Group.

Phillips, C.J. (2009). The cost of multiple sclerosis and the cost effectiveness of disease-modifying agents in its treatment. *CNS Drugs, 18*(9), 561–574,

Robbins, L. (1932). *An essay on the nature and significance of economic science.* London, England: Macmillian.

Samuelson, P. A. (1970). Prize Lecture. *Nobelprize.org.* Retrieved from http://nobelprize.org/nobel_prizes/economics/laureates/1970/samuelson-lecture.html

Shemilt, I., Mugford, M., Byford, S., Drummond, M., Eisenstein, E., Knapp, M., . . . Walker D. (2008). Chapter 15: Incorporating economics evidence. In J. P. T. Higgins, & S. Green (Eds.), *Cochrane handbook for systematic reviews of interventions.* Version 5.0.1. The Cochrane Collaboration, 2008. Available from http://www.cochrane-handbook.org

Talmor, D., Shapiro, N., Greenberg, D., Stone, P. W., & Neumann, P. J. (2006). When is critical care medicine cost-effective? A systematic review of the cost-effectiveness literature. *Critical Care Medicine, 34*(11), 2738–2747.

Wailoo, A., Tsuchiya, A., & McCabe, C. (2009). Weighting must wait: Incorporating equity concerns into cost-effectiveness analysis may take longer than expected. *PharmacoEconomics, 27*(12), 983–989

SUGGESTED READINGS

Drummond, M. (2001). Introducing economic and quality of life measurements into clinical studies. *Annals of International Medicine, 33*(5), 344–349.

Vogt, W. B., & Town, R. J. (2006). *How has hospital consolidation affected the price and quality of health care?* Princeton, NJ: Robert Woods Johnson Foundation The Synthesis Project. Retrieved from http://www.rwjf.org/publications/synthesis/ reports_and_briefs/pdf/ no9_policybrief.pdf

Wilson, T. (2000). Economic evaluation of a metropolitan wide, school-based hepatitis B vaccination program. *Public Health Nursing, 17*(3), 222–227.

PART V

Using Systematic Reviews in Practice

CHAPTER TWELVE

Systematic Reviews and Evidence-Informed Health Care Policy Making

David Anthony Forrester, Rita Musanti, and Patricia Polansky

OBJECTIVES

Upon completion of Chapter 12, you will be able to:

- Differentiate between evidence-based and evidence-informed health care policy making
- Use research evidence to define and clarify a health care policy problem
- Determine how much confidence to place in a systematic review used for health care policy making
- Assess the local applicability of the findings of a systematic review for health care policy making

IMPORTANT POINTS

- Evidence-informed health care policy making is an approach to policy decisions that aims to ensure that decision making is well informed by the best available research evidence.
- An evidence-informed approach to health care policy making better enables policy makers to have a better understanding of the evidence underlying policy decisions when they act as advocates for particular policy positions.
- Systematic reviews of health policy use the POCO pneumonic: *P*eople (e.g., elderly patients with multiple chronic conditions), *O*ption (e.g., case management), *C*omparison (e.g., routine care), *O*utcome (e.g., health-related quality of life).
- Health care policy makers need to assess health policy systematic reviews for their quality and applicability, contextual appropriateness, and equity.

INTRODUCTION

The contribution of systematic review to U.S. policy making is immense, but untapped. There are challenges to their use related to lack of familiarity about the process of systematic review and lack of understanding regarding the value of outcomes. Other challenges are related to the paucity of high-quality reviews because of meager funding and the negative perceptions of some regarding the use of a literature-based research method (Fox, 2005). Additionally, there is a limited understanding of how to implement the findings. Gray (2001) posits, however, that it is the attitude of policy makers that is most important in determining the extent to which existing evidence will be used. If the reliability of a systematic review is found to be poor, policy makers will have less confidence in the findings and will be cautious in any further use of systematic review findings to inform health care policy (Lewin, Oxman, Lavis, & Fretheim, 2009).

Some of these impediments may be because of the failure of reviewers to develop taxonomy. Oxman, Lavis, Lewin, and Fretheim (2009) differentiate between the terms *evidence-based* and *evidence-informed* health care policy making, saying that evidence-informed health care policy making "better describes the role of evidence in policy making and the aspiration of improving the extent to which decisions are well-informed by research evidence" (p. S1). They define evidence-informed health care policy making as "an approach to policy decisions that aims to ensure that decision making is well-informed by the best available research evidence" (p. S1). These approaches must be transparent so that (a) the research evidence used to inform policy decisions may be examined by others, and (b) judgments can be made about the quality of the evidence and its implications for policy making. Clearly, Oxman, et al. (2009) were describing the systematic review process.

The unfortunate reality, however, is that health care policies are often not well informed by research evidence, and poorly informed decision making is one of the reasons why health services sometimes fail to reach those most in need, health indicators may be off-track, and many countries are unlikely to be able to meet national and international health care goals (Oxman et al., 2009). Furthermore, poorly informed decision making may contribute to decreased effectiveness, efficiency (i.e., value for money), and equity of health care systems.

However, there has been some success. Legislation in Washington State mandates that decisions regarding the state government purchase of health care be made using the results from systematic review (Washington State Senate Bill 6088, Chapter 29, Laws of 2003), and in Wyoming, consumers' access to systematic review findings was assured when, in 2004, the state made access to the Cochrane Library available to all residents of Wyoming (Fox, 2005). This chapter discusses the challenges and pitfalls of using systematic reviews to make health care policy decisions. These decisions can be related to what program services should be expanded or abandoned, coverage decisions for health care plans, and the governmental constraints that need to be addressed in implementing change. According to Oxman and colleagues (2009), although research evidence is not the only type of information needed to inform health care policy decision making, strengthening the use of research evidence through well-formulated and well-disseminated systematic review, the ability of policy makers to make appropriately informed judgments about the relevance and quality of evidence, is a critical challenge that holds the promise for achieving significant health gains and better use of resources. It is imperative that the results of well-designed and well-conducted systematic reviews be used to guide policy decision to ensure the judicious use of limited resources.

An evidence-informed approach to health care policy making better enables policy makers to both manage their use of research evidence and the misuse of research evidence by lobbyists, including researchers, when they act as advocates for particular policy positions. Evidence-informed approaches allow policy makers to ask critical questions about the research evidence available to support policy making, demonstrate that they are using the best evidence as the basis for their policy decisions, and ensure that evaluations of their initiatives are appropriate and that the outcomes being measured are realistic and agreed upon in advance of policy implementation. An evidence-informed approach to health care policy making also allows policy makers to acknowledge that policies may be informed by imperfect information, thus, reducing political risk, because it offers alternative courses of action if new policies do not work as well as expected (Oxman et al., 2009). Thus, health policy decisions need to be made using the best available evidence.

EVIDENCE

In considering exactly what *evidence* is, Oxman and colleagues (2009) assert that evidence concerns facts (actual or asserted) intended for use in support policy, and that evidence alone cannot be used to make policy decisions. However, Gray (2001) believes that in the absence of resource decisions, just evidence may be sufficient to make policy decisions. Clearly, the use of evidence in decision making is a complex interplay of cost, necessary resources, and convincing evidence. Just how convincing the evidence is depends on what observations were made and the quality of these observations. Because the research process uses systematic methods to collect and analyze observations, research evidence is more convincing than mere observations, and well-designed and well-executed research is more convincing than poorly designed and executed research. Within a systematic review, judgments about the quality of research evidence are made systematically, either implicitly or explicitly, to prevent errors, resolve disagreements, facilitate critical appraisal, and communicate information (Oxman et al., 2009). The critical appraisal of evidence used in a systematic review is foundational to the review process and serves to ensure that only the highest quality evidence is included. Additionally, all evidence is context sensitive; therefore, judgments need to be made methodically and explicitly about the applicability of the evidence beyond its original context or setting. For example, use of contextual evidence implies that evidence obtained from a specific setting takes into consideration the modifying factors in specific settings such as the degree of need, the prevalence of disease or risk factors or problems with health care delivery, financial or governmental constraints, values, costs, and the availability of resources. The ultimate goal is to avoid errors and bias in making health care policy decisions and ensure that conflicts of interest do not influence policy-making decisions or any future research undertaken in support of policy making.

Using Research Evidence to Define and Clarify a Health Care Policy Issue

Debate regarding how best to define a health care policy problem is critically important to the policy-making process. The definition of a policy problem and its clarification influences *whether* and *how* policy makers take action to address the problem (Kingdon, 2003; Lavis, Wilson, Oxman, Lewin, et al., 2009).

According to Kingdon (2003), problems may come to our attention through focusing events or a change in an indicator or feedback on a current policy. Focusing events are common in health care, because poor policy decision making may lead to extreme and often high-profile events such as dramatically increased morbidity and mortality resulting, for example, from a precipitous outbreak of disease. A change in an indicator, although less dramatic than a focusing event, may gain policy makers' attention because of a special report or media attention. For example, the Institute of Medicine's (IOM; 2011) consensus report, *The Future of Nursing: Leading Change, Advancing Health*, which holds that, among other things, nurses should achieve higher levels of education and training, practice to the full extent of their education and training, and be full partners with health care professionals in redesigning health care in the United States. Feedback from the operation of a current policy or program may be informal feedback from a program manager who reports that a particular program is failing to meet its target indicators/outcomes because of limited resources or formal because of an audit.

Kingdon (2003) points out that not all policy problems brought to our attention are worthy of policy action. A potential policy problem may be defined as warranting action by (a) comparing current conditions with values related to a "more ideal" state of affairs, (b) comparing performance with other jurisdictions, and (c) framing a problem in a new way. Efforts to clarify policy problems are more likely to result in action if they reflect an understanding of concurrent developments related to policy and program options (e.g., the publication of a report demonstrating the effectiveness of a particular policy option) and are influenced by concurrent political events (e.g., a shift in political party leadership and power resulting in a change in perceptions and attitudes regarding a particular policy issue). In order to be placed on the *decision agenda*, a policy option must be seen as a viable solution, technically feasible, consistent with dominant values and the public's mood, and acceptable in terms of budgetary considerations and political support or opposition (Kingdon, 2003). Political events that might influence whether a policy option is brought forth can include swings in the public's mood, changes in levels of support or opposition from interest groups, and/or changes in the governing party or prevailing legislative priorities (Kingdon, 2003). Lavis, Wilson, Oxman, Lewin, et al. (2009) offer five questions that can be used to guide policy makers in identifying and clarifying a health care policy problem as presented in Table 12.1.

TABLE 12.1

Questions That Address a Health Care Policy Problem

Question	Considerations
What is the problem?	A health care policy problem may be related to a disease or condition, programs or services, or the current status of an agreed upon course of action (e.g., guideline).
How did the problem come to attention, and has this process influenced the prospect of it being addressed?	Policy problems can be identified through an unusual event, such as a disaster, poor results from a quality indicator, or a report.
What indicators can be used, or collected, to establish the magnitude of the problem and to measure progress in addressing it?	Information about the policy issue can be obtained from community surveys and vital registries, health care administrative data (i.e., health management information systems), monitoring and evaluation data, health care provider surveys, legislation, regulation, policies, drug formularies, and policy maker surveys for indicators about governmental considerations or health expenditure surveys and reports.
What comparisons can be made to establish the magnitude of the problem and to measure progressing in addressing it?	Comparisons that can be made include comparisons over time to determine whether a health care problem is improving or worsening; comparisons between countries and other appropriate comparators (when comparable data are available) to establish the magnitude of a health care problem and what targets might be achievable and help to mobilize support for addressing the problem; comparisons against plans (e.g., national goals and benchmarks) that may help mobilize support for addressing a health care problem; and comparisons against what policy makers and/or stakeholders predicted or wanted.
How can the problem be described in a way that will motivate different groups	The meanings that individuals or various constituent groups attach to a particular health care policy problem, the indicators used to measure it, and the comparisons made to establish its importance must be acknowledged and analyzed to determine how important a health policy is to a given constituency.

Adapted from Lavis, J. N., Wilson, M. G., Oxman, A. D., Lewin, S., & Fretheim, A. (2009). SUPPORT tools for evidence-informed health policymaking (STP) 4: Using research evidence to clarify a problem. *Health Research Policy and Systems, 7*(suppl 1), S4. Retrieved from http://www.health-policy-systems.com/content/7/S1/S4

Using Research Evidence to Frame Options to Address a Health Care Policy Problem

Health care policy makers may find themselves in one or more of the following three situations, requiring them to characterize the costs and consequences of options to address a problem (Kingdon, 2003; Lavis, Wilson, Oxman, Grimshaw, et al., 2009):

Situation 1: A health care policy decision has already been made, and the role of the policy maker is to maximize the benefits of an option, minimize its harm, optimize the impact achieved for the money spent, and, possibly, to design a monitoring and evaluation plan.

Situation 2: A health care policy-making process is already underway, and the role of the policy makers is to assess the options presented to them.

Situation 3: A health care policy-making process has not yet begun, and the role of the policy maker is to identify options, characterize the costs and consequences of these options, and look for "policy windows" of opportunity in which to act.

In any of these three situations, research evidence, particularly about benefits, potential harm, and costs, is very useful in determining if a particular health care policy option is viable. To more thoroughly address each of these situations, Lavis, Wilson, Oxman, Grimshaw, et al. (2009) offer six questions that can be used to guide policy makers in identifying health care policy and program options to address a high-priority problem and to characterize the costs and consequences of these options:

1. Has an appropriate set of options been identified to address a problem? Policy makers may be able to identify existing frameworks that enable the identification of health care policy or program options. These frameworks may be the focus of reports, may be embedded in systematic reviews, or in overviews of systematic reviews. It is important to point out that multiple competing frameworks for identifying health care policy options may exist, these may not be mutually exclusive, and there is often no empirical evidence to support the use of one framework over another.

2. What benefits are important to those who will be affected, and which benefits are likely to be achieved with each option? Health care policy makers are concerned here with determining the (a) likely benefits (or positive effects) of each policy option, (b) which benefits are likely to be important to those who will be affected by the decisions made, and (c) whether they are more interested in particular populations (e.g., children, adults, or the elderly) or particular comparisons (e.g., comparing the option of doing nothing with the option of providing standardized care).

To accomplish this, Lavis, Wilson, Oxman, Grimshaw, et al. (2009) offer the acronym *POCO* (analogous to *PICO*, discussed elsewhere in this text), which refers to the four key elements they assert must be considered in identifying research evidence about the benefits of particular health care policy options and to ensure that such evidence is used effectively:

- People (e.g., elderly patients with multiple chronic conditions)
- Option (e.g., case management)
- Comparison (e.g., routine care)
- Outcome (e.g., health-related quality of life)

3. What potential harms are there to those who will be affected? Information about potential harms is sometimes found in effectiveness studies (randomized controlled trials) and, more frequently, in observational studies that track those *exposed* to an option, whether or not the exposure was part of a particular test of the health care policy option (e.g., a large-scale drug surveillance system). Sometimes, systematic reviews of these types of studies can be found. As with all systematic reviews, health care policy makers need to assess their quality and applicability, as well as incorporate equity considerations. Once potential harms have been identified, mitigating actions should be identified to reduce these harms.

4. What are the local costs of each option, and is there local evidence about their cost-effectiveness? Because two or more policy options may be effective, one may produce better outcomes for a given cost, or it may achieve the same outcomes at less cost. It is, therefore, important to determine each health care policy option's cost, and, when possible, its relative cost-effectiveness. Just as with other types of research studies and systematic reviews, policy makers should exercise caution when interpreting results of any economic evaluation. Lavis, Wilson, Oxman, Lewin, & Fretheim (2009) remind us that economic evaluations are always written from a particular perspective (e.g., provider, payer, society at large). Similarly, health care policy makers and other stakeholders should be aware of their own particular viewpoint that they bring to any economic analysis. Refer to Chapter 11 for a discussion of economic evidence.

5. What adaptations might be made to any given option, and could they alter its benefits, potential harms, and costs? It is extremely important to determine the costs and consequences of a health care policy option and to determine whether there might be significant interest in, or even pressure, to *adapt* an option that has been tried elsewhere. Policy makers should, therefore, search specifically for qualitative studies that can help to identify how and why a particular health care policy option works. These assessments can then be very useful in informing policy makers' judgments about which elements of a particular policy option are critically important to retain, and which elements of an option are not important and should be eliminated or modified. Refer to Chapter 10 for a discussion of qualitative evidence.

6. Which stakeholder views and experiences might influence an option's acceptability and its benefits, potential harms, and costs? In considering the costs and consequences of various health care policy options, it is important to determine whether the views and experiences of potential stakeholders (e.g., health care consumers, health care providers, health care systems, policy makers, society at large) influence the acceptability and impact of the options under consideration. If influence

is likely, health care policy makers should seek out qualitative studies that specifically examine the views and experiences of such stakeholders. Refer to Chapter 10 for a discussion of qualitative evidence.

Using Research Evidence to Address How a Health Care Policy Option Will Be Implemented

The process of translating health care policy into practice is challenging and must be accomplished in an organized way using careful planning to prevent *good policies* from being poorly implemented (Fretheim, Munabi-Babigumira, Oxman, Lavis, & Lewin, 2009). Attention to potential barriers and strategies at various levels of the health care system when implementing a health care policy or program is crucial. The barriers to successful health care policy implementation vary from policy to policy and among varied contexts. Research findings regarding barriers to policy implementation in other settings and lessons learned from previous experience are helpful but, by themselves, are insufficient. Fretheim and colleagues (2009) propose a structured approach to identifying barriers to successful health care policy implementation that focuses on those who are affected by the policy—the policy stakeholders. These stakeholders are the individuals and groups who are most likely to foresee possible barriers to successful policy implementation. Several methods can be used to explore the views of stakeholder groups about new health care policies; for example, using a *mixed methods approach* that may include brainstorming, focused group discussions, interviews, and other qualitative methods, or a combination of these (Fretheim et al., 2009). According to Fretheim and colleagues (2009), well-conducted qualitative studies may provide insights into the behavior of health care consumers regarding their use of health services (e.g., underutilization, nonadherence to recommended lifestyle changes or treatment schedules). Such behaviors may be significant obstacles to successful health care policy implementation. It is important to understand why targeted populations behave in particular ways, because this behavior will influence the choices that people make in accessing and using health care services. Such activities can provide new insights into stakeholders' perceptions and identify both barriers and facilitators to health care policy implementation. Surveys that ask respondents to rate a list of potential obstacles to change and barriers to policy implementation may also be useful. Once likely barriers to health care policy implementation have been identified, strategies or interventions that address these barriers can be formulated. The choice of strategies and interventions should be guided by the available evidence of their effectiveness and costs, as well as stakeholders' views (Fretheim et al., 2009).

The Cochrane Consumer and Communication Review Group has extensively documented the effects of interventions to improve interactions between health care consumers and health care providers and systems (Santesso, Ryan, Hill, & Grimshaw, 2007) and developed a catalog of interventions that includes (a) provision of education or information, (b) support for changing behavior, (c) support for developing skills and competencies, (d) personal support, (e) facilitation of communication and decision making, and (f) system participation (Santesso et al., 2007).

A systematic review conducted by Cabana and colleagues (1999) addressed barriers to guideline adherence among physicians and identified seven main categories of barriers. These can be used as well in identifying barriers to health care policy implementation among health professionals: (a) lack of awareness, (b) lack of familiarity, (c) lack of agreement, (d) lack of self-efficacy, (e) lack of outcome expectancy, (f) inertia of previous practice, and (g) external barriers (Cabana et al., 1999; Fretheim et al., 2009).

The Effective Practice and Organisation of Care (EPOC) Review Group in the Cochrane Collaboration has developed an arrangement of provider-targeted interventions, which provides an overview of the types of health interventions that may be considered for implementation purposes (Cochrane EPOC Review Group, 2002; Fretheim et al., 2009). These include (a) educational materials, (b) educational meetings, (c) educational outreach visits, (d) local opinion leaders, (e) local consensus processes, (f) peer review, (g) audit and feedback, (h) reminders and prompts, (i) tailored interventions, (j) patient-mediated interventions, and (k) multifaceted interventions.

Moderately effective strategies designed to achieve behavioral changes include (a) evaluation of health care professionals' health care policy guideline implementation, (b) educational outreach visits and multifaceted interventions that specifically target identified barriers, (c) circulation of health care policy guidelines, and (d) hosting of educational meetings (Fretheim et al., 2009). More effective strategies in influencing health professional behavior include (a) financial incentives, although these may lead to potentially negative consequences in terms of cost-effectiveness, and (b) regulatory measures that are inexpensive but may be poorly received by professional groups (Fretheim et al., 2009). Additional research and systematic reviews of existing research are needed to identify more effective strategies for changing the behavior of health care professionals regarding successful policy implementation.

Many organizational change strategies attempt to identify the steps in a process that leads to change, define why there is a need for change, and identify barriers to change (Fretheim et al., 2009). Most of these are based almost entirely on theory, or on singular applications and opinion. Evidence to support the effectiveness of these strategies is lacking, thus, making it difficult to predict whether or not a specific strategic method is likely to result in the desired organizational change. Fretheim and colleagues (2009), however, point out that although the impacts of such change management strategies are uncertain, they may still be useful in encouraging active reflection on how organizational change may be facilitated.

According to Fretheim and colleagues (2009), changes in the overall health system may be necessary to implement a new health care policy. These may include changes to governmental systems, financial systems, and health care delivery systems. The body of evidence on how to implement such changes is small, and those making policy decisions may have to draw on case studies and policy implementation experiences in other jurisdictions. For particular health care policy implementation issues, systematic reviews may be useful, such as those related to the costs of scaling up interventions or factors that may affect the sustainability of health care programs.

DETERMINING HOW MUCH CONFIDENCE TO PLACE IN A SYSTEMATIC REVIEW USED FOR THE PURPOSE OF HEALTH CARE POLICY MAKING

The reliability of systematic reviews regarding the effects of health care interventions are variable and, therefore, when making policy decisions based on these reviews, health care policy makers need to assess how much confidence can be placed in such evidence (Lewin et al., 2009). As recommended throughout this chapter, using systematic and transparent processes in making health care policy decisions may help prevent the introduction of errors and bias in these important decisions. When making health care policy decisions informed by the evidence presented in a review, policy makers need to consider assessments of the reliability of a systematic review along with other information, such as the usefulness of the review in relation to the policy question and evidence on formulation of health care policy in the local context (Lewin et al., 2009).

Lewin and colleagues (2009) suggest five questions that should be considered when deciding how much confidence to place in the findings of a systematic review of the effects of an intervention and policy making based on these findings. These are as follows:

1. Did the review explicitly address an appropriate policy or management question?
2. Were appropriate criteria used when considering studies for the review?
3. Was the search for relevant studies detailed and reasonably comprehensive?
4. Were assessments of the studies' relevance to the review topic and of their risk of bias reproducible?
5. Were the results similar from study to study?

ASSESSING THE LOCAL APPLICABILITY OF THE FINDINGS OF A SYSTEMATIC REVIEW FOR HEALTH CARE POLICY MAKING

Differences between health care settings often result in a policy or program option that, although may be useful in one setting, is not feasible or acceptable in another, or simply will not work the same way or may even achieve a different impact in another setting. Health care policy makers, therefore, face the challenge of determining whether research evidence about a particular health care policy option is applicable in their local setting. According to Lavis, Oxman, et al. (2009), systematic reviews make the challenge of health care policy making easier, because they offer a systematic summary and appraisal of research studies conducted in different *settings* (e.g., political/country jurisdictions), *sectors* (e.g., primary care, acute care), and *locales* (e.g., rural, urban). Systematic reviews are also helpful in making judgments about the applicability of the evidence to specific settings by providing a framework for understanding and research evidence that can be useful in identifying the essential factors needed for a health care policy option to work or that may modify its impact (Lavis, Oxman, et al., 2009).

It should be pointed out, however, that many systematic reviews do not provide adequate descriptions of the features of the actual settings in which the original studies were conducted. Many systematic reviews do *not* do the following: (a) adequately describe the settings in which research studies were conducted, particularly those factors that might modify the impact of a health care policy option; (b) provide a framework for identifying potential modifying factors; or (c) provide research evidence about modifying factors (Lavis, Oxman, et al., 2009). In such instances, articles that analyze policies or narrative reviews may provide more helpful frameworks that can be useful to inform judgments about the applicability of the evidence in a systematic review (Lavis, Oxman, et al., 2009). Systematic reviews of administrative database studies and of community surveys may be helpful in understanding health care problems from a comparative perspective. Reviews of observational studies may be useful in characterizing a health care policy option's potential harms. As indicated earlier, reviews of qualitative studies may assist in gaining insights into the meanings that individuals or groups assign to particular health care problems, how and why particular policy options work, and the stakeholder's views about experiences with particular health care policy options (Lavis, Oxman, et al., 2009).

Lavis, Oxman, et al. (2009) offer five questions to guide health care policy makers in assessing the applicability of the findings of a systematic review to a specific (local) setting:

1. Were the studies included in a systematic review conducted in the same setting, or were the findings consistent across settings or periods?
2. Are there important differences in actual realities and constraints that might substantially alter the feasibility and acceptability of a policy option?
3. Are there significant differences in health care systems that may mean that an option could not work in the same way?
4. Are there important differences in the baseline conditions that might yield different absolute effects even if the relative effectiveness is the same?
5. What insights can be drawn about health care policy options, implementation, monitoring, and evaluation?

There may be little reason to be concerned about the local applicability of the findings of a systematic review, if the studies included in the review were conducted in the *same* or *very similar* settings as the policy maker or the findings have been shown to be consistent across settings or periods and a similar impact may be expected (Lavis, Oxman, et al., 2009). The following information in systematic reviews can be used by health care policy makers to inform judgments regarding the local applicability of review findings: (a) information about the settings of studies and specifications regarding the periods over which the studies were conducted—usually found in a section of the review entitled "Characteristics of Included Studies" (or similar); and (b) information about the consistency of findings—usually found in the review abstract or in the *results* section (Lavis, Oxman, et al., 2009).

If information about settings and periods is missing in a systematic review, health care policy makers may wish to contact the authors of the review to see whether they have this information and will make it available. Alternatively, if this is a sufficiently high priority, policy makers may wish to retrieve the original studies included in the review if, of course, resources and time allow. Lavis, Oxman, et al. (2009) point out that one potential benefit of establishing direct contact with review authors is that it may encourage them to give attention to information regarding local applicability assessments and considerations in future reviews.

Systematic reviews rarely include information about resource and capacity constraints or stakeholder influence. Instead, most reviews focus on describing the health care policy options (e.g., programs, services, drugs) that were studied. Health care policy makers in settings with very significant resource and capacity constraints have to carefully consider the feasibility of available policy options (Lavis, Oxman, et al., 2009). For example, in a local setting where there is an extreme shortage of advanced practice nurses (APNs), a health care policy option requiring a significant role for APNs might not be feasible, at least in the short term. It is possible, however, that such a constraint could be addressed over time; expanding APN educational programs could produce sufficient number of graduates to meet the present and future local need for their services.

If a systematic review does not provide the information necessary to determine whether the characteristics of a particular health care system might result in a policy option not working in the same way it has worked in other systems, policy makers could look for (a) policy analysis articles or narrative reviews incorporating helpful frameworks that could be used to identify factors that might modify the impact of a health care policy option, and (b) detailed descriptions of the health care system, specifically those characteristics that might substantially alter the potential impact of a policy option (Lavis, Oxman, et al., 2009).

Unlike the possibility of change over time discussed in the previous question regarding realities and constraints, there is far less chance that health care systems can be modified. Health care systems are difficult to change, and typically, the underlying rationale for change would need to be considerably more compelling than simply the *possibility* that the proposed change will enhance the impact of a single health care policy option (Lavis, Oxman, et al., 2009).

Information about baseline conditions can often be found in systematic reviews in a section titled "Characteristics of Included Studies." Alternatively, this information may have to be retrieved from the original studies included in the review. Local evidence about baseline conditions, oftentimes, is available in the policy maker's own health care setting (Lavis, Oxman, et al., 2009).

Health care policy makers in settings with *different* baseline conditions may expect a very different absolute impact. The link between baseline conditions and absolute effects is relevant in clinical settings in which the relative effectiveness of a clinical intervention is often the same across patients but where patients' baseline risks may vary quite dramatically. This link is also relevant in public health settings where, for example, immunization programs might be introduced in countries with very different baseline conditions (Lavis, Oxman, et al., 2009).

Even if the findings from systematic reviews are not directly applicable to a given local setting, important lessons can still be learned. Policy makers may (a) discover an idea for a health care policy option that they might otherwise not have considered; (b) may gain insight into how various health care policy options have been implemented in other settings; and (c) draw directly on the systematic review

TABLE 12.2

Suggested Questions When Using a Systematic Review to Make Policy Decisions

Does the question relate to your context, constituents and/or capacity?

Are the outcomes examined in the review the ones necessary to make a policy decision?

Are the methods used in the review, i.e., the search strategy, transparent and easy to understand?

Would you be easily able to find the original documents or papers if necessary?

Were adequate attempts made to find evidence other than published papers and research studies?

Is it evident that only high quality studies were used in the review? Are the methods of quality assessment provided?

Has the evidence been displayed and discussed in a manner that is helpful to your decision making?

Have the policy implications of the review been presented?

itself in developing a monitoring and evaluation plan (Lavis, Oxman, et al., 2009). Table 12.2 provides a list of questions to ask when examining systematic reviews related to policy decisions.

SUMMARY

Evidence-informed health care policy making is an approach to policy decisions that aims to ensure that decision making is well informed by the best available research evidence. It is characterized by the systematic and transparent access to, and appraisal of, evidence as an input into the policy-making process (Oxman et al., 2009). This chapter has provided readers with the opportunity to differentiate between evidence-based and evidence-informed health care policy making and explore the importance of systematic reviews in formulating evidence-informed health care policies. Information has been provided to guide health care policy makers in using research evidence to (a) define and clarify a health care policy problem, (b) frame options to address a health care policy problem, and (c) address how a health care policy option will be implemented. Parameters for determining how much confidence to place in systematic reviews used for the purpose of health care policy making and the local applicability of the findings of systematic reviews for health care policy making have been discussed.

EXERCISES

Read the front page of your local newspaper every day for 1 week. Write down the health-related issues that are in the news. What are people in your area concerned about? Choose one of the current issues and determine what evidence there is to support best practice change. Write a letter to the editor of the newspaper regarding the chosen issue, with emphasis on the way in which evidence can inform policy making regarding this issue.

REFERENCES

Cabana, M. D., Rand, C. S., Powe, N. R., Wu, A. W., Wilson, M. H., Abboud, P. A., & Rubin, H. R. (1999). Why don't physicians follow clinical practice guidelines? A framework for improvement. *Journal of the American Medical Association, 282*(15), 1458–1465.

Cochrane Effective Practice and Organisation of Care Review Group. (2002). Data collection check list. Retrieved from http://www.epoc.cochrane.org//sites/epoc.cochrane.org/files/uploads/datacollectionchecklist.pdf

Fox, D. M. (2005). Evidence of evidence-based health policy: The politics of systematic reviews in coverage decisions. *Health Affairs, 24*(1), 114–122. doi:10.1377/hlthaff.24.1.114

Fretheim, A., Munabi-Babigumira, S., Oxman, A. D, Lavis, J. N., & Lewin, S. (2009). SUPPORT tools for evidence-informed policymaking in health 6: Using research evidence to address how an option will be implemented. *Health Research Policy and Systems, 7*(Suppl 1), S6. Retrieved from http://www.health-policy-systems.com/content/7/S1/S6

Gray, J. A. M. (2001). Using systematic reviews for evidence based policy making. In M. Egger, G. D. Smith, & D. G. Altman (Eds.), *Systematic reviews in health care: Meta-analysis in context* (2nd ed., pp. 410–418). London, UK: BMJ.

Institute of Medicine. (2011). *The future of nursing: Leading change, advancing health.* Washington, DC: The National Academies Press.

Kingdon, J. W. (2003). *Agendas, alternatives, and public policies* (2nd ed.). New York, NY: Longman.

Lavis, J. N., Oxman, A. D., Souza, N. M., Lewin, S., Gruen, R. L., & Fretheim, A. (2009). SUPPORT tools for evidence-informed health policymaking (STP) 9: Assessing the applicability of the findings of a systematic review. *Health Research Policy and Systems, 7*(Suppl 1), S9. Retrieved from http://www.health-policy-systems.com/content/7/S1/S9

Lavis, J. N., Wilson, M. G., Oxman, A. D., Grimshaw, J., Lewin, S., & Fretheim, A. (2009). Support tools for evidence-informed health policymaking (STP) 5: Using research evidence to frame options to address a problem. *Health Research Policy and Systems, 7*(Suppl 1), S5. Retrieved from http://www.health-policy-systems.com/content/7/S1/S5

Lavis, J. N., Wilson, M. G., Oxman, A. D., Lewin, S., & Fretheim, A. (2009). SUPPORT tools for evidence-informed health policymaking (STP) 4: Using research evidence to clarify a problem. *Health Research Policy and Systems, 7*(Suppl 1), S4. Retrieved from http://www.health-policy-systems.com/content/7/S1/S4

Lewin, S., Oxman, A. D., Lavis, J. N., & Fretheim, A. (2009). SUPPORT tools for evidence-informed health policymaking (STP) 8: Deciding how much confidence to place in a systematic review. *Health Research Policy and Systems, 7*(Suppl 1), S8. Retrieved from http://www.health-policy-systems.com/content/7/S1/S8

Oxman, A. D., Lavis, J. N., Lewin, S., & Fretheim, A. (2009). SUPPORT tools for evidence-informed health policymaking (STP) 1: What is evidence-informed policymaking? *Health Research Policy and Systems, 7*(Suppl 1), S1. Retrieved from http://www.health-policy-systems.com/content/7/S1/S1

Santesso, N., Ryan, R., Hill, S., & Grimshaw, J. (2007). *A taxonomy of interventions directed at consumers to promote evidence-based prescribing and drug use.* Poster presented at the Canadian Agency for Drugs and Technologies in Health symposium. Retrieved from http://www.latrobe.edu.au/chcp/assets/downloads/CADTH07_poster.pdf

Washington State Senate Bill 6088, Chapter 29, Laws of 2003; House Bill 1299, Chapter 276, Laws of 2003, signed by Governor Gary Locke, effective 27 July 2003.

SUGGESTED READINGS

The Bamako call to action on research for health: Strengthening research for health, development, and equity. (2008). Paper presented at the Global Ministerial Forum on Research for Health, Bamako, Mali. Retrieved from http://www.who.int/rpc/news/BAMAKOCALL-TOACTIONFinalNov24.pdf

Chalmers, I. (2005). If evidence-informed policy works in practice, does it matter if it doesn't work in theory? *Evidence & Policy, 1*(2), 227–242. Retrieved form http://www.ingentaconnect.com/content/tpp/ep/2005/00000001/00000002/art00006

Fretheim, A., Schünemann, H. J., & Oxman, A. D. (2006). Improving the use of research evidence in guideline development: 15. Disseminating and implementing guidelines. *Health Research Policy and Systems, 4*, 27. Retrieved from http://www.health-policy-systems.com/content/4/1/27

Iles, V., & Sutherland, K. (2001). *Managing change in the NHS. Organisational change: A review for health care managers, professionals, and researchers.* London, UK: National Co-ordinating Centre for NHS Service Delivery and Organisation R & D. Retrieved from http://www.sdo.nihr.ac.uk/files/adhoc/change-management-review.pdf

Isaacs, D., & Fitzgerald, D. (1999). Seven alternatives to evidence based medicine. *British Medical Journal, 319*(7225), 1618. Retrieved from http://www.bmj.com/cgi/content/full/319/7225/1618

Macintyre, S., & Petticrew, M. (2000). Good intentions and received wisdom are not enough. *Journal of Epidemiology and Community Health, 54*(11), 802–803. Retrieved from http://www.jech.bmj.com/cgi/content/full/54/11/802

The Mexico statement on health research: Knowledge for better health: Strengthening health systems. (2004). Paper presented at the Ministerial Summit on Health Research, Mexico City, Mexico. Retrieved from http://www.who.int/rpc/summit/agenda/Mexico_Statement-English.pdf

Moynihan, R. (2004). *Using health research in policy and practice: Case studies from nine countries* (Milbank Memorial Fund Report). Retrieved form http://www.milbank.org/reports/04 09Moynihan/0409Moynihan.html

World Health Assembly (2005). *World Health Assembly Resolution.* Paper presented at the 58th meeting of the World Health Assembly, Geneva, Switzerland. Retrieved from http://www.who.int/rpc/meetings/58th_WHA_resolution.pdf

CHAPTER THIRTEEN

Using Systematic Reviews at the Point of Care

Ronell Kirkley

OBJECTIVES

Upon completion of Chapter 13, you will be able to:

- Describe the use of clinical guidelines in clinical decision making
- Locate clinical guidelines using various electronic sources
- Critically appraise clinical guidelines
- State ways to increase the use of clinical guidelines

IMPORTANT POINTS

- The aim of a clinical practice guideline (CPG) is to improve quality health care by providing health care professionals with evidence-based recommendations for the treatment of clients.
- Evidence-based CPGs can reduce the delivery of inappropriate care and support the introduction of new knowledge into clinical practice.
- Guidelines should be developed by a multidisciplinary team, be based on a systematic review, and explicitly link the recommendations to the evidence. The level of evidence is determined by the question type and considers both the type of design and methodological quality. Strength of the recommendation is influenced by the level of evidence, the balance of benefits to risks, the client's values and preferences, and the resource use.
- Because most health care organizations do not have the ability/resources to develop their own CPGs, specialty organizations have attempted to locate, critically appraise, and adapt these guidelines for use in specific clinical situations.
- Multiple strategies for dissemination and implementation of CPGs are more effective than a single strategy.

INTRODUCTION

Globally, anywhere from 30%–40% of clients do not get treatment of proven effectiveness, and a great number (25%) receive unnecessary care or care that is potentially harmful (Grol, 2001; Schuster, McGlynn, & Brook, 1998). There is growing consensus that health care services in the United States have greater variance, are enormously expensive, and, overall, fall short of expectations than other developed countries (The Commonwealth Fund Commission on a High Performance Health System, 2008). According to The Commonwealth Fund Commission on a High Performance Health System (2008), the United States falls woefully short when compared with other countries in comparison with quality indicators such as infant mortality. In fact, a very common finding from health services researchers is the failure to translate research findings into point of care practice. Consequently, there is a tremendous push for clinicians, researchers, and, ultimately, policy makers to generate, synthesize, and critically appraise high-quality research that is unbiased in an effort to make strides in decreasing these disparities, improving outcomes, and, ultimately, in making heath care more cost effective. CPGs have the potential to meet this mandate and should be an integral tool in the armamentarium of clinicians delivering services at the point of care.

CPGs are an attempt to support implementation of evidence into practice. They are "systematically developed statements formulated to assist practitioner's decisions about appropriate health care and interventions for specific clinical scenarios" (Grimshaw & Russell, 1993a, p. 243). Guidelines should be an outgrowth of a rigorous systematic identification and appraisal of relevant research (Turner, Misso, Harris, & Green, 2008) with the statements linking recommended practice to underlying scientific research, client input, and expert opinion. They provide a resource for practitioner and clients in decision making about how to prevent, diagnose, and/or treat presenting symptoms (Hoffman, Bennett, & Del Mar, 2010).

The aim of CPGs is to improve quality health care, reduce the delivery of inappropriate care, and support the introduction of new knowledge into clinical practice (Shiffman et al., 2003). An overarching goal of guidelines is the translation of often complex research findings into recommendations that caregivers and clients can use for clinical care decisions. In addition, guidelines can be used to develop standards to assess current clinical practice of health providers as well as in the education and training of health professionals. They can also serve to improve communication between patient and health professional, as well as communication between health professionals across disciplines (National Institute for Health and Clinical Excellence, 2010).

Eddy (1990) used the terms *standards*, *guidelines*, and *options* in his attempt to illustrate the importance of linking the scientific evidence, patient's care, and condition with the desired outcome. He defined standards as appropriate care that should be followed in all circumstances, with no flexibility for the clinician; guidelines should be followed in most circumstances, but they do allow for flexibility in some circumstances; whereas options are so flexible that they really provide almost no guidance at all. Those elements, which are well founded scientifically and are classified with the highest levels of evidence and have, therefore, been found to have important implications for increasing positive outcomes, should be linked to the evidence in the CPGs as a standard of care and it should be followed in all circumstances with no flexibility for the clinician. For example, in a susceptible patient who is exposed to certain agents commonly used in the administration of general anesthesia, a malignant hypertensive (MH) episode can occur. Prompt diagnosis, rapid and early discontinuation of the triggering agent, and administration of a skeletal muscle relaxant (dantrolene sodium) has been shown conclusively to reduce subsequent mortality (The Malignant Hyperthermia Association of the United States, 2010). The administration of dantrolene is an example of a time-tested element of a clinical guideline that is, in fact, a standard of care and one that has a consensus of vested stakeholders and the supporting evidence that this treatment must be administered by clinicians in all circumstances.

Clinical guidelines are not meant to provide an algorithmic approach to patient care in all circumstances and for all clients (Buie, 2010). The use of clinical guidelines are, in their broadest interpretation, *guides* that should not replace the clinical skill or critical thinking germane to all sound clinical care. They help direct suitable behavior without mandating that the recommendation be followed without fail (Alpert, 2010). Based on both evidence and opinion, guidelines are "neither infallible nor a substitute for clinical judgment" (Manchikanti, 2008, p. 172). Guideline recommendations must be applied with careful consideration about the clinical context and attention to any potential contraindications for the individual patient.

Guidelines cover a wide range of topics of interest and cater to a wide variety of end users, including health care providers, purchasers, health plans, educators, policy makers, and integrated delivery systems. Topics include diseases and mental disorders, as well as topics relevant to behavioral disciplines, guidelines on the uses of chemicals and drugs, as well as analytical, diagnostic, and therapeutic techniques, and equipment use (Agency for Healthcare Research and Quality [AHRQ], 2010).

A large number of organizations support the development of CPGs including specialty societies (i.e., American Academy of Sleep Medicine, American College of Chest Physicians, and American Diabetes Association) and national groups such as the U.S. Preventive Services Task Force, Centers for Disease Control and Prevention (CDC), National Institute for Health and Clinical Excellence (NICE) in the United Kingdom, the Scottish Intercollegiate Guideline Network (SIGN), the World Health Organization (WHO), and the National Health and Medical Research Council of Australia (NHMRC). There are now nearly 2,500 guidelines currently registered with the National Guideline Clearinghouse (NGC).

CLINICAL GUIDELINE DEVELOPMENT AND CHARACTERISTICS

Attributes of Guidelines

The SIGN identifies three core principles for guidelines development. First, guidelines should be developed by a nationally representative, multidisciplinary team with clearly identified expertise in both the topic area and the methodology (i.e., systematic review and guideline development). Second, a systematic review is the foundation for linking recommendations with research. To this end, a systematic review must be completed to identify and critically appraise the evidence, a process described in preceding chapters. The third principle is that in the actual guideline, recommendations must be explicitly linked to the supporting evidence (http://www.sign.ac.uk/methodology/index.html).

Attention to the development of guidelines is critical if the product is to be viewed as trustworthy and usable. The 1992 Institute of Medicine Report, *Guidelines for Clinical Practice: From Development to Use*, identified desirable attributes of CPGs to assure its trustworthiness and usefulness (Field & Lohr, 1992). These attributes continue to be the cornerstone of guideline development for most groups with adaptations over the years. The attributes of validity, reliability, clinical applicability, and clinical flexibility contribute to the substantive content and credibility of the guidelines. Clarity, reproducibility, representative development, scheduled review, and documentation focus on assuring accountability in the process of guideline development. (See Table 13.1 for a list of the attributes of a good clinical guideline.)

Levels of Evidence

Credible guidelines provide linkages to the scientific evidence accompanying it. Grading the level of evidence and strength of the recommendations is done to provide the practitioner a way to determine the quality and strength of the guideline. Generally, scientific and clinical evidence should take precedence over expert judgment. Although there are various systems for defining the level of evidence in this way, most use a numerical approach with the highest level of evidence as a Level I. It must be pointed out that quality of evidence is a continuum and that schemes with discrete categorization do involve some degrees of arbitrariness (Guyatt et al., 2008a).

Levels of evidence are a hierarchical rating systems used to qualify study quality. Quality of evidence captures the "extent of confidence that an estimate of effect is correct" (Terracciano, Brozek, Compalati, & Schünemann, 2010) and is based on ranking according to the level of bias associated with the different study designs, thus, a focus on internal validity. There has been significant controversy over levels

TABLE 13.1
Attributes of Good Clinical Guidelines

Valid
Reproducible
Reliable
Representative
Population-based
Unambiguous and precise
User-friendly format
Transparent as to evidence and methods used to develop the guideline and experts who reviewed the guideline

Based on Grimshaw and Russell (1993a).

of evidence, in part because they have been primarily focused on effectiveness or treatment questions with randomized controlled trials as the highest level of evidence. Not all questions can be answered by randomized controlled trials but rely on other designs that provide quality evidence for recommendations. For the malignant hyperthermia guideline presented as an example earlier in this chapter, the recommendation for administration of dantrolene in a suspected MH episode is not supported by the highest level of evidence (Level I). Administration of dantrolene, substantiated with lower levels of evidence, has been a standard of care for more than 30 years. Designing a prospective randomized trial to test this would be, at best, difficult and, at worst, unethical. Retrospectively, this treatment has been shown to save lives numerous times using studies that are considered lower levels of evidence (Gurunluoglu, Swanson, & Haeck, 2009), but clearly, the treatment *ought* to be done.

More recently, there has been a move to consider hierarchies of evidence according to question type. Table 13.2 presents a quantitative evidence hierarchy developed by the NHMRC in Australia. This framework designates levels of evidence according to type of question, capturing questions related to intervention, diagnostic accuracy, prognosis, etiology, and screening intervention. As can be seen, systematic reviews of high-quality studies are at the high end of the hierarchy for all question types. There is variation among the question types as to the strongest level of evidence. For intervention studies, randomized controlled trials are the highest level of evidence and case series studies are at the lower rung. As randomized controlled trials are not feasible for many nonintervention question types, the highest level of evidence will vary according to whether the question addresses diagnostic accuracy, prognosis, etiology, or screening. For each outcome in the clinical guideline, a rating of evidence should be apparent.

The Grading of Recommendations Assessment, Development and Evaluation (short GRADE) Working Group was developed to examine better approaches to grading guidelines. The working group recognized the limitations of leveling by study design alone and considered it essential that methodological quality of individual studies be examined in determining levels of evidence. To this end, they consider factors that can reduce or increase the quality of evidence for a particular study design in rating the quality of evidence. Thus, evidence from randomized controlled trials may begin as high-quality evidence but can be moved to a lower quality rating in the presence of significant study limitations (major deficiencies that are likely to result in a biased assessment of the treatment effect), inconsistency of results (several randomized controlled trials yield widely differing estimates of treatment effect), imprecision, and indirectness of evidence (evidence from randomized controlled trials is derived from similar, but not identical, populations to those of interest to the practitioner). Similarly, observational studies may begin with a "low-quality" rating but be upgraded if the magnitude of the treatment effect is very large, if there is evidence of a dose–response relation, or if all plausible biases are working to underestimate the magnitude of an apparent treatment effect such that the actual treatment effect is very likely to be larger than what the data suggest (http://www.gradeworkinggroup.org).

Quality of evidence in the GRADE framework is presented as high, moderate, low, and very low. High-level evidence is where further research is very unlikely

TABLE 13.2

National Health and Medical Research Council Evidence Hierarchy: Designations of "Levels of Evidence" According to Type of Research Question

Level	Intervention	Diagnostic Accuracy	Prognosis	Etiology	Screening Intervention
I	A systematic review of level II studies	A systematic review of level II studies	A systematic review of level II studies	A systematic review of level II studies	A systematic review of level II studies
II	A randomized controlled trial	A study of test accuracy with: an independent, blinded comparison with a valid reference standard, among consecutive persons with a defined clinical presentation	A prospective cohort study	A prospective cohort study	A randomized controlled trial
III-1	A pseudorandomized controlled trial (i.e., alternate allocation or some other method)	A study of test accuracy with: an independent, blinded comparison with a valid reference standard, among nonconsecutive persons with a defined clinical presentation	All or none	All or none	A pseudorandomized controlled trial (i.e., alternate allocation or some other method)
III-2	A comparative study with concurrent controls: ■ Nonrandomized experimental trial ■ Cohort study ■ Case-control study ■ Interrupted time series with a control group	A comparison with reference standard that does not meet the criteria required for Level II and III-1 evidence	Analysis of prognostic factors among person in a single arm of a randomized controlled trial	A retrospective cohort study	A comparative study with concurrent controls: ■ Nonrandomized, experimental trial ■ Cohort study ■ Case-control study

(Continued)

TABLE 13.2

National Health and Medical Research Council Evidence Hierarchy: Designations of "Levels of Evidence" According to Type of Research Question *(Continued)*

Level	Intervention	Diagnostic Accuracy	Prognosis	Etiology	Screening Intervention
III-3	A comparative study without concurrent controls: ■ Historical control study ■ Two or more single-arm study ■ Interrupted time series without a parallel control group	Diagnostic case-control study	A retrospective cohort study	A case-control study	A comparative study without concurrent controls ■ Historical control study ■ Two or more single-arm studies
IV	Case series with either posttest or pretest/ posttest outcomes	Study of diagnostic yield (no reference standard)	Case series, or cohort study of persons at different stages of disease	A cross-sectional study or case series	Case series

Source: Based on Coleman et al. (2009).

to change confidence in the estimate of effect. Very low evidence is when any estimate of effect is very uncertain (Terracciano et al., 2010). GRADE guidelines have been adopted by many professional medical societies, health-related branches of government health care regulatory bodies. Kavanagh (2009) highlights the need for validation of this schema.

Qualitative evidence is missing from these hierarchies and, as grounded in a different paradigm, would need its own typology. The Joanna Briggs Institute with its pluralistic approach to evidence identifies a hierarchy of evidence for studies addressing feasibility, appropriateness, and meaningfulness, as well as effectiveness research and economic evidence. Thus, they embrace research about the extent to which an activity or intervention is practical (feasibility), ethically or culturally appropriate (appropriateness), as well as the meaningfulness to the individual or population of interest. This knowledge is critical to the decision to adopt recommendations. This hierarchy is presented in Table 13.3. It should be noted that the expert opinion in this schema is considered a form of evidence, whereas in other frameworks, expert opinion is not a category of quality of evidence but is "considered an interpretation of existing evidence and necessary to integrate and contextualize evidence, either from a clinical or a methodological viewpoint" (Terracciano et al., 2010, p. 379).

TABLE 13.3

Joanna Briggs Institute Levels of Evidence

Level of Evidence	Feasibility F (1–4)	Appropriateness A (1–4)	Meaningfulness M (1–4)	Effectiveness E (1–4)	Economic Evidence EE (1–4)
1	Metasynthesis of research with unequivocal synthesized findings	Metasynthesis of research with unequivocal synthesized findings	Metasynthesis of research with unequivocal synthesized findings	Meta-analysis (with homogeneity) of experimental studies (e.g., RCT with concealed randomization) or One or more large experimental studies with narrow confidence intervals	Metasynthesis (with homogeneity) of evaluations of important alternative interventions comparing all clinically relevant outcomes against appropriate cost measurement and including a clinically sensible sensitivity analysis
2	Metasynthesis of research with credible synthesized findings	Metasynthesis of research with credible synthesized findings	Metasynthesis of research with credible synthesized findings	One or more smaller RCTs with wider confidence intervals or Quasi-experimental studies (without randomization)	Evaluations of important alternative interventions comparing all clinically relevant outcomes against appropriate cost measurement and including a clinically sensible sensitivity analysis
3	a. Metasynthesis of text/opinion with credible synthesized finding b. One or more single research studies of high quality	a. Metasynthesis of text/opinion with credible synthesized findings b. One or more single research studies of high quality	a. Metasynthesis of text/opinion with credible synthesized findings b. One or more single research studies of high quality	a. Cohort studies (with control group) b. Case controlled c. Observational studies (without control group)	Evaluations of important alternative interventions comparing a limited number of appropriate cost measurement, without a clinically sensible sensitivity analysis
4	Expert opinion	Expert opinion	Expert opinion	Expert opinion, or physiology bench research, or consensus	Expert opinion, or based on economic theory

Source: The Joanna Briggs Institute (2008).

Strength of Recommendations

Level of evidence will influence but is not the only factor in considering the *strength* (grade) of the recommendations. Guyatt and colleagues (2008a) recommend that decisions regarding the quality of evidence (level) be separate from the strength of recommendations, and highlight that high-quality evidence does not equate automatically with strong recommendations.

The strength of the recommendation is a reflection of the degree of confidence that the desirable effects (i.e., reduction in mortality and morbidity, improved quality of life, reduction in the burden of treatment and lower costs) of an intervention outweigh the undesirable effects (Guyatt et al., 2008b). The undesirable effects similarly capture risks, burden, and cost. When it is very clear that benefits do, or do not, outweigh the risks and burdens, then a strong recommendation may be made. In addition to quality of evidence and the balance between desirable and undesirable consequences of alternative management strategies, other factors to consider in the strength of a recommendation are client's values and preferences and resource use. Table 13.4 presents some questions to ask to determine the strength of recommendations provided by a clinical guideline.

Determinants of Strength of Recommendation

In rating the strength of recommendations in clinical guidelines, the strength of recommendation is generally given with a letter designation, with A being the strongest support for the recommendation. The grade recommendation should be listed alongside a given recommendation within a CPG. Level A recommendations indicate that there is strong empirical support, which merits implementation; level B indicates moderate support where the recommendation should be considered; and level C indicates that there is no empirical support for the recommendation (The Joanna Briggs Institute, 2008). The GRADE work group has developed a binary classification of evidence as strong and weak, where weak indicates that a debate and discussion needs to occur before a decision is made and strong indicates that the recommendation can be implemented as stated. The GRADE software is free and can be obtained from the work group website.

The GRADE working group website (http://www.gradeworkinggroup.org/index.htm) provides an example of a strong recommendation—use of short-term

TABLE 13.4
Questions to Ask when Assessing the Strength of CPG Recommendation

Is there a balance between desirable and undesirable effects?

Is the evidence of high quality? What are the levels of evidence?

Are patient preferences considered in the guideline?

Is the context of the guideline similar to yours?

How much will it cost to implement the recommendations in terms of both economic and opportunity costs?

Do you have the resources to allocate to implementation of this guideline?

Source: Based on Guyatt et al. (2008a).

aspirin for clients experiencing a myocardial infarction (MI). It is believed that short-term aspirin therapy reduces relative risk of death after MI by about 25%. The risks of this intervention are minimal and the cost is low. Additionally, it is quite certain that clients suffering from a MI would, if they understood the choice they were making, opt to receive aspirin. Clinicians can, therefore, offer clients a strong recommendation for this therapy. In contrast, when available evidence shows that benefits and risks/burdens are finely balanced or there is considerable uncertainty about the magnitude of the benefits and risks, then clinicians provide a weak recommendation to clients. In considering these balances, consider an adult who develops idiopathic deep vein thrombosis (DVT). After taking an adjusted dose of warfarin for 1 year, should the clinician recommend its continuation? Continuance of the regimen decreases the risk of recurrent DVT by about 10% per year. However, there are ongoing burdens of persistent warfarin therapy including daily medication, keeping dietary intake of vitamin K constant, monitoring the intensity of anticoagulation with blood tests, and living with the increased risk of both minor and major bleeding. When fully informed by the clinician, some clients are likely to consider the downsides worth it, whereas others may consider the benefit not worth the risks and inconvenience (http://www.gradeworkinggroup.org).

As is clear from these examples, patient values and preferences must be considered along with the strength of the recommendations. The role of the clinician is to fully inform clients about the benefits and risks and assist them to weigh these in context with their values and preferences. It is likely that fully informed clients may make different choices congruent with what is important to them. Clinicians may find the use of decision aids valuable in assisting clients to become fully informed so that evidence can be balanced with preferences and values. Decision aids are designed to complement, rather than replace, counseling from a health practitioner.

Decision aids, whether in print, video, audio, or interactive media format, provide information about treatment options and their associated relevant outcomes. It allows the patient and family to become involved in choosing among different options, appreciate the scientific uncertainties inherent in that choice, clarify personal value or desirability of potential benefits relative to potential harms, as well as provide recommendations for communicating their values to clinicians (Elwyn et al., 2006). Elwyn estimates that well more than 500 decision aids are available, produced largely by a mix of not-for-profit and commercial organizations. As with any systematic review or clinical guideline, the quality of decision aids varies and should be evaluated for methods used, for strategies to avoid bias, and whether valid evidence sources are provided. A good website for guiding personal decisions regarding health-related or social decisions is the Ottawa Personal Decision Guide (OPDG; http://www.decisionaid.ohri.ca/decguide.html).

Where to Find Guidelines

National Guideline Clearinghouse

The NGC database (www.guideline.gov) was created by the AHRQ, U.S. Department of Health and Human Services in partnership with the American Medical Association

(AMA), and America's Health Insurance Plans (AHIP), formerly American Association of Health Plans. The mission of the clearinghouse database is to provide health professionals and others access to "objective, detailed information on CPGs and to further their dissemination, implementation and use" (AHRQ, 2010). As of August 2009, NGC contained 2,422 individual summaries and 406 guidelines in progress. Table 13.5 provides the criteria for inclusion of a guideline in the NGC.

NGC information is gathered from Federal Register posts; searches performed in databases, annual directories, and through hand-searching techniques; as well as recommendations from users. NGC offers summaries of guidelines, with a feature allowing for side-by-side comparison of selected guidelines of one's choice. Within each guideline summary, a link or information can help an investigator obtain the full text of the guideline. Some guideline full-text documents are free, whereas others are available for a fee. Guidelines included as part of NGC are current, with the most recent version of a guideline often occurring in the last 5 years.

Search for NGC content using the search box on the home page. If a searcher types more than one word in the search box, it will be processed with *AND*, the default connecting word, or Boolean operator for NGC database. If the words typed in the search box fit in something called the Unified Medical Language System (UMLS), NGC will search the words in the *disease/condition* and/or *treatment/intervention* fields and as potential text words in an NGC summary. Otherwise, the word(s) typed are searched for in the text or body of the NGC summary.

TABLE 13.5
Criteria for Inclusion of Clinical Practice Guidelines in National Guideline Clearinghouse

All of the following criteria must be met for a clinical practice guideline to be included in National Guideline Clearinghouse (NGC):

1. The clinical practice guideline contains systematically developed statements that include recommendations, strategies, or information that assists physicians and/or other health care practitioners and patients to make decisions about appropriate health care for specific clinical circumstances.

2. The clinical practice guideline was produced under the auspices of medical specialty associations; relevant professional societies, public or private organizations, government agencies at the federal, state, or local level; or health care organizations or plans. A clinical practice guideline developed and issued by an individual not officially sponsored or supported by one of the aforementioned types of organizations does not meet the inclusion criteria for NGC.

3. Corroborating documentation can be produced and verified that a systematic literature search and review of existing scientific evidence published in peer reviewed journals was performed during the guideline development. A guideline is not excluded from NGC if corroborating documentation can be produced and verified detailing specific gaps in scientific evidence for some of the guideline's recommendations.

4. The full text guideline is available upon request in print or electronic format (for free or for a fee) in the English language. The guideline is current and the most recent version produced. Documented evidence can be produced or verified that the guideline was developed, reviewed, or revised within the last 5 years.

NGC offers a link under the search box on the main page entitled "Search Help," and that section is a short one, worth visiting for tips on how to use truncation and perform phrase searching in NGC.

NGC also offers "Detailed Search," which allows one to set search limits, making use of available search filters before performing a search. An example of a limit that one can apply to a search for a guideline is "Chart Documentation/Checklists/Forms" located under the Implementation Tools section. Another limit is to allow a guideline search to retrieve guidelines for an intended user such as advance practice nurses. Really simple syndication (RSS) feed or e-mail service can be used for keeping current on the latest/newest guidelines but cannot be used for creating feeds from a search. Feeds cannot be restricted for sending an investigator's information on a sole guideline topic of interest.

Other Sources for Guidelines

There are many national and international sources for clinical guidelines. Some of these are governmental sources and, others, such as OpenClinical, are not-for-profit organizations committed to development and dissemination of clinical guidelines. Some of these can be found in the Appendix B.

In addition to national organizations, there are many specialty medical organizations that have developed clinical guidelines. The American Academy of Orthopedic Surgeons, the American Academy of Family Physicians, the American College of Physicians, the Registered Nurses' Association of Ontario (RNAO), and the National Comprehensive Cancer Network are a few examples of hundreds of such websites. Furthermore, universities, health care organizations, and institutes can all produce guidelines.

There are other sources of evidence-based care summaries that provide best practice information, which guides practice. The CINAHL Plus evidence system (http://www.ebscohost.com/biomedical-libraries/cinahl-plus) provides a valuable tool for locating summaries for various conditions with references to published studies and other supporting evidence. This database provides indexing for approximately 3,802 journals and contains over 300 evidence-based care sheets, which can be used in the development of clinical guidelines (Washington University in St. Louis School of Medicine, 2010). The Joanna Briggs Institute's website provides best practice sheets accompanying systematic reviews (www.joannabriggs.edu.au). The Cochrane Library (http://www.cochrane.org/) can be used to locate high-quality, independent evidence for informing decisions in the clinical arena. This database provides resources such as systematic reviews, abstracts, economic evaluations, as well as individual clinical trials, which can be used for the development of CPGs.

Searching for Guidelines in Databases

It is possible to search for and/or narrow search results to guidelines in some databases. Below are a few tips for locating guidelines in CINAHL (*EBSCOhost*) and MEDLINE (*U.S. National Library of Medicine*) databases: two major systematic review resources that are of value for nursing.

For CINAHL (on EBSCOhost search retrieval system), use the advanced search option. Opt for subject terms such as *practice guidelines, decision support systems*, and *clinical* to locate guidelines and combine those results with results from a topic search. Another alternative is after performing a search in CINAHL on a topic, use the CINAHL limits feature in the area labeled "Refine your results" to narrow search results to the publication type: *practice guidelines*.

Using MEDLINE, the publication type format terms: *practice guideline, consensus development conference* and *consensus development conference, NIH* could be used to focus a search toward retrieving guidelines on a topic. MEDLINE also offers non-publication-type related medical subject headings (MeSH) phrases such as *practice guidelines as topic, consensus development conferences as topic*, and *consensus development conferences, NIH as topic*, which could be employed as part of a search to highlight results mentioning guidelines.

Appraising Guidelines

There has been significant concern over the inherent weakness of many published guidelines. Some studies have shown a lack of documentation of the strength of the recommendations (Newhouse, 2010). In a review of 1,275 recommendations by Hussain, Michel, and Shiffman (2008), strength of recommendations was not included in 52.7% of recommendations or was found to be inaccurate in 6.6% of the recommendations reviewed. Grilli, Magrini, Penna, Mura, and Liberati (2000), as cited in Shiffman et al. (2003), similarly found in their review of 431 published guidelines, 82% did not cite specific criteria that could be used to grade the scientific evidence supporting their recommendations.

Another weakness in guidelines occurs when appropriate methodological standards are not followed. Shaneyfelt, Mayo-Smith, & Rothwangl (1999), as cited in Shiffman et al. (2003), found in their evaluation of 279 guidelines published by various U.S. medical associations in peer reviewed publications that many do not adhere to methodological standards. Grilli et al. (2000), as cited in Shiffman et al. (2003), reported that out of 431 published guidelines reviewed, 87% of those guidelines did not state whether a systematic review was conducted, and 67% did not describe which type of professionals were involved in the development of a given guideline.

Another problem found in translating research into practice is recommendations based on low-level evidence. In an assessment of American College of Cardiology and the American Heart Association guidelines by Tricoci, Allen, Kramer, Califf, & Smith (2009), 48% of the 2,711 recommendations made (compiled from 16 guidelines where levels of evidence were reported) were based on level C evidence. Level C evidence is evidence that is composed via consensus of expert opinion, case studies, or standards of care (Buie, 2010). Although the value of expert opinion is acknowledged as a key component of evidence-based practice, the accompanying confidence in the recommendation is limited.

It is clear that the quality of clinical guidelines can vary considerably. It is critical that guidelines be critically appraised prior to adoption. Chou (2008) provides an efficient, straightforward approach for the clinician to use in reviewing guidelines. Five questions need to be answered in the appraisal:

- Were all relevant perspectives considered when developing the guidelines?
- Are potential conflicts of interests adequately described?
- Are the guidelines current?
- Were appropriate methods used to synthesize evidence?
- Were appropriate methods used to grade strength of recommendations?

More detailed appraisal instruments are available. Two commonly used ones include the Appraisal of Guidelines Research and Evaluation (AGREE) instrument and the Conference on Guideline Standardization (COGS) checklist.

The AGREE instrument can be used to appraise new, existing, or updated guidelines. This instrument can be used by a team of reviewers to calculate domain scores, which would ultimately represent the quality of the CPGs. These domains include *scope and purpose* (overall aim of the guideline, the specific clinical questions, and the target patient population); *stakeholder involvement* (extent to which the guideline represents the views of its intended users); *rigor of development* (process used to gather and synthesize the evidence); the methods to formulate the recommendations and to update them, *clarity and presentation* (language and format of the guideline); *applicability* (organizational, behavioral, and cost implications of applying the guideline); and *editorial independence* (independence of the recommendations and acknowledgement of possible conflicts of interest from the guideline developers; The AGREE Collaboration, 2001). Visit the AGREE Collaboration website (http://www.agreecollaboration.org).

The COGS checklist emerged from a 2002 conference convened to define standards for guideline reporting and implementation of CPGs (Shiffman et al., 2003). The 18 topics listed in the COGS checklist serve to specify the nature of the information that should be included in a given CPG but does not specify the specific content that should be in the guideline. An overarching goal of the checklist, according to Shiffman et al. (2003), is to supply the components necessary to be used in evaluating the validity and ultimate usability of a CPG. Table 13.6 provides an overview of the essential elements of a clinical guideline.

How to Implement Guidelines

Over the course of this chapter and in the text thus far, the benefits of effectively translating the best available evidence into practice and the role of CPGs to that end have been highlighted. Unfortunately, the development of high-quality CPGs do not ensure their use in practice. The goal of this portion of the chapter is to identify effective ways in which health care organizations and individual practitioners can effectively implement CPG in their practices, as well as to present methods of disseminating and implementing CPG that have been shown by the literature to be effective.

There is no single way to ensure the use of guidelines in practice; organizations and policy makers should use multidimensional approaches to implement

TABLE 13.6

Outline for Reporting Clinical Guidelines

Discuss the clinical focus of the guideline (e.g., Heart Failure).

Describe the clinical setting where the guideline is suggested for use.

Explain goals and outcomes to be achieved by using the guideline.

Describe the target patient population. Describe any exclusion criteria.

Identify any funding sources or interested parties used when developing the guidelines.

Disclose any conflict of interest.

Provide a description of the methods used to gather, appraise, and synthesize the evidence used in the development of the guideline.

Explain data analysis methods (e.g., meta-analysis, narrative summary, evidence tables).

Relate how the guideline was evaluated (e.g., using a panel of experts).

Describe the plan for review and update of the guideline.

Discuss the anticipated benefits and any potential harm.

Describe anticipated benefits, potential risks, any barriers associated with implementation.

Describe the role of patient preferences.

Provide references.

Suggest audit criteria for performance improvement evaluations.

Source: Based on Shiffman et al. (2003).

guidelines (Feder, Eccles, Grol, Griffiths, & Grimshaw, 1999). Familiarity with the theoretical basis of changing behavior among health care professionals as well as the observed evidence surrounding the efficacy of various implementation approaches must be considered in translating CPGs into practice. Various organizational strategies have been identified for overcoming barriers for effectively implementing CPG. The strategy used is dependent on a keen knowledge of the given organization, whether there are barriers related to the health care professional's knowledge, whether the given group of professionals is aware of suboptimal practice, and whether the barriers are related to the existing routines and culture of a given group of professionals or are seen more with the processing of information within consultations (Feder et al., 1999).

Various theories have been put forth by the behavioral and social science communities to help guide policy makers and key stakeholders to most effectively implement change, in general, and, in particular, change in clinical practice. Implementation research, as it has been coined, "consists of the scientific investigation that supports movement of evidence-based, effective health care approaches (e.g., as embodied in guidelines) from the clinical knowledge base into routine use . . . implementation science consists of a body of knowledge on methods to promote systematic uptake of new or underused scientific findings into usual activities of regional and national care and community organizations" (Rubenstein & Pugh, 2006, p. S58). In other words, implementation science as it is applied to the dissemination and implementation of CPGs is the science of translating evidence-based best practices from their *published* form to the point of care.

A systematic review conducted in Canada by Davis and Taylor-Vaisey (1997) examining the adoption of CPGs, showed mixed efficacy of several potential change initiatives for improving implementation of CPGs. Intervention strategies, which were shown to be weak, included didactic, traditional continuing medical education and mailings. Audit and feedback (especially when done concurrently) was found to be moderately effective when delivered by peers or opinion leaders. The findings reminder systems, academic detailing (face-to-face education of a clinician regarding treatments—their consistency with evidence, support of patient safety, and cost), and multiple interventions, in general, were found to be relatively strong by the authors of this review.

An overview of 41 systematic reviews by Michie and Johnston (2004) found that approaches, which showed the most promise, used several interventions including audit and feedback, reminders, and educational outreach. In other words, no clear single approach or strategy has been shown to work best in all situations, and a multifaceted approach may be most effective. That said, one single intervention, which is inexpensive and relatively simple, has been demonstrated to be effective in increasing the use of CPGs—rewording (Michie & Johnston, 2004). Research has shown that using concrete statements increased the extent to which information was understood (Ley, 1988). In a study conducted in Great Britain of 10 national clinical guidelines, physicians followed guidelines 36% of the time when they were vague and not particularly specific. This number increased to 67 % when guidelines were both concrete and precise (Grol et al., 1998). Part of any evaluation and reevaluation of current CPGs should include an in-depth review of the language used in the guideline in an attempt to produce a guideline that is as concise and concrete as possible. Without this, CPGs run the risk of being ignored if they are too vague. Rewriting guidelines at various intervals may be a simple and hopefully effective way to increase implementation of CPGs.

Moulding, Silagy, and Weller (1999) identified eight key theoretical concepts for encouraging and maintaining guideline adoption. The importance of one of their concepts, "environmental support is crucial to the initiation and maintenance of change," should not be minimized. Even if health care providers are aware of the evidence and are willing to implement recommendations from CPGs into their practice, they will not be able to if the environment (practical, political, ethical, and litigious) is not amenable to change. In other words, policy makers must continue to evaluate not only incentives for implementation, but also an examination of the tools readily available.

The goal of all these implementation strategies discussed remains the same—to decrease the gap between what researchers have shown to be best practices (based on a critical review of all available research) and the care that clients receive. This has implications most importantly, not only for increasing the safety and efficacy of interventions, but also toward providing care that is cost effective.

It is an unfortunate reality that far too many clients do not receive appropriate care, or receive care that is unnecessary, or in worst cases, unsafe. Systematic reviews play an important role in linking high quality, critically appraised evidence with recommendations in the form of CPGs.

SUMMARY

This chapter defined CPGs and described the various types of guidelines available. Approaches to the leveling of evidence and determination of strength of recommendations were provided. Strategies for locating guidelines were given as well as methods for critically appraising CPGs were summarized. Basic tenets for implementing guidelines into practice were reviewed.

EXERCISES

Review the presentation: *The GRADE approach and Summary of Findings Tables—and Introduction* by Dr. Schünemann. Available at: http://www.gradeworkinggroup.org/toolbox/index.htm

REFERENCES

Agency for Healthcare Research and Quality. (2010). *U.S. Department of Health & Human Services. National Guideline Clearing House.* Retrieved from http://www.guideline.gov

The AGREE Collaboration. (2001). Appraisal of Guidelines for Research & Evaluation (AGREE) Instrument. London, UK: St George's Hospital Medical School.

Alpert, J. S. (2010). Why are we ignoring guideline recommendations? *American Journal of Medicine, 123*(2), 97–98.

Buie, W. D. (2010). Clinical practice guidelines: Appraising the evidence. *Diseases of the Colon and Rectum, 53*(8), 1107–1109.

Chou, R. (2008). Using evidence in pain practice: Part 1: Assessing quality of systematic reviews and clinical practice guidelines. *Pain Medicine, 9*(5), 518–530.

Coleman, K., Norris, S., Weston, A., Grimmer-Somers, K., Hillier, S., Merlin, T., . . . Salisbury, J. (2009). NHMRC additional levels of evidence and grades for recommendations for developers of guidelines: Stage 2 consultation. *National Health and Research Council.* Retrieved from http://www.nhmrc.gov.au/_files_nhmrc/file/guidelines/Stage%202%20Consultation%20Levels%20and%20Grades.pdf

The Commonwealth Fund Commission on a High Performance Health System. (2008). *Why not the best? Results from the national scorecard on U.S. health system performance, 2008.* Retrieved from http://www.commonwealthfund.org/content/publications/fund-reports/2008/Jul/Why-not-the-best-results-from-the-national-scorecard-on-U-S-Health-System-Performance-2008.aspx#/

Davis, D. A., & Taylor-Vaisey, A. (1997). Translating guidelines into practice. A systematic review of theoretic concepts, practical experience and research evidence in the adoption of clinical practice guidelines. *Canadian Medical Association Journal, 157*(4), 408–416.

Eddy, D. M. (1990). Clinical decision making: From theory to practice. Practice policies—what are they? *Journal of the American Medical Association, 263*(6), 877–878, 880.

Elwyn, G., O'Connor, A., Stacey, D., Volk, R., Edwards, A., Coulter, A., . . . Whelan, T. (2006). Developing a quality criteria framework for patient decision aids: Online international Delphi consensus process. *British Medical Journal, 333*(7565), 417.

Feder, G., Eccles, M., Grol, R., Griffiths, C., & Grimshaw, J. (1999). Clinical guidelines: Using clinical guidelines. *British Medical Journal, 318*(7185), 728–730.

Field, M. J., & Lohr, K. N. (Eds.). (1992). *Guidelines for clinical practice: From development to use.* Washington, DC: National Academy Press.

Grilli, R., Magrini, N., Penna, A., Mura, G., & Liberati, A. (2000). Practice guidelines developed by specialty societies: The need for a critical appraisal. *Lancet, 355*(9198), 103–106.

Grimshaw, J., & Russell, I. (1993a). Achieving health gain through clinical guidelines. I: Developing scientifically valid guidelines. *Quality in Health Care, 2*(4), 243–248.

GRADE Working Group. (2008). Grading of recommendations, assessment development and evaluation. Available at http://www.gradeworkinggroup.org

Grol, R. (2001). Successes and failures in the implementation of evidence-based guidelines for clinical practice. *Medical Care, 39*(8 Suppl 2), II46–II54.

Grol, R., Dalhuijsen, J., Thomas, S., Veld, C., Rutten, G., & Mokkink, H. (1998). Attributes of clinical guidelines that influence use of guidelines in general practice: Observational study. *British Medical Journal, 317*(7162), 858–861.

Gurunluoglu, R., Swanson, J. A., & Haeck, P. C. (2009). Evidence-based patient safety advisory: Malignant hyperthermia. *Plastic and Reconstructive Surgery, 124*(4 Suppl), 68S–81S.

Guyatt, G. H., Oxman, A. D., Kunz, R., Falck-Ytter, Y., Vist, G. E., Liberati, A., & Schünemann, H. J. (2008a). Going from evidence to recommendations. *British Medical Journal, 336*(7652), 1049–1051.

Guyatt, G. H., Oxman, A. D., Vist, G. E., Kunz, R., Falck-Ytter, Y., Alonso-Coello, P., & Schünemann, H. J. (2008b). GRADE: An emerging consensus on rating quality of evidence and strength of recommendations. *British Medical Journal, 336*(7650), 924–926.

Hoffman, T., Bennett, S., Del Mar, C. (2010). Introduction to evidence based practice. In T. Hoffman, S. Bennett, & C. Del Mar (Eds.), *Evidence Based Practice Across the Health Professions* (pp. 1–15). Sydney: Elsevier.

Hussain, T., Michel, G., & Shiffman, R. N. (2008). How often is strength of recommendation indicated in guidelines? Analysis of the Yale Guideline Recommendation Corpus. *American Medical Informatics Association Annual Symposium Proceedings*, 984.

The Joanna Briggs Institute. (2008). Levels of evidence FAME. Retrieved from: http://www.joannabriggs.edu.au

Kavanagh, B. (2009). The GRADE system for rating clinical guidelines. *PLoSMED, 6*(9), e1000094

Ley, P. (1988). *Communicating with patients: Improving communication, satisfaction, and compliance.* London, UK: Croom Helm.

The Malignant Hypertension Association of the United States. (2010). Medical professionals frequently asked questions—dantrolene. Retrieved from http://medical.mhaus.org/index.cfm/fuseaction/Content.Display/PagePK/MedicalFAQs.cfm

Manchikanti, L. (2008). Evidence-based medicine, systematic reviews, and guidelines in interventional pain management, part I: Introduction and general considerations. *Pain Physician, 11*(2), 161–186.

Michie, S., & Johnston, M. (2004). Changing clinical behaviour by making guidelines specific. *British Medical Journal, 328*(7435), 343–345.

Moulding, N. T., Silagy, C. A., & Weller, D. P. (1999). A framework for effective management of change in clinical practice: Dissemination and implementation of clinical practice guidelines. *Quality in Health Care, 8*(3), 177–183.

National Institute for Health and Clinical Excellence. (2010). *Aim of clinical guidelines.* Retrieved from http://guidance.nice.org.uk/CG

Newhouse, R. P. (2010). Clinical guidelines for nursing practice: Are we there yet? *Journal of Nursing Administration, 40*(2), 57–59.

Rubenstein, L. V., & Pugh, J. (2006). Strategies for promoting organizational and practice change by advancing implementation research. *Journal of General Internal Medicine, 21*(Suppl 2), S58–S64.

Schünemann, H., & Santesso, N. (2010). The GRADE approach to summarizing findings (Video). Available at: http://www.gradeworkinggroup.org/toolbox/index.htm

Schuster, M. A., McGlynn, E. A., & Brook, R. H. (1998). How good is the quality of health care in the United States? *Milbank Quarterly, 76*(4), 517–563, 509.

Shaneyfelt, T. M., Mayo-Smith, M. F., & Rothwangl, J. (1999). Are guidelines following guidelines? The methodological quality of clinical practice guidelines in the peer-reviewed medical literature. *Journal of the American Medical Association, 281*(20), 1900–1905.

Shiffman, R. N., Shekelle, P., Overhage, J. M., Slutsky, J., Grimshaw, J., & Deshpande, A. M. (2003). Standardized reporting of clinical practice guidelines: A proposal from the Conference on Guideline Standardization. *Annals of Internal Medicine, 139*(6), 493–498.

Terracciano, L., Brozek, J., Compalati, E., & Schünemann, H. (2010). GRADE system: New paradigm. *Current Opinion in Allergy and Clinical Immunology, 10*(4), 377–383.

Tricoci, P., Allen, J. M., Kramer, J. M., Califf, R. M., & Smith, S. C., Jr. (2009). Scientific evidence underlying the ACC/AHA clinical practice guidelines. *Journal of the American Medical Association, 301*(8), 831–841.

Turner, T., Misso, M., Harris, C., & Green, S. (2008). Development of evidence-based clinical guidelines (CPGs): Comparing approaches. *Implementation Science, 3,* 45. doi:10.1186/1748-5908-3-45

Washington University in St. Louis School of Medicine. (2010). Assessing the impact of research: Clinical practice guidelines. *Becker Medical Library.* Retrieved from http://www.becker.wustl.edu/impact/assessment/clin/guidelines.html

SUGGESTED READINGS

DI Pietro, T. L., Doran, D. M., & McArthur, G. (2010). Supportive decision making at the point of care: Refinement of a case-based reasoning application for use in nursing practice. *Computers, Informatics, Nursing. 28*(4), 235–240. doi:10.1097/NCN.0b013e3181e1e77a

Grimshaw, J. M., & Russell, I. T. (1993b). Effect of clinical guidelines on medical practice: A systematic review of rigorous evaluations. *Lancet, 342*(8883), 1317–1322.

Shaneyfelt, T. M., & Centor, R. M. (2009). Reassessment of clinical practice guidelines: Go gently into that good night. *Journal of the American Medical Association, 301*(8), 868–869.

Wright, J. G. (2007). A practical guide to assigning levels of evidence. *The Journal of Bone and Joint Surgery. American Volume. 89*(5), 1128–1130.

CHAPTER FOURTEEN

Future Developments of Systematic Reviews and Evidence-Based Medicine*

Jos Kleijnen

Jos Kleijnen is a physician (University of Maastricht, Netherlands) and is specialized as a clinical epidemiologist. Currently, he is director of an independent company, Kleijnen Systematic Reviews Ltd, which prepares systematic reviews and health technology assessments for various commissioners and provides training courses in these areas. Previously, he was professor and director of the Centre for Reviews and Dissemination at the University of York and director of the Dutch Cochrane Centre at the University of Amsterdam. His interests include methodology of patient-related research, health technology assessment, placebo effects, diagnostic and screening procedures, dissemination and implementation of research-based evidence, evidence-based medicine, systematic reviews, and the Cochrane Collaboration.

INTRODUCTION

In this lecture, I would like to address several issues that in my view are relevant or will become relevant in the next few years in the playing field of systematic reviews and evidence-based medicine (EBM). A lot has happened since in 1992, Gordon Guyatt and others at McMaster University in Hamilton, Ontario, Canada, coined the term *evidence-based medicine* (Guyatt, Cairns, & Churchill, 1992). At about the same time, the term *systematic review* appeared, and in fact, there was considerable overlap between the early champions of EBM and those of systematic reviews. The practice of EBM, or broader, evidence-based health care, depends on readily available information, which has been critically appraised and summarized in an easily digestible way.

There have been several factors that have driven the steep rise of EBM and systematic reviews. One of the main factors was the emergence of information technology, which has greatly facilitated access to information for health care professionals and, perhaps, more importantly, for the patients and the public. If doctors can't keep up to date with developments, patients will. Another main factor is the rising costs of health care, being felt in all countries, even the very richest. This has

*This paper is based on the 2007 Joanna Briggs Oration, a biennial event initiated by the Joanna Briggs Institute to serve as an occasion of celebration of the evidence-based health care movement, its accomplishments, and to focus on visioning the future. This discourse brings together health professionals from a diverse range of backgrounds to celebrate achievements and anticipate the further evolution of evidence-based health care in the future.

resulted in rationing of what is covered in health insurance or national health services. Very difficult and often unpopular choices have to be made everywhere, and several countries have established institutes that evaluate effects and cost effectiveness of interventions. Cornerstones in such evaluations are systematic reviews and economic decision analytic models integrating costs and effects.

In epidemiology, medical research in patients is often divided into the areas of etiology, diagnosis, prevention and therapy, and prognosis. I would like to address some recent developments and some future developments relevant to EBM and systematic reviews in each of these areas. I will end with some thoughts about making decisions in the era of EBM.

ETIOLOGY

Although there have been early champions of clinical epidemiology such as Alvan Feinstein and David Sackett who focused on patient care, a lot of what epidemiologist were investigating from the 1950s until very recently was in the domain of etiology (Spitzer, Feinstein, & Sackett, 1975). Major new insights emerged about the etiology of cardiovascular diseases and cancer, and in the areas of hygiene, diet, and nutrition. However, the new concept of systematic reviews was not taken up as readily in etiological epidemiology as it was in clinical epidemiology. Perhaps, the complications of having to deal with observational study designs and problems with meta-analysis of such studies, as opposed to randomized trials, go some way to explaining this slow take-up.

However, in recent years, this has been changing and, in this context, I would like to bring to your attention the efforts of the World Cancer Research Fund (WCRF) in trying to provide an overview of what is known about diet, nutrition, physical activity, and the prevention of cancer. The WCRF has succeeded in bringing together some of the world's leading nutritional and cancer epidemiologists over a period of some seven years and to develop a complete overview of all studies addressing the relationship between our dietary and physical activity habits and the occurrence of cancer. And it did all of this by means of systematic reviews.

At their website, one can read:

> . . . in 2001, WCRF/[American Institute for Cancer Research] AICR set itself a new objective: to systematically review and assess the body of evidence on diet, physical activity, and cancer and to publish a second-expert report. This report is the largest study of its kind, and its conclusions are as definitive as the available evidence allows. The WCRF network is committed to interpreting scientific evidence in this field and has set up a continuous review project to update the report on an ongoing basis.

I highly recommend that you visit their website (http://www.wcrf.org/about_us/index.php#history) and view and download the report.

DIAGNOSIS

Arguably, diagnosis is a field doctors have even more uncertainties about than therapy. Tools to help clinicians interpret the findings of diagnostic test-accuracy studies have been around since the 1980s, but one problem is that the accuracy of diagnosis of a certain state of health or disease is only one element of diagnostic research.

For example, diagnostic research may aim to assess whether a new test finds additional cases on top of those found by an existing test. A lot of testing is also done for monitoring purposes, be it for clinical or for legal reasons. Screening is a special case of using diagnostic tests. Furthermore, diagnostic research may aim to assess whether a new test should replace an existing one; whether a test can play a role as a triage instrument for possible further (invasive) testing; or what the most efficient order is in which multiple tests should be used. Finally, tests may help to decide whether a treatment should be given and, if so, to predict who will respond to treatment and who will get the adverse effects. The latter examples make the link with prognostic research, which essentially could be considered as diagnostic but linked to outcomes after follow-up rather than to a gold standard.

Different diagnostic questions call for different study designs to address them. In addition, diagnosis by nature is a multivariable process, and this should be taken into account in diagnostic research. Evaluations of single tests are rarely clinically useful unless meaningful subgroup analyses are possible. Diagnostic research is, thus, complicated, and systematic reviews of diagnostic research are not for the fainthearted. In general, it is recommended to get a methodologist with experience in diagnostic research on board of any team trying to prepare a diagnostic systematic review. The Cochrane Collaboration is in the process of putting such support in place.

The Cochrane Diagnostic Test Accuracy Working Group was constituted to develop and implement reviews of diagnostic test accuracy within the Cochrane Collaboration. To be able to give authors and review groups all the support they may need, four regional support units are to be created. Two of these are already active: the UK Support Unit (UKSU) and the Continental Europe Support Unit (CESU). In October 2007, during the colloquium in São Paulo, the implementation of systematic reviews of diagnostic test accuracy was officially launched. The new version of Review Manager, RevMan 5, will allow the preparation of reviews of diagnostic accuracy studies. In addition, a *Cochrane Handbook for Diagnostic Test Accuracy Reviews* is being developed. The working group members are doing their best to get all processes ready as soon as possible and will keep everyone *up to date* through the following website: http://srdta.cochrane.org

Diagnostic systematic reviews will remain in high demand.

PROGNOSIS

I have already mentioned when talking about diagnosis that what doctors, patients, and fourth-hurdle institutes such as the National Institute for Health and Clinical Excellence (NICE) in the United Kingdom ideally want to know is to predict who will respond to treatment and who will get the adverse effects. NICE recently approved two drugs for the National Health Service (NHS) under a deal with the drug company that the NHS will pay the drug bill for responders and the company will pay for the patients who do not respond. In genetic research, investigators are aiming for similar goals.

However, it currently is extremely difficult to do meaningful subgroup analyses in systematic reviews; ideally, one would need the individual patients' data to be able to do such analyses. In the long run, we also need new guidance about subgroup analyses both in primary studies and in systematic reviews, because these will become increasingly important in answering the questions of the previous paragraph. Current guidance from methodologists and statisticians about subgroup analyses is in my view, similar to treating symptoms instead of the underlying disease.

Imagine the following ideal situation: We have resolved the issue of selective reporting of outcomes in randomized trials; for all trials, there is a registry with their protocols, and it has become mandatory for authors to make the findings for all outcomes and all subgroups evaluated and available in the public domain. Furthermore, we do not make our inferences based on an arbitrary p value at the cutoff of $p < .05$ anymore. Instead, results are reported as point estimates with 95% confidence intervals, and readers of medical research have undergone a mandatory course about Bayesian inference. In this course, they have learned to express their prior belief about hypotheses to be investigated as a percentage with a *credibility interval* (similar to a confidence interval); they have also learned to change their prior belief to a posterior belief after having seen the study results for each subgroup. Silly examples of star signs significantly related to an outcome will be swiftly dealt with in such an ideal situation, because for most readers, their prior belief will be so low that the findings of a single study will not change their posterior belief to a level that has any consequence. With accumulating evidence, true effects will, in due time, lead to similar posterior beliefs among most health care professionals. We will also have gotten rid of the silly effect of current guidance about subgroup analyses, which pretends that data are somehow truer when a hypothesis has been defined in advance than they are with a post-hoc hypothesis. The data are exactly the same in both situations.

PREVENTATIVE AND THERAPEUTIC INTERVENTIONS

Systematic reviews of preventative and therapeutic interventions have undergone a great development to the good side in the past 20 years. They are becoming higher quality pieces of research, and recommendations from systematic reviews may also have had an impact on the quality of primary research.

However, developments will also continue in this area. One development will be that we will pay even more attention to head-to-head comparisons of different treatment alternatives. Fourth-hurdle institutes such as NICE base their conclusions on such comparisons, whether a new drug is better than placebo when an effective other treatment is available, is of limited importance. I predict that even the Food and Drug Administration (FDA) in the United States, in the near future, will be permitted by Congress to demand head-to-head comparisons with existing effective treatments before licensing a new drug. It is unethical, anyway, to do a placebo-controlled trial when an effective treatment is available, isn't it?

Another development will be a more differentiated approach to the inclusion criteria concerning study design in systematic reviews. We will see fewer reviews that just include randomized trials; instead, we will see separate inclusion criteria for addressing different outcomes. For example, in a systematic review of an analgesic, randomized (and double blinded) trials will be demanded to assess the effects on pain, and controlled observational studies will be demanded to address rare but important (adverse) effects. Qualitative studies might be included to clarify reasons for noncompliance.

Attention to adverse effects will become much more prominent. Different study designs may be needed for different questions. For the early recognition of rare but important adverse effects, case reports will be the means of identification. Controlled observational studies such as case-control studies will confirm or refute suspicions raised by case reports. Cohort studies and, sometimes (meta-analyses of) randomized trials will allow a precise estimate of harm.

We will move further away from surrogate outcomes and go toward outcomes relevant to patients and reported by patients. Deveraux and colleagues showed in the *British Medical Journal* (BMJ; 2001, 24 November) that patients and physicians may have very different perceptions about the importance of certain outcomes, as demonstrated by different judgments about serious bleedings, as opposed to having a stroke. In addition, fourth-hurdle institutes are instrumental in setting the scene; they tend to insist on patient-relevant outcomes and, by doing that, are most likely influencing the research stakeholders planning to support their claims.

DECISION MAKING

I am determined that no matter how much I trust my treating doctors, I want to be assured that the decisions we make together are based on as much evidence as is in existence at the time. I believe that is my fundamental right, and a right of others in a similar situation.

The challenge I face in getting the evidence I need to make informed decisions is almost overwhelming.

I also believe it is my right to determine the value that I place on different outcomes, to express my own treatment preferences (and have these taken into account), and to feel that my treating doctors are prepared to respect my experiences as a valid and important input when we come to make decisions.

—*Chris Silagy (1999)*

I find these quotes by Chris Silagy very powerful, and I thank one of the champions of consumer input into research, Gill Gyte, for drawing my attention to them.

On the individual level, priorities, needs, values, and preferences come into play; on the organizational and national level, costs, resources, equity, and innovation are other factors that may come into the decision-making process on top of those of the individual level. Interplay between the patients and the health care professional is crucial, and the professional should be conscious of the possibility that a patient's values and preferences may be very different from their own, as shown by Deveraux and collegaues.

Barriers to getting the evidence needed for decision making are slowly being discovered and addressed, and information needed is increasingly becoming available. In fact, the broader area of knowledge transfer between basic and clinical research on one hand and between clinical research and practice on the other hand, is being better recognized as crucially important; for example, in the United Kingdom, The Medical Research Council (MRC) and the National Institute for Health Research (NIHR) have announced a new joint arrangement for clinical trials. The initiative forms a key part of the developing MRC–NIHR joint strategy for translational research. Its aims include clinical trials and evaluative studies that add significantly to the understanding of biological or behavioral mechanisms and processes, exploring new scientific or clinical principles, evaluating clinical efficacy of interventions where proof of concept in humans has already been achieved, and the development or testing of new methodologies. The new strategy will ensure that promising technologies are carried from the efficacy and safety stage through to being assessed for clinical and cost effectiveness, and then to the NHS. The Cochrane Effective Practice and Organization of Care group provides systematic reviews of the evidence concerning "getting evidence into practice."

Evidence is increasingly used and made a mandatory component of health care decision making around the world. In Germany, EBM has been written into law, and in Brazil, a law was passed (11.108/05) stipulating the right for women in labor to have an accompanying person with them based on a systematic review.

SUMMARY

Systematic reviews are currently being used in all areas of patient-based research: etiology, diagnosis, prevention and therapy, and prognosis.

Diagnostic research is complicated and, when preparing systematic reviews of diagnostic research, it is recommended to get help from a methodologist with experience in diagnostic research. Diagnostic systematic reviews will be in high demand.

Prognostic research will focus on finding out who will respond to treatment and who will get the adverse effects. Guidance about subgroup analyses will need to be rewritten.

Preventative and therapeutic reviews will focus more on head-to-head comparisons, address adverse effects, and consider a range of study designs addressing different aspects of systematic reviews. Emphasis will shift further to patient-relevant and patient-reported outcomes.

Priorities, needs, values, preferences, costs, resources, equity, and innovation are all factors that are part of decision making, in addition to the evidence of effects. Different parties may well have different views about several of these factors.

Barriers to knowledge transfer are being investigated, and EBM is becoming part of the law.

REFERENCES

Devereaux, P. J., Anderson, D. R., Gardner, M. J., Putnam, W., Flowerdew, G. J., Brownell, B. F., . . . Cox, J. L. (2001). Differences between perspectives of physicians and patients on anticoagulation in patients with atrial fibrillation: observational study. *British Medical Journal, 323*(7323), 1218–1222.

Guyatt, G., Cairns, J., & Churchill, D. (1992). Evidence-based medicine. A new approach to teaching the practice of medicine. *Journal of the American Medical Association, 268*, 2420–2425.

Silagy, C. (1999). Introduction to the new edition: The post-Cochrane agenda: consumers and evidence. In A. L. Cochrane, *Effectiveness and efficiency: Random reflections on health services* (pp. xix–xxx and xxvii). London: Royal Society of Medicine Press Ltd.

Spitzer, W. O., Feinstein, A. R., & Sackett, D. L. (1975). What is a health care trial? *Journal of the American Medical Association, 233*(2), 161–163.

A Toolkit for Systematic Review

This appendix provides a compilation of useful resources for conducting a systematic review. The resources provided here are neither all inclusive, nor are they meant to be. These are selected resources that have proved useful in the authors' work in conducting and in teaching systematic review. Most of these resources have been referred to throughout this book and are presented here for easy access.

SYSTEMATIC REVIEW TOOLKIT

General Systematic Review Resources

Select Resources Including Systematic Reviews

The Campbell Collaboration (C2)
- http://www.campbellcollaboration.org

The Cochrane Collaboration
- http://www.cochrane.org/index.htm

The Joanna Briggs Institute of Evidence-Based Nursing and Midwifery
- http://www.joannabriggs.edu.au/about/home.php

PubMed Special Queries—Search for Systematic Reviews
- http://www.ncbi.nlm.nih.gov/entrez/query/static/clinical.shtml

Systematic Reviews
- http://www.york.ac.uk/inst/crd/index.htm

Resources Used to Guide Steps in Constructing a Systematic Review

Writing a Foreground Clinical Question

Asking the Right Question
- http://www.nottingham.ac.uk/toolkits/play_1067

The Well-Built Clinical Question
- http://www.hsl.unc.edu/services/tutorials/EBM/Question.htm

Writing the Proposal

Campbell Collaboration Guidelines and Protocols
- Offers guidelines at http://www.campbellcollaboration.org/guidelines.asp
- Offers protocols at http://www.campbellcollaboration.org/ECG/proto.asp

The Cochrane Collaboration: Handbook for Systematic Reviews of Interventions of Effectiveness
- http://www.cochrane.org

The Joanna Briggs Institute
- http://www.joannabriggs.edu.au

General Statistics (may be reported for more than one question domain)

Confidence Intervals
- http://www.nottingham.ac.uk/nmp/sonet/rlos/ebp/confidence_intervals/index.html

Probability
- http://www.nottingham.ac.uk/nmp/sonet/rlos/statistics/probability/index.html

Sensitivity and Specificity
- http://www.nottingham.ac.uk/nmp/sonet/rlos/ebp/sensitivity_specificity/

Clinically Significant Statistics per Question Domain/Type

Numbers Needed to Treat
- http://www.nottingham.ac.uk/nmp/sonet/rlos/ebp/nnt_nnh/

Numbers Needed to Treat and Numbers Needed to Harm
- http://www.nottingham.ac.uk/nmp/sonet/rlos/ebp/nnt_nnh/

Identifying and Learning About Study Designs

Cohort and Case-Control Studies
- http://www.nottingham.ac.uk/toolkits/play_1083

How to Conduct a Meta-Analysis
- http://www.pitt.edu/~super1/lecture/lec1171/index.htm

Meta-Analysis Research Methodology
- http://www.wilderdom.com/research/meta-analysis

Nursing Research Series
- http://www.nursingpathways.kp.org/scal/research/resources/researchseries/index.html

What Is Research?
- http://www.linguistics.byu.edu/faculty/henrichsenl/researchmethods/RM_1_01.html

Qualitative Research Methods

- http://www.wilderdom.com/qualitative.html

Constructing Search Strategies

- http://www.lib.monash.edu.au/vl/sstrat/sstrcon.htm
- http://www.lib.utk.edu/instruction/learnhow/searchstrategy.html
- http://www.nlm.nih.gov/bsd/disted/pubmedtutorial/020_020.html

Searching Online Bibliographic Databases

- http://www.uic.edu/classes/bhis/bhis510/lim3/orgknow.htm

Searching for Grey Literature

Grey Literature
- http://www.scirus.com
GreyNet
- http://www.greynet.org/
For an annotated, more extensive listing of Grey Literature resources see Appendix C.

Searching for Health Policies

Agency for Healthcare Research and Quality
- http://www.ahrq.gov
Georgetown University Health Policy Institute
- http://www.ihcrp.georgetown.edu/

Search Citation Management Tools (Check with your health care or academic institution for availability before purchasing personal subscriptions)

Citeulike
- http://www.citeulike.org
EndNote
- http://www.endnote.com
RefWorks
- http://www.refworks.com

Critical Appraisal Tools for Individual Studies for Systematic Reviews

Critical Appraisal Checklists
- http://www.ebbp.org/appraisal.html
- http://www.phru.nhs.uk/Pages/PHD/resources.htm
Critical Appraisal Tools
- http://www.unisa.edu.au/cahe/CAHECATS
Why Is Appraisal Necessary?
- http://www.nottingham.ac.uk/nmp/sonet/rlos/ebp/research_critique/index.html

Analysis and Synthesis Tools for Individual Studies for Systematic Reviews

Database Tutorials: A Step-by-Step Guide to Using Databases
- http://www.geekgirls.com/menu_databases.htm

Determining the Importance of Clinical Trial Results
- http://www.nottingham.ac.uk/nmp/sonet/rlos/ebp/trial_results/

Meta-Analysis Software

- http://www.meta-analysis.com
- Comprehensive meta-analysis (commercial software; product endorsement is not intended)

Tutorials on Databases, Spreadsheets, and Excel for Statistics
- www.ats.ucla.edu/stat/spss

Resources for Learning and Using Statistical Package for Social Sciences
- http://www.distdell4.ad.stat.tamu.edu/spss_1/DescriptiveStatsSPSS.html

Metasynthesis Software

- http://www.qsrinternational.com/#tab_you
- NIVO (commercial software; product endorsement is not intended)

Resources for Displaying Data

Creating Graphs
- http://www.nces.ed.gov/nceskids/graphing/classic

Writing General Review Links

Writing a Literature Review
- http://www.unc.edu/depts/wcweb/handouts/literature_review.html#4

Writing Systematic Review Background/Significance Section

Agency for Healthcare Research and Quality
- http://www.ahrq.gov

Health Research Projects in Progress
- http://wwwcf.nlm.nih.gov/hsr_project/home_proj.cfm

Health Services/Technology Assessment Text
- http://www.ncbi.nlm.nih.gov/books/bv.fcgi?rid=hstat

Health Technology Assessment Database
- http://www.york.ac.uk/inst/crd/htadbase.htm

National Institutes of Health
- http://www.nih.gov

Office of Health Care Statistics
- http://hlunix.ex.state.ut.us/hda/

U.S. National Library of Medicine
- http://www.nlm.nih.gov

Resources for Systematic Review Application in Practice

Knowledge Translation

Cochrane Nursing Care Field
- http://cncf.cochrane.org/home

Evidence-Based Decision Making
- http://www.health-evidence.ca/

Evidenced-Based Practice
- http://hsl.lib.umn.edu/learn/ebp/mod01/index.html

Knowledge Translation Clearinghouse
- http://ktclearinghouse.ca/cebm/resources/web

Open Access Journal on Translational Science
- http://www.implementationscience.com/

Translating Knowledge to Practice
- http://www.cihr-irsc.gc.ca/e/29529.html

Prefiltered Best Evidence Resources

Systematic Review Portals

The Campbell Collaboration (C2)
- http://www.campbellcollaboration.org

The Cochrane Collaboration
- http://www.cochrane.org/index.htm

The Joanna Briggs Institute of Evidence-Based Nursing and Midwifery
- http://www.joannabriggs.edu.au/about/home.php

Guideline Resources

National Guideline Clearinghouse
- http://www.guideline.gov/

National Institutes for Health and Clinical Excellence (NICE) Clinical Guidelines
- http://guidance.nice.org.uk/CG
- http://www.gin.net/index.cfm?fuseaction=membersarea&fusesubaction=docs&documentID=33

New York State Department of Health
- http://www.health.state.ny.us/professionals/protocols_and_guidelines/

Registered Nurses of Ontario: Implementation of Clinical Practice Guidelines
- http://www.rnao.org/Page.asp?PageID=924&ContentID=823

U.S. Preventive Services Task Force
- http://www.uspreventiveservicestaskforce.org/recommendations.html

For an annotated, more extensive listing of Guideline resources see Appendix B.

Organization Resources

Academy of Medical-Surgical Nurses
- http://amsn.inurse.com

Agency for Healthcare Research and Quality
- http://www.ahrq.gov

Agency for Healthcare Research and Quality Indicators
- http://www.qualityindicators.ahrq.gov

American Academy of Ambulatory Care Nursing
- http://www.aaacn.org

American Academy of Nurse Practitioners
- http://www.aanp.org

American Association of Occupational Health Nurses
- http://www.aaohn.org

American Hospital Association
- http://www.aha.org/resource/

American Nurses Association
- http://www.ana.org

American Organization of Nurse Executives
- http://www.aone.org/

American Psychiatric Nurses Association
- http://www.apna.org

Association of Nurses in AIDS Care
- http://www.anacnet.org

Association for Professionals in Infection Control and Epidemiology
- http://www.apic.org

Association of Rehabilitation Nurses
- http://www.rehabnurse.org

Association of Women's Health, Obstetric and Neonatal Nurses
- http://www.awhonn.org

Center for Health Care Ethics
- http://www.chce.org

Centers for Medicare & Medicaid Services
- http://www.cms.gov/medicarereform/

Clinical Reflection
- http://www.nottingham.ac.uk/nmp/sonet/rlos/placs/critical_reflection/

Comparative Health Systems, Services, and Economics
- http://www.lib.umich.edu/libhome/PubHealth.lib/bib/compare.html

Council of States Governments Health Policy Group
- http://www.csg.org/CSG/Policy/health/default.htm

Emergency Nurses Association
- http://www.ena.org

Evidence-Based Decision Making
- http://health-evidence.ca/

Health Resources and Services Administration's Center for Health Services Financing and Managed Care
- http://www.hrsa.gov/financeMC/

Home Health Nurses Association
- http://www.hhna.org

Integrated Health Care Delivery Systems
- http://www.kurtsalmon.com/KSA_library/libraryindex.html

Institute for Healthcare Improvement
- http://www.ihi.org

Institute for Safe Medication Practices
- http://www.ismp.org

Institute of Medicine
- http://www.iom.edu

Joint Commission Annotated Resources for Sentinel Events
- http://www. jointcommission.org

Joint Commission on Accreditation of Healthcare Organizations
- http://www.jointcommission.org/

Legislative Information on the Internet
- http://thomas.loc.gov/

Library of Congress
- http://www.loc.gov

Managed Care Information Center
- http://www.themcic.com

Medscape
- http://www.medscape.com/

National Association of Orthopaedic Nurses
- http://www.orthonurse.org

National Association of Pediatric Nurse Practitioners
- http://www.napnap.org

National Association of School Nurses
- http://www.nasn.org

National Center for Health Statistics
- http://www.cdc.gov/nchs/

National Coalition on Health Care
- http://www.nchc.org

National Conference of State Legislatures
- http://www.ncsl.org/public/ncsl/nav_statefedissues.htm

National Institute of Nursing Research
- http://www.ni-component_of_the_national_institutes_of_health.the_us.h.gov

National Library of Medicine: National Institutes of Health
- http://www.nlm.nih.gov/

National Patient Safety Foundation
- http://www.npsf.org

National Quality Forum
- http://www.qualityforum.org/home.html

National Women's Health Information Center
- http://www.womenshealth.gov/

Nursing Journals—University of Texas Medical Branch
- http://www.son.utmb.edu/catalog/catalog.htm

Pan American Health Organization
- http://www.paho.org/

Reference Desk/Health and Medicine
- http://www.refdesk.com/health.html

Statistical Abstracts of the United States
- http://www.census.gov/compendia/statab/

U.S. Agency for International Development, Population, Health, and Nutrition Links
- http://www.info.usaid.gov/pop_health/

U.S. Department of Health and Human Services
- http://www.hhs.gov/

University of Wisconsin Extension: Health Policy Information Updates
- http://www.uwex.edu/ces/flp/health/updates.html

World Health Organization
- http://www.who.ch/

Resources for Systematic Review in Health Policy

Agency for Healthcare Research and Quality
- http://www.ahrq.gov

Alliance for Health Policy and Systems Research
- http://www.who.int/alliance-hpsr/en/

American Association of Retired Persons
- http://www.aarp.org

American Enterprise Institute
- http://www.aei.org

Brookings Institution
- http://www.brookings.edu

Canadian Health Services Research Foundation
- http://www.chsrf.ca/home.aspx

Changing Professional Practice (Edited by: Thorsen, T., Mäkelä, M.) Copenhagen:
Cochrane Consumers and Communication Review Group Resource Bank
- http://www.latrobe.edu.au/chcp/cochrane/resourcebank/index.html

Cochrane Effective Practice and Organization of Care (EPOC) Review Group
- http://www.epoc.cochrane.org/en/index.html

The Commonwealth Fund
- http://www.commonwealthfund.org

Evidence-Informed Policy Network
- http://www.who.int/rpc/evipnet/en/
- http://evipnet.bvsalud.org/php/index.php

Finding and Applying for Grants
- http://www.grants.gov

The Henry J. Kaiser Family Foundation
- http://www.kff.org

The Heritage Foundation
- http://www.heritage.org

National Association of State Units on Aging and Disabilities
- http://www.nasuad.org

National Health Policy Forum
- http://www.nhpf.org

New Jersey Department of Health and Senior Services
- http://www.state.nj.us/health

Program in Policy Decision-Making/Canadian Cochrane Network and Centre Database
- http://www.researchtopolicy.ca/search/reviews.aspx

PubMed Health Services Research Queries
- http://www.nlm.nih.gov/nichsr/hedges/search.html

U.K. Government's Policy Hub
- http://www.nationalschool.gov.uk/policyhub/

U.S. Department of Health and Human Services
- http://www.hhs.gov
- http://www.hhs.gov/recovery

Video

Health Care Policy Making Video Case Studies
- http://www.kunnskapssenteret.no/Publikasjoner/469.cms

These video documentaries tell the stories of eight case studies across six continents, where people are trying to improve health systems by using research evidence to inform decision making.

Health Care Policy Making Video Documentaries
- http://www.kunnskapssenteret.no/Artikler/2061.cms

These compelling video documentaries are part of a report on more than 150 organizations that are building bridges between evidence and policy.

Guidelines Sources

East Kent Hospitals University National Health Service (NHS) Foundation Trust
- http://www.ekhut.nhs.uk/home-page/for-staff/a-z-departments/clinical-quality-patient-safety/nurse-practice-development/nursing-guidelines-and-policies/

Institute for Clinical Systems Improvement (ICSI)
- http://www.icsi.org/
- includes guidelines, order sets, and protocols that affect practice.

McGill University Health Centre, Nursing Research, Clinical and Professional Staff Development Research, and Clinical Resources for Evidence-Based Nursing Guidelines
- http://muhc-ebn.mcgill.ca/guidelines.htm
- This website is an initiative of the McGill University Health Care (MUHC) Department of Nursing, Nursing Research, Academic Practice, and Professional Development, and an example of a library-based guideline page.

National Health Service Clinical Guidelines: Nursing and Midwifery Guidelines
- http://www.clinicalguidelines.scot.nhs.uk/N&M%20Guidelines.htm

National Institute for Health and Clinical Excellence (NICE)
- http://www.nice.org.uk/
- NICE is an independent organization that is responsible for providing health promotion and treatment guidance in the United Kingdom.
- NICE develops guidelines that are focusing on three main areas: public health, technology, and clinical care.

Registered Nurses' Association of Ontario (RNAO) Clinical Practice Guidelines Program
- http://www.rnao.org/
- RNAO, currently, has 40 published guidelines, as well as the *educator's resources* and a *toolkit* that support the incorporation of guidelines into the academic milieu and the implementation of guidelines in clinical areas.
- Clinical practice guidelines and supporting materials such as the educator's resources are available for download on the RNAO website, with numerous materials in both English and French.

Registered Nurses' Association of Ontario (RNAO) Nurse Guideline Network
- http://nursegn.ca/
- This is a website where individuals and organizations share their guideline implementation experiences and related resources. Users can search the network to see the guidelines that the other organizations are implementing, and they can join the groups related to specific guidelines or areas of focus.

Rutgers University Libraries: Subject Research Guides Nursing Clinical Practice Guidelines

- http://www.libraries.rutgers.edu/rul/rr_gateway/research_guides/nursing/clinical.shtml

The Guide to Community Preventive Services

- http://www.thecommunityguide.org/index.html
- Centers for Disease Control and Prevention website offering guides based on evidence on various community health topics from diabetes, obesity, sexually transmitted diseases (STDs), and vaccines.

The National Kidney Foundation Kidney Disease Outcomes Quality Initiative (NKF KDOQI)

- http://www.kidney.org/professionals/kdoqi/guidelines_commentaries.cfm
- The National Kidney Foundation, a major voluntary nonprofit health organization, is dedicated to preventing kidney and urinary tract diseases, improving the health and well-being of individuals and families affected by kidney disease, and increasing the availability of all organs for transplantation.
- NKF KDOQI provides evidence-based clinical practice guidelines for all stages of chronic kidney disease (CKD) and related complications since 1997.

Social Science and Biomedical Science Grey Literature

AcademyHealth
- http://www.academyhealth.org/index.cfm
- This includes links to websites and journals about advancing research toward policy and practice.

American Association of Retired Persons (AARP) Public Policy Institute
- http://www.aarp.org/research/ppi/
- This is a part of AARP's nonprofit and nonpartisan organization.
- This includes information on health issues and policies of importance to adults older than 50 years of age in the United States.

British Education Index
- http://www.leeds.ac.uk/bei/index.html
- This allows search to Education-line grey literature database.
- Includes full-text working papers and conference papers to support education research, policy making, and practice.

Center for Evidence in Ethnicity, Health, and Diversity (CEEHD)
- http://www2.warwick.ac.uk/fac/med/research/csri/ethnicityhealth/

DIRLINE: Directory of Health Organizations and Health Hotlines
- http://dirline.nlm.nih.gov/

Grey Source: A Selection of Web-Based Resources in Grey Literature
- http://www.greynet.org/greysourceindex.html
- Resources are grouped by classifications such as social science and biological/medical science grey literature.

HealthyNJ
- This provides a local and limited national consumer health information useful for lay persons, health professionals, and health policy makers.
- Many states have a similar consumer health product. See New York Online Access to Health (NOAH) at http://www.noah-health.org/.

Kaiser Permanente Institute for Health Policy
- http://www.kpinstituteforhealthpolicy.org/kpihp/default.aspx

MedlinePlus
- http://www.nlm.nih.gov/medlineplus/
- This is a source of consumer health information from the U.S. National Library of Medicine (NLM) and the National Institutes of Health (NIH).
- Updated daily

- This contains trusted sources of more than 570 diseases and conditions.
- It also contains lists of hospitals and physicians, medical encyclopedia and dictionaries, health information in Spanish, extensive information on prescription and nonprescription drugs, health information from the media, and links to thousands of clinical trials.

National Center for Complementary and Alternative Medicine (NCCAM)
- http://nccam.nih.gov/
- One of the 27 institutes and centers that make up the NIH.
- NCCAM supports rigorous research on complementary and alternative medicine (CAM), trains researchers in CAM, and disseminates information to the public.
- NCCAM publications are high quality and follow the rules of scientific inquiry.

OAIster
- http://oaister.org/
- Used in locating grey literature worldwide in various formats such as books, statistics datasets, theses, and video/audio files.

OpenSIGLE: System for Information on Grey Literature in Europe
- http://opensigle.inist.fr/

Partners in Information Access for the Public Health Workforce
- http://phpartners.org/guide.html
- This contains government, public health organizations, and health science libraries' pool of links in public health.

Research and Development (RAND) Corporation
- http://www.rand.org/
- This is a nonprofit and a nonpartisan institution that started in 1940s.
- This contains objective reports, including review of public policy that can impact health, and social and economic policies.

SCIRUS
- http://www.scirus.com/srsapp/
- This is a free resource that can assist in locating scientific information for various topics in many formats.
- This includes traditional as well as grey literature search results.

Virtual Health Library
- http://regional.bvsalud.org/php/index.php?lang=en
- This allows search of LILACS, the Latin American and Caribbean Health Science Literature database and other portals that may contain grey literature.

WorldCat
- http://www.worldcat.org/
- This includes information of holdings of many libraries worldwide.
- Use WorldCat's advanced search feature to search for the term *grey literature* and choose "Limit Results by Internet Resource" to see a list of more than 1,800 entries on grey literature.

World Health Organization
- http://www.who.int/about/en/
- This contains information on health statistics, health topics, and health policies.

APPENDIX D

Dissertations and Theses Databases

Agence Bibliographique de l'Enseignement Supérieur
- http://www.abes.fr/abes/DesktopDefault.aspx?Loupe=Moin
- Resource from France.

Australasian Digital Theses Program
- http://adt.caul.edu.au

Center for Research Libraries Foreign Dissertations
- http://www-apps.crl.edu/catalog/dissertationSearch.asp

Cybertesis.net
- http://www.cybertesis.net/index-en.html
- The University of Chile provides an access to 27,000 theses from 35 world universities.

DART-Europe E-theses Portal (DEEP)
- http://www.dart-europe.eu/basic-search.php

Digital Library and Archives
- http://scholar.lib.vt.edu/theses/
- This allows searching for citations and abstracts of more than 6,700 theses and dissertations.
- Free full-text access is provided for more than 4,500 of these items.

Directory of Dissertations in Progress
- http://www.historians.org/pubs/dissertations/index.cfm
- This provides an access to approximately 3,804 in-progress dissertations in the subject area of history.
- Dissertations came from Canada and the United States, representing approximately 170 academic institutions.

Dissertation.com
- http://www.dissertation.com
- This contains a collection of a few hundred dissertations and theses.
- This is also a free, full-text access to the first 25 pages of each item.

Dissertation Express
- http://disexpress.umi.com
- This is an online version of dissertation abstracts from UMI ProQuest, useful for locating theses from the United States.
- This is a free database, but a fee of about $34 each to order full text of dissertations.
- Digital Dissertations are a subset of UMI ProQuest dissertation databases comprising of all dissertations in the Dissertation Abstracts database with a degree date of the current and previous year. It is easier to search and browse, and one also gets to preview 24 pages before considering buying the whole dissertation.

Doctoral Dissertations in Musicology
- http://www.chmtl.indiana.edu/ddm/
- This is an international database that contains more than 12,000 dissertation citations in musicology.
- Dissertations are approximately from 1950s to present.
- This source may lead to dissertations on use of music in patient care.

Education Resources Information Center (ERIC)
- http://www.eric.ed.gov

Electronic Theses and Dissertations (UVa)
- http://www.lib.virginia.edu/etd/home.html

E-Theses
- http://ethesis.helsinki.fi/en
- Resource is from Finland.

EThOS
- http://ethos.bl.uk/Home.do
- This is a beta application with full-text theses from the British Library.

European Working Group of the Networked Digital Library of Theses and Dissertations (NDLTD)
- This provides an access to 106,000 doctoral theses.

Index to Theses
- http://www.theses.com
- This is a fee-based or subscription resource.

Le Fichier Central des Thèses
- http://fct.u-paris10.fr/index.jsp
- French dissertations in progress

Massachusetts Institute of Technology (MIT) Theses
- http://dspace.mit.edu

Networked Digital Library of Theses and Dissertations (NDLTD)
- http://www.ndltd.org
- Provides an access to citations from thousands of digital dissertations and theses that are in PDF format.
- Significant number of these resources are freely available in full text and can be viewed online.

OhioLINK Electronic Theses and Dissertations Center
- http://www.ohiolink.edu/etd/faq.html#who-can-use
- http://etd.ohiolink.edu/
- http://etd.ohiolink.edu/world.cgi

PhdData: The Universal Index of Dissertations in Progress
- http://www.phddata.org
- This contains citations from several thousand in-progress dissertations from various parts of the world.

Registry of Open Access Repositories (ROAR)
- http://roar.eprints.org/?action=home&country=&version=&type=theses&order=name&submit=Filter

Research in Ministry (RIM) Online
- http://rim.atla.com/star/rimonline_login.htm
- This is a free access database.
- Indexing dates back to 1981 from doctor of ministry (DMin) and doctor of missiology (DMiss) projects that were submitted by accredited schools of theology.

Rutgers Electronic Theses and Dissertations (RUetd)
- http://rucore.libraries.rutgers.edu/etd/

Theological Research Exchange Network (TREN)
- http://www.tren.com
- This contains 6,800 citations about theological theses/dissertations and conference papers.
- Items can tbe purchased.

Theses Canada Portal
- http://www.collectionscanada.gc.ca/thesescanada/index-e.html
- This provides an access to citations for all the theses in the National Library of Canada Theses Collection that were published between January 1, 1998, and August 31, 2002.

Thèses de l'Université de Lumière Lyon 2
- http://theses.univ-lyon2.fr

Thèses en Ligne (TEL)
- http://tel.archives-ouvertes.fr
- This contains multidisciplinary theses.

University of Miami Electronic Theses and Dissertations
- http://etd.library.miami.edu/

Vidyanidhi: Digital Library and E-Scholarship Portal
- http://www.vidyanidhi.org.in/
- Resource is from India.

WorldCat Dissertations and Theses
- http://firstsearch.oclc.org/WebZ/FSPrefs?entityjsdetect=:javascript=true:screensize=large:sessionid=fsapp7-42444-fybv4c0t-cxbxbo:entitypagenum=1:0
- WorldCat dissertations and theses database is only available by subscription through the OCLC product called FirstSearch.
- The larger database of WorldCat is available for free and has an advanced search screen that allows one to limit the content to "thesis/dissertation." Here is the direct link to access the advanced search page in WorldCat: http://www.worldcat.org/advancedsearch

Answer Keys to Chapter Exercises

CHAPTER 4, EXERCISE 2: FOREGROUND QUESTIONS AND SYSTEMATIC REVIEW

Foreground Research Question #1	PICO #1	Type of Systematic Review
Does use of nurse practitioners in nursing homes impact the decreasing rate of nursing home patient hospitalizations (Christian & Baker, 2009, p. 1333)?	**P** = congestive heart failure patients	
	I = medication compliance	
	C = noncompliance with medications	
	O = return or no return to the emergency department	*Interventional*

Foreground Research Question #2	PICO #2	
What is the best available "evidence related to terminally ill patients' experiences of using music therapy in the palliative setting" (Mabel-Leow, Drury, Poon, & Hong, 2010, p. 344)?	**P** = terminally ill patients	*Therapeutic intervention*
	I = music therapy	
	C = usual care	
	O = experiences	

Foreground Research Question #3	PICO #3	
What is the cost of supporting self-monitoring of blood glucose by Type 2 diabetes mellitus patients to improve glycemic control (Verteuil & Tan, 2010, p. 302)?	**P** = patients with Type 2 diabetes mellitus	*Economic evaluation*
	I = self-monitoring of blood glucose	
	C = usual care	
	O = cost of glycemic control	

(Continued)

Chapter 4, Exercise 2 (*Continued*)

Foreground Research Question #4	PICO #4	
What is the impact of hospital visiting hours on patients and their visitors (Smith, Medves, Harrison, Tranmer, & Waytuck, 2009, p. 2293)?	**P** = pregnant women in high risk pregnancies	*Interventional or meaning*
	I = bed rest	
	C = N/A	
	O = pregnancy outcomes	

Foreground Research Question #5	PICO #5	
What are the spiritual experiences of elderly individuals recovering from stroke (Lamb, Buchanan, Godfrey, Harrison, & Oakley, 2008, p. 173)?	**P** = pregnant women in high risk pregnancies	*Meaning*
	I = bed rest	
	C = N/A	
	O = coping	

Note. PICO = patient/problem, intervention, comparison, outcome.

REFERENCES

Christian, R., & Baker, K. (2009). Effectiveness of nurse practitioners in nursing homes: A systematic review. *JBI Library of Systematic Reviews, 7*(30), 1333–1352. JBL000254

Lamb, M., Buchanan, D., Godfrey, C., Harrison, M., & Oakley, P. (2008). The psychosocial spiritual experience of elderly individuals recovering from stroke: A systematic review. *International Journal of Evidence-Based Healthcare, 2,* 173–205.

Mabel-Leow, Q. H., Drury, V., Poon, W., & Hong, E. (2010) Patient's experiences of music therapy in a Singaporean hospice. *International Journal of Palliative Nursing, 16*(7), 344–350.

Smith, L., Medves, J., Harrison, M., Tranmer, J., & Waytuck, B. (2009). The impact of hospital visiting hour policies on paediatric and adult patients and their families. *Journal of Advanced Nursing, 65*(11), 2293–2298.

Verteuil, R., & Tan, W. (2010). Self-monitoring of blood glucose in type 2 diabetes mellitus: Systematic review of economic evidence. *JBI Library of Systematic Reviews, 8,* 302–342.

CHAPTER 4, EXERCISE 3: PLACING FOREGROUND RESEARCH QUESTIONS INTO THE PICO FRAMEWORK

Foreground Research Question	PICO
What is the effect of open visiting hours on family members of ICU patients? **Question category:** *Qualitative*	**P** = family members of ICU patients **I** = open visiting hours **C** = (not stated in question: could be usual ICU visiting hours *or* restricted visiting hours) **O** = effect of open visiting hours *or* favorable or nonfavorable impression on families
What is the impact of open versus restricted visiting hours on nurse and patient satisfaction on medical-surgical units? **Question category:** *Qualitative*	**P** = nurses and patients on medical surgical units **I** = open visiting hours **C** = restricted visiting hours **O** = nurse and patient satisfaction
What is the effect of an ICU residency program for recent (past 6 months) baccalaureate nursing school graduates on ICU nurse retention? **Question category:** *Qualitative*	**P** = recent (past 6 months) baccalaureate nursing graduates **I** = ICU residency program **C** = no ICU residency program offering **O** = ICU nurse retention
Does discharge teaching on medications decrease CHF patient readmission to the emergency room related to medication noncompliance? **Question category:** *Prognosis*	**P** = CHF patients **I** = discharge teaching on CHF medications **C** = no discharge teaching on CHF medications **O** = readmission of CHF patients to the emergency department
Does bed rounding contribute to a decrease of accidental patient falls in medical-surgical units? **Question category:** *Prognosis*	**P** = medical-surgical patients at risk for accidental falls **I** = bed rounding **C** = no bed rounding or similar intervention **O** = decrease, increase, or no change in patient falls

(Continued)

Chapter 4, Exercise 3 (*Continued*)

Foreground Research Question	PICO
Does use of advance practice nurses in long-term care facilities decrease patient hospitalizations? **Question category:** *Prognosis*	**P** = long-term care institutions **I** = use of APNs **C** = no use of APNs **O** = decrease in patient hospitalizations
Is there a relationship between nurse–patient ratios and nurse burnout? **Question category:** *Qualitative*	**P** = nurse–patient ratios **I** = a specific nurse–patient ratio figure **C** = another specific nurse–patient ratio figure **O** = nurse burnout
Is there any impact or change in bloodstream-related infection when a CVAD dressing is changed in 3 days versus 7 days? **Question category:** *Therapeutic Intervention*	**P** = bloodstream-related infection **I** = CVAD dressing change every 3 days **C** = CVAD dressing change every 7 days **O** = decrease or increase in bloodstream-related infection
Do magnet hospitals experience higher rates of nurse retention compared to non-magnet hospitals? **Question category:** *Qualitative*	**P** = nurses **I** = magnet hospitals **C** = non-magnet hospitals **O** = nurse retention
What is the occurrence of relocation stress or transfer anxiety in patients and their families upon transfer of the patient from an ICU to a non-ICU? **Question category:** *Qualitative*	**P** = ICU patients and families of ICU patients **I** = patient transfer to a non-ICU floor **C** = not stated **O** = relocation stress or transfer anxiety
What are the most effective strategies for decreasing transfer anxiety in hospital patients? **Question category:** *Therapeutic Intervention*	**P** = hospital patients being transferred from one floor/unit to another **I** = most effective strategies **C** = all strategies to decrease transfer anxiety **O** = decrease in transfer stress/anxiety

(Continued)

Chapter 4, Exercise 3 (*Continued*)

Foreground Research Question	PICO
Does education of ICU nurses on oral care and implementation of a *vent bundle* decrease ventilator-associated pneumonia? **Question category:** *Therapeutic Intervention*	**P** = ICU nurses
	I = oral care education *and* vent bundle implementation
	C = usual or standard care for ventilator patients
	O = decrease in VAP
In children living in an urban environment, does the presence of open spaces such as parks lead to positive health outcomes? **Question category:** *Prognosis*	**P** = children living in urban areas
	I = open spaces (e.g., parks)
	C = not applicable
	O = positive health outcomes
What is the relationship between patient repositioning and pressure ulcer prevention? **Question category:** *Therapeutic Intervention*	**P** = patients
	I = repositioning
	C = not stated in the question, but could be a type of repositioning *or* timing for repositioning *or* no repositioning
	O = pressure ulcer prevention

Note. APN = advanced practice nurses; CHF = congestive heart failure; CVAD = central vascular access device; ICU = intensive care unit; PICO = patient/problem, intervention, comparison, outcome; VAP = ventilator-associated pneumonia.

CHAPTER 5, EXERCISE 1: CONTROLLED VOCABULARY OR SUBJECT HEADINGS FOR TEXT WORDS/PHRASES

Text Word/ Phrase	MEDLINE (*Ovid*) MeSH Terms	CINAHL (*EBSCOhost*) Subject Terms	Comments on Discoveries
AIDS	Acquired immunodeficiency syndrome	Acquired immunodeficiency syndrome	
Alternative therapy	Complementary therapies	Alternative therapies	
Anti-inflammatory	Anti-inflammatory agents	■ Anti-inflammatory agents ■ Anti-inflammatory agents, nonsteroidal ■ Anti-inflammatory agents, steroidal ■ Anti-inflammatory agents, topical	
Aspirin	Aspirin	■ Aspirin ■ Anti-inflammatory agents, nonsteroidal	
Bed rest	Bed rest	Bed rest	
Cardiac catheterization	Heart catheterization	Heart catheterization	
Clinical ladder	Career mobility	Clinical ladder	
Cot death	Sudden infant death	Sudden infant death	
CPOE	Medical order entry systems	Electronic order entry	In MEDLINE, if you type *computerized prescriber order entry* instead of CPOE, you will get different list of *MeSH* terms
Hospital readmission	Patient readmission	Readmission	In CINAHL, no exact *subject term* match for hospital read-mission, but try typing the text phrase *patient readmission*, and you will retrieve the *subject term readmission*

(Continued)

Chapter 5, Exercise 1 (*Continued*)

Text Word/ Phrase	MEDLINE (*Ovid*) MeSH Terms	CINAHL (*EBSCOhost*) Subject Terms	Comments on Discoveries
Kangaroo care	Infant care	Kangaroo care	
Metabolic syndrome	Metabolic syndrome X	Metabolic syndrome X	
Nurse burnout	Burnout, professional	Burnout, professional	
PT time	Prothrombin time	■ Bleeding time ■ Prothrombin time	In MEDLINE, type out *prothrombin time* as text word instead of PT time to retrieve the *MeSH* term *prothrombin time*
Qualitative	Qualitative research	Qualitative studies	MEDLINE also offers the *MeSH* term *nursing methodology research*
Swine flu	■ Influenza, human ■ Influenza A virus, H1N1 subtype	■ Influenza, swine ■ Influenza A virus	

CINAHL = Cumulative Index to Nursing and Allied Health Literature; CPOE = computerized practitioner order entry; PT = prothrombin time.

CHAPTER 5, EXERCISE 2: ALTERNATE SPELLING FOR TERMS IN DATABASES

American Spelling	British Spelling
anesthesia	**anaesthesia**
aging	ageing
analyze	**analyse**
center	**centre**
favor	favour
fetal	**foetal**
hemorrhage	**haemorrhage**
esophagus	oesophagus
pediatrics	**paediatrics**

Index